BETWEEN HELLO & GOODBYE

BETWEEN HELLO & GOODBYE

A Life-Affirming Story of Courage in the Face of Tragedy

JEAN CRAIG

JEREMY P. TARCHER, INC.
Los Angeles

To Deirdre, Chris, Erin, and Maureen,
who were there, too.

Library of Congress Cataloging in Publication Data

Craig, Jean, 1937–
     Between hello and goodbye / Jean Craig.
          p. cm.
     ISBN 0-87477-604-X
     1. McNeilly, Edward R.–Health.   2. Cancer–Patients–California–
          Biography.   I. Title.
RC265.6.M35C73 1991
362.1'96994'0092–dc20   90-39721
[B]   CIP

The events, people, and places in this book are real. The names of all doctors
and certain other medical professionals have been changed, however, with the
exception of Alan M. Fogelman, M.D.

Epigraph on page vi: "HELLO & GOODBYE" from the motion picture FROM
NOON TILL THREE, words by Alan and Marilyn Bergman, music by Elmer
Bernstein, © 1975 UNITED ARTISTS MUSIC CO., INC. and UNART MUSIC
CORPORATION. Rights assigned to EMI CATALOGUE PARTNERSHIP. All rights
controlled and administered by EMI U CATALOG INC. and EMI UNART CATALOG
INC. All rights reserved. International copyright secured. Used by permission.

Jeremy P. Tarcher, Inc.
5858 Wilshire Blvd., Suite 200
Los Angeles, CA 90036

Distributed by St. Martin's Press, New York

Design by Susan Shankin

Manufactured in the United States of America

BOMC offers recordings and compact discs, cassettes
and records. For information and catalog write to
BOMR, Camp Hill, PA 17012.

Acknowledgments

A first book, when you're past the bravado of youth, is a shy and tentative undertaking. These are the people who gave me confidence

Bob Schulberg, an old friend who put me in touch with his cousin Budd's agent. Alyss Dorese, Budd's agent and now mine, who read the first draft and told me, "Put more of yourself in it." Ann King, my good friend, who suggested I send the finished manuscript to Norman Cousins. Norman Cousins, who read it, phoned, had lunch with me and provided enormous encouragement. John O'Toole, a mentor and friend, who also read it early on, and helped me believe I had a book. Andrea Stein, a wonderful editor and gentle guide into the world of publishing. And Jeremy Tarcher, an extraordinary publisher because he can also read the heart of a writer.

Some have a lifetime, some just a day
Love isn't something you measure that way.
Nothing's ever for ever
Forever's a lie.
All we have is
Between Hello and Good-bye

ALAN AND MARILYN BERGMAN

August *26, 1986*

CEDARS-SINAI IS THE HIGH-TECH HOSPITAL in Los Angeles. Huge. Polished. Crowded. Gurneys. Lasers. CAT-scans. Scopes. All the fancy stuff. All the fancy doctors.

We got there at two in the afternoon. My husband Ed and myself. And my son, Chris. Chris had a map he'd pulled out of a brochure rack and was studying it with the steady eye of a person who knows topography.

"We're on the wrong floor," he said. "We're not even in the right building."

"Well, let's get it figured out," said Ed. "I don't want the champagne to get warm." He'd hidden a bottle of Domaine Chandon in his overnight bag. He was going to have surgery the next day and had been on a clear-liquid diet for forty-eight hours. "Champagne is a clear liquid," he'd said as he shoved the bottle in his bag, amongst the slippers and jammies.

Chris, in the Levis, T-shirt, and beat-up Nikes that were the mainstay not only of his job with the Corps of Engineers but of his entire persona, led us through the corridors, their walls covered with a zillion-dollar art collection. Ed had hold of my hand and kept pulling me along. "Look at that machine," he'd say. "Look at that nurse," he'd say. "I don't like the look of that doctor," he'd say.

Chris finally found Admitting. The process was computerized and quick. They already knew my name. They already knew the insurance carrier. They already knew Ed's doctor. It all came up instantly on the computer screen.

Ed got his plastic bracelet. "Let it hang loose," he smiled at the Admitting lady. She didn't smile back. Then a technician came and took Ed with him for blood tests, X-rays, to piddle in the bottle—all the stuff you do before operations.

Chris and I went into an anteroom to wait. "I don't like hospitals," he said, which I knew, and I smiled at him, because I was grateful he'd taken an afternoon off from work to be my buddy. He plopped down like a teenager, which he wasn't, on a deep hospital-waiting-room chair, then stuck his slightly sunburned nose into a 1972 issue of *National Geographic*. I picked up a 1983 *Newsweek*. But I didn't really look at it as I turned the pages.

A couple of weeks earlier, Ed had noticed a tiny spot of blood on his undershorts and subsequently in his stool. With characteristic aggressiveness, he was at the doctor's by nine the next morning, and before twenty-four hours had passed he knew he had a tumor in his colon and that it was malignant. "But don't panic," the doctor had said. "It's the same thing Ronald Reagan had. It's localized. We got it early. We'll snip it out and you'll go on with the rest of your life."

Tomorrow it would be snipped. In ten days, he'd be home and this would be over. It won't be bad, I said to myself. We can still go to Tahiti in November, I said to myself.

It was a couple of hours before Ed came from Admitting, and the three of us went up to his room. They gave him hospital standard issue: the wash basin, the spit tray, the plastic cup, the plastic pitcher, the urinal bottle, the box of Kleenex, one thin towel, one thin washcloth, the brochure that says "Welcome to Cedars," and the pale-yellow hospital gown with the three ties up the back. Ed looked at it and laughed. "I need hospital gowns from Omar the Tentmaker," he said to the nurse. Ed was a big man. Six foot two. Two hundred and forty pounds. A big man.

Instead of the gown, he pulled on a pair of white cotton drawstring pants he'd taken on island vacations and left on the soft V-necked T-shirt that let little gnarls of salt-and-pepper hair fringe the edges of the V. He had Mexican huaraches on his feet, a champagne bottle in his hand, and with his bright white mustache against a head of dark hair he looked like pictures I'd seen of Papa Hemingway pub-crawling the streets of Key West in the 1940s.

As soon as the nurse left, Ed shut the door and popped the bottle of Domaine Chandon. "I think I'll go get a Coke," said Chris. At twenty-four, my son was still shy and didn't feel comfortable with a lot of things Ed did, like drinking champagne in hospitals, although he did see the humor in it. Ed didn't drink very much. But I did. And I was feeling a little silly around six o'clock in the evening when the two doctors walked into the room.

It's Dr. Mutt and Dr. Jeff, my silly head said to myself, noticing that one of the doctors was very tall and one was very short. Ed introduced the tall one as Dr. Phillip Richmond and the short one as Dr. Robert Kraft. I knew who they were—internists Ed had seen off and on over the years—but I'd never met them. Dr. Richmond was now Ed's personal physician and Dr. Kraft, who specialized in disorders of the colon, was consulting on the case.

Dr. Kraft had a paper bag in his hand with a cup of coffee in it. As he put it down on the table beside the bed, his hand was shaking. Aha, my silly head continued the dialogue with itself, he's been into the champagne too. Ed was cracking jokes about the indignities he'd been put through in the Admitting process. Chris was grinning a silly grin. But I suddenly found myself detached from the conversation, as if I was outside looking in. I followed Dr. Kraft's trembling hand as he lifted the cup of coffee to his lips. I saw that his face was ashen.

"Ed." Dr. Richmond interrupted the joking. "We need to discuss something with you, Ed."

The room went into slow motion all the while my head fast-forwarded to stone, cold sober. Chris heard the doctor's tone and looked at me. Ed coughed and ran his hand through his pewter-colored hair. I was fixated on Dr. Kraft and watched the paper cup shake again as he put it back down on the table.

"You might want privacy," Dr. Richmond said softly, nodding in the direction of me and Chris.

I was startled that the doctor implied I should leave and heard Ed asking me to stay. Then, with a sense of discomfort and some confusion, I asked Chris to step outside, because he was my son, not Ed's. As soon as Chris shut the door, Dr. Kraft began.

"Ed, do you smoke?"

"No, I quit twenty years ago."

"Before you quit, how much did you smoke?"

"A couple of packs a day."

"Have you noticed shortness of breath or a lot of coughing?"

I said, "What's going on?"

Dr. Richmond sat down beside Ed on the edge of the bed. I noticed he wore loafers and argyle socks. There was pink in the socks to match his pink pullover sweater. I liked the way he didn't dress like a doctor.

"When we took the chest X-rays this afternoon, we found some spots on Ed's lungs," he said.

"Some spots. What do you mean, 'spots'?"

"Just that," said Dr. Kraft. "We won't know what they are until we do some further tests."

"Well, what do you think they are?"

"Well, they could be an infection. They could be TB. They could be tumors." Dr. Kraft's voice cracked ever so slightly.

"What are you trying to tell us?" I asked. "Are you trying to tell us the cancer has spread?"

"We're not trying to tell you anything definite right now," said Dr. Richmond. "It could be that. But you shouldn't speculate until we do further tests. In the meantime, we've canceled tomorrow's surgery."

Ed was dumbfounded and mute. I was confused and babbling. "You've canceled tomorrow's surgery?"

Dr. Kraft and Dr. Richmond were taking turns answering. "We don't want to do the surgery until we find out about the spots," said one. "There's no need to panic," said the other.

"But what do spots on the lungs have to do with surgery on the colon?"

"We need to get a fuller picture before we do anything," Dr. Richmond said. There was a lot of emotion in his voice. "Listen," he continued, "none of us should speculate. We need to run tests tomorrow, instead of doing surgery. We'll find out what the spots are. And then we'll know what to do next. In the meantime, try not to guess."

We talked a while longer. Ed found his voice and asked a few questions, but his brain, like mine, had gone into paralysis and we were just repeating ourselves. Dr. Kraft ordered Ed some food. He could eat, since there would be no surgery. Then the doctor left. It seemed to me as if he ran from the room.

Dr. Richmond stayed a long time. He asked Chris to come back in and nodded while Ed told him about the spots. He changed the subject and told some dumb doctor jokes. He sat on the edge of the bed and talked about his profession. "Nobody practices medicine anymore," he said.

Dr. Richmond finally left. And then Chris, wearing the embarrassed grin that always overtook his features when he didn't know what to do with his feelings. I stayed until close to midnight. Since Ed had first told me the tumor was malignant, over dinner at Valentino's a couple of weeks before, I hadn't really worried. Indeed, when he'd said the word *malignant* I'd sort of laughed and said, "You don't mean 'malignant malignant' do you?" It was as if this couldn't possibly be happening to Ed and certainly not to me.

It wasn't real. It was a moment out of context with the rest of our lives, and it would soon go away. Neither of us used the word *cancer.* What we had was a growth in the colon, like Ronald Reagan had. And these spots on the lungs were certainly something, but they weren't dire. His thoughts and mine flew together and fluttered around that idea like moths fluttering around a light bulb. But the idea was quickly rejected.

The mind rejects what it can't possibly bear.

I sat on the edge of Ed's bed until midnight, swinging my feet and talking about important things like whether or not he'd be out of the hospital in time for Lem Hall's jazz party.

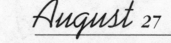 *August* 27

I HEARD DR. JOHN KRAKEWSKI'S name on the loudspeaker as I walked through the halls of Cedars on my way back to Ed's room. He's available, I said to myself. He's not doing Ed's surgery.

They ran the tests on Ed early in the day. An abdominal CAT-scan. They also stuck a needle into his chest to pull a sample, so they could do a biopsy. "Biopsy is a loaded word," Ed commented.

The tests didn't take very long and Ed was finished by noon, when Dr. Richmond came to see us in the room. He said Ed could go home and that he'd made an appointment for him with a Dr. Bornstein for three o'clock Friday afternoon.

I said, "Who's Dr. Bornstein?"

"He's an oncologist."

"What's an oncologist?" I had never heard the word before.

"It's a cancer specialist."

"So you think it's more cancer in the lungs?"

"I don't know what it is in the lungs, yet. I don't think we should speculate."

"And we're canceling the surgery entirely?"

"Yes."

I still didn't understand. Even if there was cancer in the lungs, why wouldn't they take out the cancer in the colon? As we continued talking, Dr. Kraft joined us in the room.

"Dr. Bornstein is the best person we know of," both doctors chimed in. "He'll have the test results back by Friday afternoon and will be able to tell you your options."

"Options?"

"Yes."

Suddenly we had options, and with that word, I felt the responsibility for the situation shift ever so subtly from the two doctors to the patient and his wife.

There didn't seem to be much more to do or say, so we checked out of the hospital. As we drove home, one piece of advice seemed more comforting than any other. "Don't speculate." So we didn't. Ed hadn't had a lot to eat since he went on his clear-liquid diet, so we stopped at the Hughes Market to get something for dinner and began the forty-eight-hour wait until Friday.

August 29

ED AND I LIVED IN MALIBU. Malibu, California. Home of Gidget, the Beach Boys, surfers lost in the eternal quest for the endless summer, movie stars in million-dollar beach cottages behind the gates of the Malibu Colony, the *Wall Street Journal* and *Daily Variety* on the newsstand at the am/pm mini market. You know about Malibu. Glitz. The good life. Swimming pools a stone's throw from the beach.

But there's more, and the unlikely place to find it is Hughes—the supermarket that anchors the shopping center.

The whole eclectic mess of humanity that lives, or hangs out, in Malibu rubs elbows at the Hughes Market. I've seen Dustin Hoffman thumping cantaloupes next to somebody's maid. The remnants from the various '60s subcultures that still hang on in nearby Topanga Canyon, or up Decker Canyon, or way back in the Santa Monica mountains come down to the Hughes Market to shop. They still buy lots of yeast and wheat germ. They still wear Birkenstocks on their feet. They never stopped tie-dying.

There's a good surfing beach right off the Malibu point, and that crowd drips its way in wet suits to the phones outside the Hughes Market. Somebody's always calling, saying they'll be late. Or calling to say there's a four-foot surf.

And then there's the local color provided by the nonlocals. The Malibums. People who drift in, stay a while, then drift out. A lot of construction workers. A lot of waiters and waitresses. Gas-station attendants. A lot of young men and women (or old men and women) in a place where you can just hang out. Do some odd jobs. A little bit of this. A little bit of that. House sit. Baby sit. Dog sit. Pick up some change. Make a few bucks. When you're not working, you drink Coronas at the Malibu Inn and watch one of the most celebrated places in the world go by.

You don't find Malibums in celebrated places like Beverly Hills, Palm Springs, or Grosse Point. But you do find them in celebrated places like Key West, Newport, Fire Island, St. Tropez, Bora Bora, St. John, St. Thomas, St. Croix, Turtle Island, Melanos, and Majorca.

What it takes is a beach. The beach makes it okay to walk barefoot through the Hughes Market, and that's why Ed and I, along with the Malibums, migrated to Malibu in the first place.

This Friday was a barefoot day and our house was a barefoot house. Easy and comfortable. A Cape-Cod-style cottage on a little street that turned off Pacific Coast Highway just as it began to saunter through the long but narrow strip of beachfront that was Malibu. The house was surprising, because you'd walk past the unpretentious façade into a living room full of wicker and overstuffed couches covered in canvas duck to be startled by a view of the Pacific Ocean that must rival the views in Monte Carlo, the south of France, or the Greek Islands. It's a white-water view, which in real-estate language means you can see not only the endless expanse of water sometimes as far as Catalina Island but also the surf rolling toward the beach.

We could stand on our deck and watch the languorous traffic on Pacific Coast Highway in rhythm with the lazy summer surf. The ocean looks different every single day. On that day, it was a deep, denim blue and had about as much energy as an old man in overalls on the porch of a general store.

On that day, our deck was spilling over with flowers. I love plants that bloom in what the gardening books describe as a "riot of color." Showy annuals like zinnias and marigolds. Gaudy perennials like Bougainvillea, hibiscus, and azaleas.

We were having lunch on the deck with the surf in the background and the flowers in the foreground, passing the time until the scheduled appointment with the oncologist, when the phone rang. It was Dr. Bornstein's office. They wanted us to come at two instead of three. There was some urgency. They had the results back. The nurse said, "Why don't you come right away."

We put on our shoes and drove the forty-five minutes to Dr. Bornstein's office, in West LA. We were concerned. But this wasn't real, so we weren't alarmed. In fact, we were laughing when we walked into the waiting room. The swishing, high-tech elevator doors had closed too fast and left me behind.

There were no other patients waiting. "The doctor wants to leave early," I thought to myself, "because it's the Labor Day weekend. That's why they wanted us to hurry." Then I amended my own opinion. "Don't be such a cynic."

We waited what seemed like a long time. It was probably about fifteen minutes. Ed filled out some forms. Finally, the nurse called him. They wanted to do an examination first. So I waited.

After about half an hour, the nurse asked me to join Ed in Dr. Bornstein's office. It was a tiny, cramped room with no outside windows. It was dark and stuffy. Ed was there by himself.

I said, "What did he say?"

"He hasn't said anything yet," Ed answered. "They took my weight, listened to my chest, and I peed into a bottle."

So we sat there. Five long minutes went by. Dr. Bornstein came in. Bearded. Bookish. Steel-rimmed glasses. Long lab coat. Austere. Serious. He finally began to talk.

"The results of the biopsy are back. The spots on your lungs are cancer."

The moment froze forever in time.

"This is a very grave situation," he continued. "I'm very sorry."

"Well...," my mind was racing... "can't we operate?"

"No." Dr. Bornstein put long pauses between his sentences. "It wouldn't do any good. The cancer is in both lungs. We could take one lung, and he might live, but he's already got it in the other."

"What about radiation?" I was asking the questions. Ed was stunned into silence.

"I'm afraid it's too widespread for that. This is a very grave situation." He paused again. "There is chemotherapy."

I said that my impression of chemotherapy was that it didn't work very well.

He said, "That's right."

I couldn't believe what I was hearing. Dr. Bornstein began fumbling around his desk until he found a green book, which he opened. "There is a drug we can start. But it's only palliative. It won't cure. It will only arrest for a time."

"Well, how much time?"

"I don't like to speculate."

There was that phrase again. Don't speculate.

"Listen," I said, feeling an old anger swell up that I thought I'd forgotten. "We have a life. We have children. And jobs. We have a business we're about to buy. We have decisions to make. We have a right to know anything you know."

Dr. Bornstein didn't look up. "Six months. Maybe a year."

"Good God." My mind spun so fast it sucked my mouth dry and the words strangled in my throat. I suddenly wondered why we were hearing this from a man we hadn't met until an hour before. Where was Dr. Richmond? Where was Dr. Kraft? Had they known all along?

Ed began firing questions about chemotherapy. But the doctor remained slow and deliberate. He said Ed could start it next week. Or the week after. There was no hurry. He began saying things like "we want you to be comfortable."

He kept repeating, "This is a very grave situation."

He turned down a corner of a page in the green book he'd been rummaging for on his desk and handed the book to Ed. "This will describe the chemotherapy and prepare you for the side effects. We hope they'll be mild."

Suddenly, neither Ed nor I could breathe. We just wanted out of there. Ed told the doctor he'd phone him on Tuesday, the day after Labor Day, and headed for the door.

As I followed Ed out through the waiting room toward the elevator, struggling for composure, I saw the nurse staring at us. She had the look of morbid curiosity people get on their faces when they stare at things like auto accidents.

She's known all along, I thought to myself, and she's looking at us to see the hurt.

I clapped my hand across my mouth and swallowed hard to keep from throwing up, then ran after Ed out the door.

❧ *It was the second time in my life I'd been told my husband had a terminal illness.*

The first time was twenty-two years earlier. It was my first husband, Kevin. But when I was told that day, about Kevin, I didn't get it. I sat there listening to the doctor, but in a conversation saturated with euphemisms and leaking from half-truths, I didn't understand what he was telling me.

The doctor's name was Bracco. I can't remember his first name anymore. He was part of a team at the UCLA Medical Center that had performed surgery on Kevin.

Kevin had atherosclerosis, the disease that causes arteries to harden and become clogged with cholesterol deposits. By the time we discovered he had the disease, when he was thirty-three, his arteries were already severely narrowed and, in some cases, blocked. We were to learn later that his condition was hereditary and that his brothers and sisters and their children and our children shared the problem.

Dr. Bracco operated on Kevin to clear his right carotid artery, the one that branches out from the aorta and goes to the brain. I remember that the surgery lasted twelve hours. I was pregnant with Maureen, our fourth child, and waited the whole twelve hours by myself. I was twenty-six years old and very shy. I was new in Los Angeles. I tended to shrink into the woodwork when dealing with doctors.

What really went on during those twelve hours of surgery, I'll never know. I do know it was a medical drama in its own right. It was never supposed to last that long. Kevin had a vague, perhaps faulty memory of reentering consciousness sometime during the procedure and being quickly put back under. He carried a huge, ugly scar across his neck for the rest of his life, because the doctors didn't take the time to cosmetically close the incision. I can only guess they thought he was a goner, and why bother. Or he'd been under too long and they were in a hurry. Either way, it was an unseemly thing to do. About all I know for sure is that the operation was a failure. They did not clear the artery.

They didn't tell us much about why. I've learned since that doctors never tell you much. They precisely answer the precise questions you ask, and that's all. They never offer information. They never explain anything, unless you press. And you have to learn how to press, which puts the taste of steel in my mouth every time I walk into a doctor's office.

Indeed, the noninformation syndrome is so bad I think there must be a required course in every medical school in America entitled "How to Tell Your Patients as Little as Possible."

I'm sure doctors have their reasons. Divulge too much information and you open yourself to malpractice. Giving information takes time, and little if anything is as important to a doctor and his staff as protecting the doctor's time. Mainly, I think they think people wouldn't understand anyway; that a little learning is a dangerous thing; and that people are better off not knowing.

What they told Kevin and me was the blockage in the carotid artery went too deep into the brain and they couldn't get it out. I was never completely satisfied with that answer. There was more, and whatever it was, we were never told. Today, I'd ask to see the X-rays and the records. People have a right to see their own X-rays. I'd ask for a debriefing from the head surgeon. Full disclosure has been passed into law for every business and profession in America except medicine. You know more about what a mechanic does to your car than what a surgeon does to your body. You get a computer printout from your Chevrolet dealer, detailing what was done. From your surgeon you get something sweeping like, "We patched the hole in his heart and he's fine."

At any rate, they told us the surgery had failed, they sewed Kevin's neck shut like you'd sew together the top of a burlap bag, and they sent us home. A couple of weeks later, Dr. Bracco phoned and asked us to come over to UCLA to meet with him.

In retrospect, the two of us must have seemed pitiful, although we certainly didn't perceive ourselves that way. I was eight months pregnant and working part-time as an advertising copywriter and had three small children already at home. There wasn't much money. Kevin, despite his brains, his good schooling, and his cultivated upbringing, was a postal clerk. He worked for the U.S. Post Office in Beverly Hills.

Dr. Bracco met with us in a lounge at the UCLA Medical Center. He said things like "we've done all we can do." Or "you know the other carotid is in bad shape too." I asked him how long it would take it to clog up. He said about six months, maybe a year. He said, looking at me, "You have a big family and a lot of responsibilities."

I recalled the conversation from time to time, because Dr. Bracco was so poignant. But it wasn't until months later that it snapped together in my brain. He was trying to tell me that when the other artery went, Kevin was going to die. But by the time I figured this out, Kevin had blown all the theories to hell anyway.

Kevin lived thirteen more years. It took three years, not six months, for the other artery to go. But by the time it did, surgical techniques had improved and Kevin's collateral circulation had built up. The doctors were able to successfully remove the diseased left carotid and replace it with a vein they took from his leg. He lived ten years more after that.

But Dr. Alan Fogelman, the highly regarded coronary researcher at UCLA who became Kevin's doctor and friend, told me the real reason Kevin lived so long was because "he decided to."

The ability of the human spirit to "decide to live" is extraordinary. In his book The Healing Heart, Norman Cousins writes of the "doctor inside every one of us who has the power to heal."

Kevin put that doctor to work. He walked around for thirteen years with what must have been wax, not blood, running through his arteries. A normal cholesterol count for an adult male is around 200, and 300 is high. Kevin's count was in the 700s. By the time he died, he'd lost

90 percent of the circulation in the carotid artery they'd replaced and Lord knows how much elsewhere. You can't live with the amount of circulation Kevin lost. Yet he did live.

I remember one summer evening in 1974. We'd just bought our home on Benecia in West Los Angeles. And Kevin, who hadn't been able to get life insurance for years, decided that a homeowner's policy on our new house might be a way for him to get coverage.

I said, "Kevin, you're crazy. You'll never pass the physical."

But Kevin didn't always listen to me. So, that balmy summer evening, a young medical technician came to the door. He told me he was there to give my husband an insurance examination.

I muttered twenty-seven curses toward Kevin under my breath, but I let the young man in and he proceeded to give Kevin the routine exam. At that time, Kevin was in his early forties and was working full time. He looked fine; there were no physical signs that anything was wrong except the scar on his neck, which was easy to hide under a shirt.

The technician started his exam and took hold of Kevin's wrist to take his pulse. But he couldn't get a pulse. He was startled, so he tried to get one in the neck. But, of course, Kevin hadn't had a pulse you could read in the neck for years. The technician started to look tense and act flustered. Kevin was trying to be cool. He was muttering about having low blood pressure and about how they had had trouble getting his pulse back when he was in the Army. I couldn't stand it. I left the room.

The technician checked Kevin's chest and the heartbeat was there. His color was okay. The technician looked at the veins. They were there. And there was blood in them. So he left and came back about a week later.

This time he was very smug, because he had a machine with him designed to pick up a faint pulse. The look on his face said, "I'm going to get your pulse this time, baby."

Kevin just sat there drinking a beer and chewing the fat while the man worked. The technician hooked him up to the machine and stepped back as if he'd just set the clock on a time bomb.

But he still didn't get a pulse. He fiddled with dials and knobs. He set gauges and tried again but still didn't get a pulse.

He finally left, looking sort of terrified. Of course, we didn't get the insurance.

The point is, Kevin had a circulatory system so badly clogged even a machine couldn't pick up a pulse. Yet he was walking around. Going to work. Raising kids. Bitching at me. Caring for me. Living.

The American medical profession neither understands nor recognizes the doctor inside every one of us. Most physicians do precious little to put that doctor to work. They are medical engineers who treat the body but do not engage the spirit. Those who refer to themselves as "compassionate" and who have reputations for being "good people doctors" do it, by and large, for the wrong reason.

They do it to be nice people, not out of a belief that a biological link exists between human emotions and healing.

They are so wrong. ❧

I don't know how to describe the twenty-four hours after Ed and I left Dr. Bornstein's office. But one thing's for sure. This time I got it. There was no doubt I understood what Dr. Bornstein had said. It was as if Ed had walked in front of a truck and been killed. Except he was living. I kept looking at him with my mouth open. I kept saying to myself, "This can't be happening."

How could Ed be a person with terminal cancer? It wasn't possible. Not Ed. It just didn't fit. It didn't make any sense.

And how could it be happening to me? It'd already happened to me, for Christ's sake. How could it be happening *again*?

My life with Kevin had made me so skittish that the first time Ed took me to dinner, three full years after Kevin's death, I asked him, "How's your health?" I didn't want to be around illness. I didn't want to be with someone who couldn't do things. I didn't want to be around a person who couldn't run with me down the beach. I was afraid of somebody who got too many colds, for God's sake. Now, here we were with cancer. Jesus Christ.

Was I being punished? What had I done? What had Ed done? What in the name of God was bringing this down on us?

We drove out to Malibu and everything we saw made a hot, slashing pain in the pit of my stomach. "Islands" where we liked to meet for lunch. The beach at Temescal Canyon where we went for Sunday-morning picnics. The marigolds and petunias spilling all over our front yard. I'd wanted to mix the colors of the petunias—reds and pinks and blues. Ed had said, "No. No. No." He insisted on all white ones. Then he showed me how to plant them too close together so they made an explosion when they bloomed. He was right. They were beautiful.

We went into the house. Ed yelled. He screamed at the sky and the sea. He kept saying, "Three years,... it's only been three years. It's not fair. It's too short."

Ed and I were married, three years before, on November 25, 1983, in a small but beautiful wedding on the deck of our own home. We'd met in the advertising business where I'd been working since the first month I'd arrived in Los Angeles in 1961–first as a copywriter, then as Creative Director, finally as an agency principal–all the while the children were being born and growing up, all the while Kevin was sick. Indeed, Kevin's illness cinched my commitment to a career as well as to children.

Ed was in the advertising business too, and we met in a circle of mutual business associates after Kevin's death. I caught him staring at me over drinks after work one evening and when I asked him why, he said, "Because you're part tycoon and part shy child and I can't figure that out." He was right, and I can't figure it out myself. But the insight was the shoot that made a relationship take root.

Our wedding day three years later was like a page from a lovesick novel. My four children were there, along with my brothers and my sisters-in-law and a few close friends. We were married right at the second when the sun slips into the sea and you think the water's going to sizzle. Ed was fifty-six years old that day in November, I was forty-six, and I thought my life had turned toward my own private Camelot.

Edward R. McNeilly was a strong personality. A powerful and successful marketing executive. A photographer, architect, automobile enthusiast, antique collector, and flamboyant cook. He loved the ocean, like I did. He loved old movies, like I did. And he loved the hell out of me. He thundered into my life, threw his big bear hug around me, and began to take care of me as no one ever had and to love me with an intensity that was almost scary.

Once when he flew home from a business trip he stopped at a bank of phones at LAX to call me, and when three phones in a row were out of order, he angrily tried to pull the last one out of the wall, wrecking it forever for Ma Bell.

I said, "Ed, why did you do that?"

He said, only a little sheepishly, "I wanted to talk to you."

When we decided to get married and move to Malibu, I found myself using dumb expressions like "my heart sings" until my friend Annie suggested I was sounding like Mary Poppins.

I thought about Ed's health and did calculations in my mind. I figured I could be married to him for as long as I was married to Kevin– seventeen years. I thought Ed could live into his seventies. He drank too much. He was overweight. But he was so strong. When I worried about him, it was a heart attack that came to mind. I never dreamed of cancer. Not Ed. He wasn't the type.

He was on the deck yelling, like a great, wounded bull. "How can I be doing this to you!" he roared.

There was a strange circle of agony and guilt. I think all critically ill people worry about the ones around them as much as they worry about themselves. Nobody wants to be a burden. Cancer patients have killed themselves to avoid taking their families through the illness. Ed's pain because of me was excruciating because of Kevin. Not only was he going to take me through it, he was dragging me through a second time. All the while, I felt my own customized brand of guilt. Ed was going to need me and I was dazed, absolutely dazed, at the thought of going through this again and guilty when my thoughts drifted to myself and away from him.

I sat on the deck in shock and in silence, trying to make the thoughts and feelings stop colliding in my brain. And I was trying to deal with the pain. Both my own and my husband's. I should know what to do, I thought. I've been here before.

But nothing ever prepares you for the pain in life. Each experience cuts fresh. Makes its own wound. Leaves its own scar. I had no words of real comfort for Ed. And none for myself.

We drank a lot of vodka. Finally, it was night, and "War Week" was on Channel 13. We stared at *Midway* for about the hundredth time, not really seeing the movie, not really hearing the words, but letting the sounds and images fill the brain until there wasn't room for anything else. After a long while, we went to sleep.

August 30

HOME WAS IMPOSSIBLE. We knew it the minute we got out of bed that Saturday morning, because it started all over again. Ed made coffee. He made coffee every morning. But now there was a clock ticking and a finite number of times left he'd be making coffee. I couldn't stand to watch him do it.

He said, "Let's get out of here."

I said, "We'll drive to Palm Springs or up the coast to Santa Barbara."

"No," he said. "I'll phone Beverly."

Beverly was his travel agent. He called her so often the number was programmed into the phone. He got her at home. He didn't tell her why; he just told her he wanted a flight to Hawaii. She said, "Ed, it's the Labor Day Weekend." He said, "I know."

Somehow she got us on a flight to Kauai. Somehow he got us a condominium there. Somehow we made it to the airport by eleven A.M.

By six o'clock that evening, Hawaii time, we were driving out of Lihue, in a Suzuki jeep, onto Highway 50 toward a condo on Poipu Beach.

August 31

THE PACIFIC THAT SLAPS THE SAND in Malibu is the same Pacific that slaps Kauai. Yet they're oceans apart. And there was some peace in that.

We were running from home, where a cup of coffee smelled of fear. We were also running from our thoughts. And the more we did, the less we thought, so we crammed a lot of doing into a couple of days. We climbed into a helicopter, and with its tape deck washing the air with Wagner's eerily metaphoric "Flight of the Valkyries" we viewed Waimea Canyon and Mt. Wauakeake's crater. We poked each other while the music did its swirling crescendo and laughed.

We took a boat trip to look at the cliffs and caves on the Na Pali shore. The boat eased into a lagoon and let us off to snorkel. Ed had a graceful dive for a man his size. He arched his 240 pounds into the air and slipped into the water like a porpoise. I countered with a fanny flop, splashing as much water as I could, and we laughed some more.

We took a sunset drive to Hanalei and drank too much tequila in a seedy island bar called Tahiti Nui. Ed and I had a love for dumpy bars parked on island beaches. They poured good brands of tequila and had all the great rums, like Mt. Gay, Appleton Gold, and Bacardi Superior. But the best thing was the people. You got a cast that rivaled the gang at the bar in the opening of *Star Wars*, where the Wookie seemed like a pretty normal guy. Ed and I whiled away a great evening at Tahiti Nui, swapping stories with a one-armed soldier from Bristol named Darien, a diamond trader from the Netherlands, and a blond-haired surfer from California who claimed to be the house-boy at Billy Jean King's estate, which was indeed right down the beach.

We bought dumb shirts on Kauai, had Mahi-Mahi for breakfast at a place only Hawaiians frequent, and got lost in our rinny-tinny Suzuki jeep. But what we really did was regroup.

I calmed myself and did my best to separate Kevin and Ed in my feelings as two entirely unrelated accidents of life. What happened to

Kevin and me had nothing to do with Ed and me. That was then. This was now. It was unfair to Ed to allow him to take on some additional burden because a man he'd never met had died. And I told him so. It was also unfair to myself to let my mind wander toward a connection between the two. I wasn't being punished. There was no diabolic pattern. But there was also no explanation, and that was the most difficult part.

Pain. Bad luck. Fate. They make random stops, with the furious nonsense of a tornado smashing one house into splinters while leaving another next door untouched.

"You don't deserve this, Jean," Ed said over and over and over again. I didn't. He didn't. Nobody deserves cancer. Nobody deserves a son dying in Vietnam. Or a child suffering with leukemia. Or an infant born impaired. Acceptance of the unfairness is the first step in being able to cope. Yes. It is unfair. No. I will not be defeated by that.

Ed regrouped as well. He traded fear for determination and as we climbed aboard the red-eye to fly back to Los Angeles, he told me he couldn't wait to get home. Because he'd decided to fight.

September 2

THE FIRST THING ED DID was "fire" Dr. Bornstein. He called and told the doctor he was going to get second opinions. The doctor said, "Fine. They will be the same." Ed said, "Maybe. But I want to know that for myself."

Then he phoned Dr. Richmond and asked him for two things: where to get second opinions and how to find out about experimental programs. By that time, we'd decided to go beyond conventional treatment. Maybe there was something going on experimentally that would give us a shot. When Ed phoned Dr. Richmond, I asked if he wasn't angry.

"It's not like you never go to the doctor, Ed. You were just there. And you saw Dr. Kraft in May. Aren't you angry? How could cancer of the colon that had metasticized to the lungs have gotten past both of them?"

"Don't do that, Jean," he said. "It doesn't do any good. I can't spend my energy on finding someone to blame. Besides, I avoided proctoscopes and I have to take responsibility for myself."

Dr. Richmond directed Ed to the cancer centers at UCLA and the University of Southern California for second opinions. And to the

National Cancer Institute in Bethesda, Maryland for information on experimental programs.

Ed phoned information in Bethesda to get NCI's phone number and called them cold. But he got a wonderfully warm response. He began a telephone relationship with a woman at NCI named Linda. Just Linda. I don't believe he ever asked her last name.

Linda gave Ed an education in cancer research. She used Federal Express and Overnight Mail to get information to him as quickly as possible. She answered questions and spent endless time on the phone, explaining to him how cancer research works.

First of all, it's important to know that cancer isn't one thing, like the polio virus was "one thing." There are many different kinds of cancer cells. A cell that responds to one kind of treatment won't respond to another. A drug that shrivels up breast tumors will have no effect on cancer in another part of the body, like the colon. In a way, nobody does "cancer" research. They do breast-cancer research, or lung-cancer research, or testicular-cancer research. Every kind of cancer cell requires its own treatment, its own line of defense, its own study. That's why there's little expectation for a single cure for cancer and why research has progressed so slowly. It's like the weeds in a garden. What stops a dandelion doesn't even faze a patch of crabgrass.

Linda taught Ed all of that. And she also educated him about research protocols.

The protocol is the systematized approach to research set down by NCI. There may be fifteen different institutions doing the same program. But while the institutions may be different from each other, they follow the same protocol. That way there's a constant basis for comparison of results. Generally, there are five phases to an NCI protocol. If the program has a good enough success rate at Phase I, it moves on to Phase II. And it must show a certain level of success again before it moves on to Phase III.

By the end of the week, Ed knew that he should be looking for Phase III programs. And that a 40-to-45-percent success rate was really high. That means the program has had some success with 40 to 45 percent of the people who were in it. To count, it doesn't have to have good success, just "some" success.

Perhaps the most valuable thing that Linda did for Ed was to Federal Express him a copy of PDQ.

PDQ (Physician's Data Query) is a computer printout of all the experimental programs being conducted in the United States, at any given time, under the auspices of NCI. It tells you the name and address of the institution where the research is happening and the names of the doctors in charge. It tells you what kind of cancer they're working on. It tells you what phase the program is in and the success rate that's been achieved. It tells you what kind of cancer patients are wanted in the program. Many protocols, for example, require people with previously untreated tumors. Sometimes there are age or health requirements.

PDQ is available to anybody who asks for it. But first, of course, you have to know about it. I don't believe that most oncologists are aware of it or would subscribe to it if they were, as putting a patient into a research program is not what oncologists are inclined to do. In a later conversation with Dr. Bornstein, he told Ed a bit testily, "I have PDQ, you know. I could've told you all that." But he didn't.

The mission of a doctor in private practice is to treat.

Ed's mission had become to win, and there is a world of difference between the two points of view.

Ed found twenty-nine institutions on the PDQ printout doing programs directed against colon cancer.

"I'm going to talk to them all, Jean. And I'm going to do it myself. I don't trust anyone to do this for me."

He picked up the telephone. And began calling them, one by one.

September 4

WE WENT TOGETHER TO GET the first second opinion. I can't imagine anyone with an illness that's life-threatening failing to get a second opinion. Second and third opinions are absolutely essential if you want control and if you want some degree of certainty. They're important, I believe, not only because the opinions of the problem might differ but also because the approaches to the solution might differ. Three doctors are likely to handle a problem three vastly different ways, and while it may be difficult to bring your own judgment to bear in such a situation, it's your body and your understanding of yourself that is ultimately the most reliable. If the doctors don't differ, then you're lucky and you're sure.

The notions of offending your doctor and losing sympatico with him are old hat. We live in a mobile society, in which lifelong relationships built on trust seldom exist anymore and people get multiple opinions on everything from auto repair to where to get their children educated. Also, doctors are more accustomed these days to their decisions being reviewed, because many of them are contracting with an HMO or other group that requires it. Nevertheless, if getting a second opinion offends your doctor, then offend him.

Ed's appointment was at eight-thirty in the morning at the Jonsson Cancer Center, which is part of the UCLA Medical Center, which is part of the sprawling UCLA campus in the Westwood section of Los Angeles.

I was nervous. Ed wasn't. "We're doing something," he said. "We're working on it."

We drove on Circle Drive to the Medical Center parking structure, then followed the color-coded lines that lead you through the buildings. We walked past "O" elevator, and I remembered that you take "O" elevator to the sixth floor and turn to the right to find the clinic where Kevin received his care and where Dr. Fogelman had his office. I never thought I'd be walking into UCLA again, with a sick husband again. It was eerie, but I kept my thoughts to myself and hurried to keep up with Ed.

We walked into the waiting room of the Cancer Care Center. I found myself staring at the people. Everybody here has cancer, I thought to myself, or is with someone who has cancer. There was a woman—very young, twenty or twenty-one—with a baby in her lap. I wondered if the woman had cancer. Or the baby. There was a tall man in Levis and cowboy boots talking to the receptionist. An old black woman was shaking a rattle at the baby in the woman's lap. A woman in her forties was in animated conversation with an older couple. You assumed they were her parents. But was she here with them? Or were they here with her?

The good humor I heard was surprising. There was bantering going on, like when you're waiting in line for a movie. I expected everyone with cancer to be morbid all the time and I didn't expect to hear chitchat about "my chemo." I also expected everyone to be bald, because "chemo" makes your hair fall out.

Ed and I didn't know the name of the doctor we were going to see. It was a clinic, and we'd see the doctor who was seeing patients that morning.

The nurse took us into one of the examining rooms. After about five minutes, a rumpled young man breezed in. He was wearing a brown plaid shirt, open at the neck, brown khaki-type pants, and loafers. No smock. No lab coat. No stethoscope around his neck. He introduced himself as Dr. Beckman. And I thought to myself how everybody looks like a kid to me these days.

Dr. Beckman asked Ed a lot of questions and looked over the records from Cedars. He took the X-rays to one of those special rooms where you put them on a light box. When he came back, he said, "Boy, you've got some doozies there." Then he saw my face fall and added quickly, "but you've got a lot of lung left."

Ed and Dr. Beckman talked for about fifteen minutes. I just listened. Dr. Beckman was a fighter. He said, "Ed, you've got a bad deal here, but there's plenty we can do." He criticized the conventional treatment for colon cancer, a drug called 5FU. "I wouldn't treat you with 5FU under any circumstance," he said. "It's the same as giving up." He talked about the difference, in his opinion, between doctors in research who "attack" and doctors in private practice who "treat."

He told us about an experimental program under way at UCLA. It was a program that combined a drug called Interferon with another drug called Etoposide. It was a Phase I program, about to move into Phase II.

"You're here at a good time, Ed," Dr. Beckman concluded. "We're starting a new group of people on the twenty-second of September. I feel sure you'd qualify for the program. Let me know if you're interested and we'll take the next step."

Ed said he was very interested, but he wanted to think about it. He told Dr. Beckman he'd call him.

As we left, he said to me, "It's a good program. I like it. I like him. But I don't want to commit yet. We just started."

September 7

CHRIS CAME OVER AND ED ASKED HIM to help move some big potted trees we'd just bought into the house and up the steps to the master bedroom.

"Oh, shit," I muttered when I saw Ed struggling with his half of a sixteen-inch container holding a giant fish-tailed palm. Suddenly, his lungs were full of "doozies" and things were different. I instinctively started to shout at him, "Ed, you can't do that," then changed my mind.

He could make his own decisions about what he could or couldn't do.

He and Chris paused at the foot of the stairs. The palm and the pot weighed enough to flatten a hippo. I saw a split-second decision flash through Ed's eyes. Should he? Or shouldn't he?

Damn the doozies, his eyes said. And Ed, Chris, and the palm tree went up the steps.

September 8

IT WAS SUNDAY, AND ELEVEN DAYS had passed since the chilling session with Dr. Bornstein. It was a beautiful day, out of the pale-blue palette on the water when the seam between sky and sea disappear into an endless backdrop for the pelicans, the porpoise, and the spinnaker sails. But it was also quiet, and the beauty was strangely jarring. Without the faster rhythm of the workday week, the mind slowed down to think, and it couldn't reconcile beauty and pain. How could you look out over the water and smile at the loveliness when the man standing behind you had cancer growing in his lungs?

Ed read my mind.

"Let's do something, Jean," he said. "Let's do something special and wonderful." It was as if we could no longer waste the days with ordinary things. Time was too precious. Everything took on new meaning.

"I'll make dinner," he said. "Beef Wellington. I've always wanted to try it. It'll be the most wonderful dinner of our lives, Jean."

So the two of us spent the day cooking. There were a dozen steps to Beef Wellington. Paté. Crust. Truffles. Mushrooms. We added wild rice and snow peas. Ed went to his wine cellar and brought up a 150-dollar bottle of Château Lafite Rothschild. I set the table with the good china and my mother's crystal. Neither of us spoke of cancer, but we both knew what we were doing. Drink the wine now. Do the beautiful things now. There may be no tomorrow.

But as we lifted our glasses and toasted each other, I felt a twitch at the corner of my mouth and a tightness in my throat. Halfway through the meal, I could barely eat Ed's superb Wellington and I couldn't sense the bouquet of the wine or its heady fullness. Ed asked me if the wine lived up to the occasion and I started to cry. Seconds later, I threw down my napkin and bolted out the front door to the street and the dark Malibu night. I ran until I couldn't run anymore and Ed found me sitting on the curb, watching the moon scud across the sky.

"What is it, Jean?"

"I can't be this way, Ed."

It was like a ritual. The Last Supper. A ceremony because of cancer. "I can't stand to be surrounded by it, Ed. I can't stand it."

"It's okay, Jean. You don't have to stand it." And he put his big arms around me, and the two of us sat on the curb and found the wondrous wordless comfort that two people give each other at times, just by holding on.

What we learned that night was to let go. To quit hugging the minutes. To quit trying to hoard the seconds. To let go of time. To let it pass as it had always passed. It was okay to be bored and boring. To be idle, forgetful, unaware. To let a day just go by. It was okay to smile at the loveliness of the sea. It was even okay to be happy and forget about the drama going on. We learned that we were going to find our strength, comfort, and joy in the blessed triviality of life. We were going to go to work, like always, come home, fix dinner, cuddle together on the couch and watch a movie. That was going to be our shield against desperation and despondency. Our salvation was not going to be found in the noble virtue of courage, but in the everyday succor of normalcy.

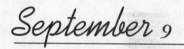

September 9

ED KEPT AN APPOINTMENT FOR his second second opinion at the University of Southern California's Norris Cancer Center. He met with Dr. Malcolm Pardo. I didn't go with him, but we met for lunch afterward.

"Pardo's got a big ego," he told me, "but I like him." He'd confirmed the original diagnosis, but the good news was they had a program starting the following week.

Ed began describing USC's program. It was the first time I heard about Interleuken 2. But it certainly wouldn't be the last.

About two years before, Interleuken 2 had come out of the research labs and into the public eye with a great deal of fanfare. The story made the cover of *Newsweek*. Interleuken 2 was looked upon as the most promising step toward the control of cancer in a decade. Maybe ever.

It was different from other cancer treatments in that it didn't attack the cancer directly but stimulated instead the body's own immune system. I read in a brochure Ed handed me: "It turns white blood cells into Samurai warriors who attack and destroy the invasive cancer cells."

"I told Pardo," Ed smiled as he nibbled at his pasta, "that the Interleuken 2 program is also being conducted at M.D. Anderson in Houston and several other places." M.D. Anderson was one of the largest cancer hospitals in the United States, second only to Sloan-Kettering in New York. Ed had learned of the program on the PDQ printout from NCI. Indeed, he'd phoned M.D. Anderson and talked to them about getting into the program.

"Pardo didn't have much good to say about the big institutions," Ed continued. "He told me they can be factories."

"Are you interested in the program?" I asked.

"Yes. But according to what I've been reading, the success of Interleuken 2 isn't holding up. I've got to find out some more."

That afternoon, Ed phoned Dr. Bornstein to ask his opinion of several of the programs he'd uncovered. The etoposide program at UCLA. Several Interleuken 2 programs—USC, Sloan-Kettering, M.D. Anderson. There was a program that looked promising at a clinic in San Jose. And another at a clinic in Virginia.

Dr. Bornstein said, with casual disdain for the effectiveness of experimental programs, "Pick the one nearest to home. The one that will be most convenient. It doesn't really make any difference. They're all about the same."

That was the last time Ed spoke to Dr. Bornstein.

September 10

ED WENT OUT AND BOUGHT A PORSCHE. A white turbo-body Cabriolet with a black top. He ordered special three-piece wheels, but he drove it home that afternoon.

Ed was a car nut, and his business career had mostly to do with cars. For fifteen years, he was Management Supervisor on the Volkswagen account at Doyle Dane Bernbach in New York. He helped introduce that car into the United States and headed the team responsible for the remarkable VW advertising in the 1960s—work that changed advertising in America, indeed all over the world.

Ed also helped introduce Porsche and Audi. And in the '80s, working for Della Femina Travisano and Partners in Los Angeles, he managed the advertising that introduced Isuzu to the U.S. market. His advertising career included a lot of other things too, like Close Up toothpaste and Gallo Wine, but mostly it was cars.

And he loved them. My God, did he love them!

He loved car races, car shows, car books, and car people. He subscribed to *Auto Week, Automobile, Automotive News, Car and Driver,*

Road & Track, and magazines only the real car guys read, like *Hemmings Motor News.*

He exposed me to a subculture built around cars that I never knew existed. The people who hang out at race tracks like Laguna Seca and Willow Springs on weekends. Who drive there in old Porsche speedsters, '56 Corvettes, and '65 Mustangs. People who know the difference between a Boxer and a Dino Ferrari. People who can recognize a MacLaren, a Siata, or a Lagonda. People who can argue over which is the more classic '30s Cabriolet, the Delahaye or the Talbot-Lago. People who know all the cars designed by Figoni and Falaschi. Who know the racing heritage of Porsche, Bugatti, Ferrari. People in their lowered Ford pickups, or their Chevies with custom-flared fenders; people who spend the weekend sitting on top of their campers watching cars race, talking about and looking at cars they can never hope to drive, much less own.

The car people.

Ed was one of them.

So when the doctors told him he had cancer, he went out and bought a Porsche.

The first afternoon he had it, he drove it to the Hughes Market. He said that several attractive young women came over to him and said, "Is that your car?"

I loved it.

September 11

WE WENT TO SEE A PRETTY YOUNG ATTORNEY, Patty McVerry, who worked for Ed's business attorney, Marty Reed, and got a will made. A simple thing. No big deal. We'd been meaning to do it anyway.

September 14

MOST PEOPLE THINK THE CLIMATE in southern California is forever spring. They're nuts. The climate in southern California is forever backwards. You can get a tan in February, but June is awful. Every year, in June, your relatives come to visit because school is out and summer is on. But for endless days, the Southern California skies are gray. The sun comes out for about fifteen minutes in the late afternoon, then promptly sets. It's chilly. Some days you feel like putting a fire in the fireplace. All your relatives are wearing their seersucker shorts, freezing to death. You tell them to bring a sweater, but nobody brings a sweater to Los Angeles. It finally starts to warm up about the Fourth of July.

But summer doesn't really start swinging until September, just when the kids are going back to school and all the relatives are leaving. September is when the desert winds blow, the skies are clear, and the nights are balmy. September is the only month when the Pacific Ocean off of Malibu is warm enough for a pantywaist, like myself, to go in past the knees.

September and October. You put Jimmy Buffett on the tape deck and sit on the beach with sand sticking to your Coppertone, your beer getting hot, your nose burning, and your serious reading—like *People* magazine—lying unread while you work up a sweat working on your tan.

It was that kind of September weekend.

Three of my children had come to Malibu: Sug (pronounced Shug), who was going to law school in San Francisco; Erin, who lived in Santa Barbara and worked there as an environmental planner; and Chris, who worked for the U.S. Army Corps of Engineers and had his own apartment in West LA. Maureen, my youngest daughter, was away at school at Wesleyan University, in Middletown, Connecticut.

Ed also had children: Robin, who lived with her husband, Michael, and their son, Matthew, in Orlando, Florida; and Kim, who was married to Mark and lived in Los Angeles. Kim was estranged from her father, however, over misunderstandings that arose out of his divorce and his marriage to me, and she hadn't been in touch with Ed for some time.

Chris, Sug, and Erin had come home for the weekend so we could talk. Ed and I both dreaded it, but Ed more so than me, because in spite of himself he'd come to love my children. And the guilt welled up again because of what he might take them through.

When I first started seeing Ed I'd been single (I've always hated the word *widowed*) long enough to be past the hard part; I'd left a twelve-year career at one of America's largest advertising agencies to become a partner in my own company, Cunningham, Root & Craig; and the children were all teenagers. Bringing a man into your life when you have four teenage children requires a finesse equal only to that required for bringing teenagers into the life of the man.

I didn't talk a lot about the kids when Ed and I first started seeing each other. Any woman who goes out to dinner with an attractive man and spends the evening talking about her sixteen-year-old daughter getting suspended for three days for telling Mr. Mulvehill to "fuck off," when she could be talking about a fascinating business meeting, is nuts.

I decided to ease Ed into the kids. When people would ask me how many I had in front of him, I'd mumble something indistinguishable. He was always getting them confused anyway.

But the reality of Ed was more immediate and quickly came into sharper focus at the Craig household. The first thing I had to do was establish a double standard, which I found perfectly fair. I could come home at two in the morning on a school night, but they could not. And there was nothing democratic about the reason why: I was forty-four years old and they were not. It was a situation single mothers run into a lot. Children, at any age, don't like to even think about their mothers having sex.

At any rate, I preferred the double standard to having my sixteen-year-old daughter or nineteen-year-old son run into Ed in the bathroom in the morning. When he first started coming to the house, he fixed things, which everybody liked. Suddenly, the back door would not only close, but lock. That was good. But it was more than a year before he stayed the night.

One of the secrets to easing a new man into a household with children, even older children, is defining roles. Who's who? is what everybody's thinking, though no one asks. How am I supposed to think about this guy? How does Mom think about this guy? So the first time Ed had Christmas dinner with us at our house on Benecia, I asked him not to sit at the head of the table—Kevin's place—but to leave that spot for Chris. A little thing, but it told everyone what they needed to know about Ed. He was for me, not for them, and he wasn't the head of our household.

And that was fine with everybody. My kids were too old for a new person to walk in and start being Father. They'd already had a father. Besides, Ed didn't want the job.

"I want to marry you, not your family," he liked to tell me as often as he could.

But I thought I'd better define roles again when Ed and I decided to get married, because that not only changed things, it turned the tables. So, when I sold the house on Benecia, I left everything in it behind. The pots and pans, the dishes, the Queen Anne desk in my bedroom, the antique stove I'd found in a field while shooting a TV commercial, the books, the bric-a-brac, the bunk beds. I said I was leaving it behind because it was wrecked by twenty years of children. And it was. The cookie sheets were so corroded Ed wouldn't use them. The dining-room table was one large, sorry attempt to cover scratch marks.

But the real reason was to make a point. To my children. To Ed. To myself. Ed and I were starting a new household, where he *would* sit at the head of the table. The rules would be changing. Ed did what he liked in his own home and expected everybody else, especially a younger generation, to do what *he* liked, as well. Cruddy tennis shoes on the kitchen counter were okay on Benecia, but they wouldn't make it in Malibu. Unless, of course, they were Ed's cruddy tennis shoes.

Before everyone came home for Christmas that first year, I wrote a letter and warned them Ed sat in front of the TV with his clicker held like a gun and switched channels every nineteen seconds, and it was irritating as hell, but they'd better not say anything to him, because it was his house now. They wouldn't have, of course. They were too scared. But he was scared too, in his way. And he went to work to make things okay.

He decorated the house to welcome them home. A tree branch covered with twinkling white lights hung from the living-room ceiling. He baked fruitcakes. He made eggnog. He bought a movie camera to film Christmas morning. He wrapped all of his own gifts. The sight of him in the middle of the living-room floor with tape, scissors, paper, and ribbons, constructing bows and getting his corners square, was enough to make a stone cry. And so, the little rivulets of affection began to turn into a stream. When the holidays were over, I heard Sug say to him, "This was the best Christmas we've had in years, Ed McNeilly, and it's all because of you."

And so it began to shift. At the beginning of our marriage, the children would introduce us by saying, "This is my Mom. And this is my Ed." But after a while, maybe a couple of years, I heard one of them say on the phone, "let me ask my parents." Eventually, I heard Sug say one day, "He isn't my father, but he might just as well be." At a family dinner one evening, she announced that someday she was naming a son Kevin Edward, and everybody else should keep their hands off that name.

That's the way it was. Nobody really intended—not Ed, not the kids —for Ed to take a father role in my children's lives. Nobody intended to love each other, either. Loving Ed was risky for my kids. They'd loved one father and lost him. Loving my kids was a pain in the ass for Ed, because when you care about kids, you find yourself doing pain-in-the-ass things like going to high-school track-team banquets, worrying because it's one A.M. and nobody's home yet, and letting a nineteen-year-old drive your Mercedes.

But it happened anyway.

And now we had to tell them just how sick he was.

They already knew there was cancer. Chris had been with us, of course, from the beginning. I'd been in constant touch with my three daughters on the phone. Indeed, there was a sixth sense of fatalism. When I first told Sug we had a problem, she asked, "Is it Ed?"

I said, "Yes."

She asked, "Is it his health?"

I said, "Yes."

And she screamed.

On this September-sunny-Sunday, with the smell of Coppertone in the air and Jimmy Buffett "wasting away in Margaritaville," we had to tell these people that once again they had a father who was very, very ill.

But one of the most admirable of human qualities is grace under pressure. People rise to occasions, and the worst of times can become the best of times.

There was a lot of tanning going on. Ed kept throwing towels over my daughters' skimpy little bikinis. "You stop that tanning," he'd say. Or he'd stand beside them and cast a shadow. "Nobody's allowed to have a better tan than mine," he'd say. He bought yellow and white helium balloons and tied them to the rail on the deck. Chris barbecued the chicken. (He was always worried Ed would burn down the deck.) Erin made one of her famous salads, with odd-ball vegetables, like kale. And Ed talked about cancer.

He didn't talk about Dr. Bornstein or twelve months or any of that. He told the children about the programs he was looking into. He talked about how good and strong he felt. He said he believed he had a good chance. He was positive, up, optimistic.

He also asked something of us. "I'd like to keep this all in the family," he said. "Except for immediate family and one or two friends of mine and your mom's, I don't see why anyone has to know."

We talked about that as much as we talked about anything. "It's a big burden to carry around secrets like that," said Erin. "It'll be hard on Mom," said Chris. "Your friends will feel shut out," said Sug.

Ed explained himself as best he could. "I think a lot of people see weakness in being sick. I've done it myself and it's especially bad with cancer. People never look at you the same again. They may treat you well. But inside, their feelings about you have changed. I don't want to be surrounded by that. I don't want the stink of cancer."

Privacy flies in the face of today's conventional wisdom about illness. Openness, sharing, letting feelings out, joining support groups are all considered important aspects of living with disease. I don't deny the value of any of the above, but I'd like to speak to the other side of it.

I fought as hard as I knew how for normalcy during the thirteen years of Kevin's illness and found myself instinctively fighting for it again with Ed. The best thing you can do when you're ill is to live as if you're not. To send messages to the billions of cells in your body that you're strong, that you're okay. To send messages to the billions of cells in your brain that you're positive and optimistic. To get your mind and body working with you, not against you.

When you're thinking about your illness all the time, and talking about it all the time, it's hard not to feel sorry for yourself. Or, at least, to set yourself apart as someone who is now different.

I believe you should fight to be the same. "Treat me the same. Act the same around me. Expect the same of me. And I will rise to those expectations."

Illness, especially dire illness, is difficult for most people to be around. And they will not—most of the time, try as they might—treat you the same.

I'm not saying illness should be a deep, dark secret, or that an ill person should become a closed personality, or that illness is anything to be ashamed of. I'm saying, rather, that you should fight for normalcy within your own self and from the people around you. Maintaining normalcy requires some discretion and doesn't allow you to wear illness as a badge. My friends knew that Kevin had a problem. But we downplayed it, seldom talked about it, and never lived as if he did.

Ed had the same attitude, as I did in regard to him. He needed to tell a friend or two, and he did confide in Eric Davison, for example, right from the start. But could he have had a normal business lunch with his colleagues, drinking too much and carrying on, if they all knew he'd just been diagnosed with lung cancer? Terminal lung cancer? I think not. Could he and I have had a dinner party and had friends in without the friends feeling as if they had to walk on eggs and screen what they said? I think not.

In the end, we agreed to do our best to keep the talk of cancer within the family.

Then we all drank too many of Ed's killer Margaritas as we watched the sun set. And we argued, like any other family ending a summer weekend, over whose turn it was to do the dishes.

September 15

"I don't like the name," Ed commented as he turned the Porsche into the entrance and drove slowly past the rose garden. "It sounds like hope-less."

"This place is huge," I said. There seemed to be acres of single-story brick buildings. A lot of cottages here and there. You certainly didn't get the whirring, purring high-tech feeling you got at Cedars. "It's like a college campus," I went on. "In Kansas."

"They told me to look for the statue and the fountain." Almost as Ed said it, there was the statue. It's a sculpture, really—a man, a woman, and a child—posed in a moment of triumph. A half-hearted fountain played at the base.

The City of Hope is a National Pilot Medical Center sprawling over 107 acres on the edge of a nondescript town called Duarte, about thirty miles from downtown Los Angeles. We had driven past miles and miles of gravel pits on the 605 Freeway to get there. Ed was trying to tell me that the Los Angeles Raiders were negotiating to build a stadium "in the pits."

"That's going to spawn a lot of pitiful jokes," I said, spawning one.

We went into the building behind the statue and found the outpatient clinic. Ed was here, not for yet another second opinion but because he'd found a promising experimental program at the City of Hope, among those on his PDQ printout. Phil Richmond, who'd kept in close touch and been a considerable comfort, helped him get the appointment.

As usual, they took Ed away for blood tests, urine tests, and X-rays. I sat down to wait and found myself smiling at two old ladies sitting across from me. They were in their seventies, with white hair you knew had once been blonde. They were wearing print dresses, of the kind my mother used to call "house dresses." They both had on white canvas shoes. Well, yes... tennis shoes. But what, indeed, riveted your attention was they were identical twins.

I tried to remember if I'd ever seen twins that old who still dressed alike. They've got to be living together, I thought to myself. How could you get up every morning, go to the phone, and call your sister to find out what she's going to wear? I wondered if they'd lived together all their lives. I wondered, as my mind continued to try to make up their story, which one of them had cancer. I was trying to overhear their chitchat when Ed came back and took me with him to an examining room to wait for the doctor.

"The doctor we're going to see," he told me, "is named Ronald Ewen."

I was pacing when Dr. Ewen entered the room. "Do sit down and stay awhile, Mrs. McNeilly," he smiled at me. "We don't bite, you know."

He was British. Thirty-fiveish. He had that reserve shot with dry wit that makes a lot of Englishmen seem puckish. He began with a question no other doctor had ever asked Ed. "What do you do for a living?" Ed told him about advertising, marketing automobiles, and that he was currently looking for a car-related business to buy.

Dr. Ewen listened. "I know nothing about commerce," he said at one point. "The business world is a mystery to me." He continued to chat with Ed, asking about me, children, where we lived.

Then he explained the clinical trials in progress at the City of Hope. They were testing an experimental drug called Leucovoran. It was a Phase III program with a 45-percent success rate. He felt confident Ed would qualify. "But you must take into consideration," he cautioned, "that we have a test group and a control group. If you choose the program, the computer randomly picks the group you go into." The control group got the standard treatment for colon cancer, the drug called 5FU.

"I don't want the control group," Ed said. "Is there any way I can be assured of the test group?"

"No," was Dr. Ewen's complete answer.

Ed told him about the programs he was investigating at UCLA and USC. At the mention of Dr. Malcolm Pardo at USC, Dr. Ewen bristled. "I know him," he said. "He likes attention." And then he added with a deep sigh. "Everybody wants to be the Jonas Salk of cancer."

Dr. Ewen then talked about the Interleuken 2 program. "I think it was appalling the first research results were published so early," he said. "There had been no clinical trials. It was unconscionable to let people think a cure might be in hand. NCI sank to new depths." In a somewhat softened tone he added, "NCI probably did it to get publicity and funding."

Ed asked him about the published success of the Interleuken 2 program at one of the big cancer hospitals. Dr. Ewen raised his eyebrows. Ed was not an ordinary patient. He knew too much. "They have a reputation," said Dr. Ewen, "for publishing positive results that cannot be duplicated elsewhere."

He means they're cheating, I thought to myself. Isn't this fascinating, I thought to myself.

The inside look at the medical community that was beginning to unfold was, indeed, fascinating. The lack of respect the doctors in research had for the doctors in private practice. The rivalries among the research institutions, as well as among individual doctors. The criticism of public agencies, like NCI. The criticism, from one doctor to another, of how and what to treat.

Dr. Ewen told us about the Interleuken 2 program at the City of Hope. "We brought people to death's door and then back again, with no clear results." Apparently, the highly touted Interleuken 2 wasn't bearing out in clinical trials. What's more, it was extremely hard on the patients. All of the blood was removed from their bodies and replaced with blood in which the white cells had been zapped with the drug. "We almost killed a couple of people here, in the process," said Dr. Ewen. "And then it didn't work." There were no further Interleuken 2 studies then under way at the City of Hope.

The conversation then turned back to Ed and his particular situation. Dr. Ewen startled us with a statement that was to throw our lives into turmoil for the next two weeks. "I think we'd do well to take a look," he said, "at removing the tumor from the colon."

Ever since Dr. Richmond, with his pink argyles, and Dr. Kraft with his shaking cup of coffee, had walked into Ed's room at Cedars, the tumor in the colon had been almost forgotten. The "doozies" in the lungs simply overshadowed it. Dr. Richmond, Dr. Kraft, and Dr. Bornstein finally explained to us that the colon surgery had been cancelled because there was no point.

"It's difficult, dangerous surgery," we'd been told. "It would be hard on Ed, and hard on the family. It won't accomplish anything. There will still be cancer in the lungs."

"But shouldn't we get out as much as we can?" I'd asked. "Doesn't it at least slow things down?"

"It doesn't help," I'd been told. "All cancer broadcasts. If you can't ultimately get all of it, there's no point in getting part of it."

Dr. Ewen knew all of that logic. But he wanted to remove the tumor anyway. "I understand that conventional medical wisdom is to leave it alone," he said. "But you can't possibly win, Mr. McNeilly, unless we take it out. Also, we theorize that chemotherapy works better when you remove the primary mass. And, the tumor may rupture."

Dr. Ewen left us alone to talk while he went to check on whether or not there was room for Ed in the City of Hope clinical trials.

I could tell that Ed had made up his mind. "It's a Phase III program," he said. "It's farther along than either USC's or UCLA's. I like that they want to fight. If there's room for me in the program, I'll tell them 'yes' right now."

"What about the surgery?" I said. "Do you want them to do the surgery?"

"Yes."

Twenty minutes later, Ed was in the program.

We drove home to Malibu elated. In only a little more than two weeks he'd taken control of his own situation. He'd made himself knowledgeable, done his own research, found his own programs, interviewed the doctors.

With control comes strength. And with knowledge comes power. Ed had gone from a man terminally ill who was going to be kept comfortable, to a man fighting, in charge, living—and, the most amazing thing of all, to a man who was happy.

September 15

ED PHONED UCLA AND USC and cancelled his involvement in their programs. Then he phoned Dr. Richmond to bring him up to date on what had happened, and to tell him about the program at the City of Hope. That's when the turmoil started.

"Ed, you're crazy to do surgery," Dr. Richmond said over the phone. "There's no evidence that removing the main mass of cancer lets chemotherapy work better. It's a difficult, debilitating, painful operation. It'll be hard on you and your wife. It's for nothing."

Ed was taken aback by the intensity of Dr. Richmond's opinion. "I like the idea of the surgery," he countered. "It means we're doing something. We're getting rid of some of it."

"I understand, Ed," Dr. Richmond continued. "You want to lash out. You want to do something. But you must keep control."

He urged Ed to ask the doctors at the City of Hope if there was clinical evidence that removing the tumor makes chemotherapy work better. Ed promised he would.

"Don't be a Steve McQueen, Ed," was Dr. Richmond's final plea. Steve McQueen had gone all over the world looking for a way to stop his cancer in his final months.

"I don't see what's the matter with what Steve McQueen did," Ed said to me later. "You can do nothing and die. Or you can do something. Maybe you still die. But you did something."

September 17

ED HAD A MEETING WITH DR. EWEN and with Dr. Andre Marcos, a surgeon at the City of Hope. (Ed always referred to his doctor's appointments as "meetings." "I don't go there, Jean, to listen," he explained, "but to discuss things." And he expected to be treated as an equal, which he was. "Actually," he said, using advertising terminology, "I'm the client and I expect to be treated that way.")

Dr. Marcos agreed with Dr. Ewen that the colon tumor should come out. Ed told them both about Dr. Richmond and, as Dr. Richmond had suggested, asked if there was clinical evidence of the surgery's benefits.

"Your doctor is correct," said Dr. Ewen. "There is no clinical evidence, no hard data. That evidence is next to impossible to gather. It is very hard to quantify, in these kinds of cases, if a particular action lengthens life." He then told Ed about the Goldman hypothesis.

"It's only a theory," he said, "an instinct. We can't prove it, but the Goldman hypothesis is that you take out as much of the main mass of tumor as possible, causing the chemotherapy to be more potent on what's left."

"In addition," Dr. Marcos added, "the tumor may cause an obstruction. Or it may rupture."

Surgery was scheduled for the following week. But the debate continued.

September 19

DR. RICHMOND PHONED. He'd consulted with several doctors and surgeons at Cedars. He continued to urge Ed to forget the surgery. He characterized the surgery as major and difficult. Dr. Marcos had described it as routine.

September 20

ED AND I WERE DAZED AND CONFUSED. How can two sets of doctors from two such highly respected institutions be 180 degrees apart on such a fundamental issue? Don't the doctors *know*?

It reminded me of how important diagnosis is to the practice of medicine. It reminded me just how big a guessing game goes on. It reminded me how fallible doctors are. It reminded me how important it is to equip yourself to make the final decision yourself. It reminded me of Kevin.

🐚 *I'll never forget the day—June 2, 1964. It was six-thirty A.M. I was in that half-sleep state you're in as you start to wake up. I could hear Erin, the cutest baby ever born, in her crib. She was seven months old and a "rocker." One of those babies who gets up on her hands and knees and rocks back and forth. She was rattling her bed from rocking so hard. Erin was my "happy" baby. She grinned and laughed and hugged and smiled and never cried.*

Chris and Sug, our twins, were two-and-a-half. I could picture them without opening my eyes. Chris, my "contemplative" baby, would be lying on his back, rubbing a ragged piece of blanket against his cheek, staring up at the ceiling, and thinking about the sandbox, potty training, Froot Loops, or whatever two-and-a-half-year-olds think about.

Sug was my "ebullient" baby. She'd go from being asleep to being wide awake in an instant and at two-and-a-half was already assistant-Mom. I knew she wasn't awake yet, because if she was, she'd be calling to me from their room, "Can we get up now? Can we get up now?"

Suddenly, Kevin, who was asleep on his side of the bed, kicked me. He kicked me really hard. And I turned over, wide awake and mad. But in a split second, anger turned to fear.

He was kicking and jerking uncontrollably. His arms were flailing. His legs were jerking. I looked at him and went white. He was flailing so violently he fell from the bed to the floor. His eyes were rolled back in his head and there was foam at the corners of his mouth. He was making guttural, animal sounds.

I had a friend in college who was an epileptic. I knew I was seeing a Grand Mal seizure.

I bolted into the kitchen, grabbed a wooden spoon, and ran back to try to jam it between his teeth so he wouldn't bite his tongue. His teeth were clenched so tight I couldn't get the spoon in. I tried to hold his arms so he wouldn't hurt himself. I didn't know what to do. He was on his back still in violent spasms. I finally laid down right on top of him and tried to bring his body quiet with the force and weight of my own.

The seizure stopped as suddenly as it began. I don't know how long it lasted. It seemed an eternity. It was probably about two minutes. His body was quiet. But he was unconscious.

His teeth were still clenched. His breathing was full of rattles. When I pulled his eyelids open, all I could see were the whites of his eyes. I ran to the phone and called an ambulance.

The ambulance came very quickly, sirens blaring. All three children were still in their beds, playing with their toys, oblivious to what was happening. The ambulance drivers (this was before paramedics) asked me what had happened. I said that my husband had had a seizure. They asked if he was an epileptic. I said no. He was still unconscious. I asked, "Where are you taking him?" They said, "UCLA Emergency." I couldn't go with him. I had three babies in their beds in the other room. It was seven in the morning. We'd lived in the house (our first) only a couple of months. I didn't know a single neighbor. Suddenly Kevin was gone, with the ambulance sirens blaring again as they drove away.

As I whirled around in a panic, a policeman came to the door. "We always follow up emergency calls," he said, inviting himself in. He saw the mess in the bedroom. A bedside table had overturned when Kevin hit the floor, upending an empty beer bottle.

True to his Irish heritage, Kevin drank Guinness Stout, a formidable black beer. The policeman saw the mess and the Guinness bottle. He asked if there had been a quarrel. A fight. Domestic violence. He talked to me for about five minutes, satisfied himself, and left. He didn't offer me any help with the children or my fear, nor did he offer me a ride to UCLA. He just left.

I remember going to the phone and standing there shaking, trying to figure out what to do. My best friend, Shirley Kittleson, from the advertising agency where I worked part-time, lived in Hollywood, which was thirty minutes away.

I thought about calling my mother in Oklahoma City. What good would that do? Then I heard a knock at the front door. I opened it to a white-haired woman about seventy years old. Her hair was pulled back in a tidy bun. She was rosy-faced and plump. She was wearing an apron. "I'm Mary Canova," she said. "I live across the street. I saw the ambulance and the policeman. I know you have small children. I thought you might need some help."

To this day, I cry when I remember Mary Canova. She helped me get my three babies dressed and took them to her apartment so I could go find my husband at UCLA Emergency.

By the time I got there, Kevin was conscious and sitting up. He'd begun to come out of the epileptic state in the ambulance and seemed perfectly fine now. He remembered the previous night. He was lucid, but he didn't remember a thing about the morning. He was laughing— chagrined that I didn't think to bring him clothes—and ready to go home.

But UCLA Emergency wouldn't release him. "A thirty-three-year-old man with no history of epilepsy doesn't have a seizure for no reason," they said. They began tests that very morning. When I went home to rescue Mary Canova from Chris, Sug, and Erin, she was pooped and quite happy to see me. "I had to give them Cheerios for breakfast and lunch," she said. "It was all I had in."

Kevin spent the next two months as an outpatient at UCLA's Neuropsychiatric Institute, or NPI as it's called. They ran every test known to man trying to find out why he had had a seizure.

They looked for a tumor or an aneurysm in the brain. They checked for multiple sclerosis. They did spinal taps and brain scans. They looked for nerve damage. They ran tests for neurological disorders I'd never heard of. They did electroencephelograms. They ran into a blank wall every place they turned. Tests would begin to indicate a direction, but a further test wouldn't bear it out. Kevin routinely failed the most simple neurological tests that doctors do—like the one in which they run a nail across your foot, or the one in which they ask you to bring two fingers together in front of your nose. Yet the more complex tests showed that there was no neurological problem. I remember how blown away they all were when they did a spinal tap. They were expecting to find an indicator of neurological dysfunction in his spinal fluid, but it was normal. They did three spinal taps before they finally believed the results.

About the middle of August, they decided to hospitalize Kevin, because outpatient diagnosis wasn't getting anywhere. So Kevin checked into NPI. When I went to see him the first time, I remember how sick everyone else was. When something goes wrong with the brain, it's always something dreadful. Like multiple sclerosis. Or tumors. Yet he seemed so well.

Then, one day after he'd been in the hospital about two weeks, I went to visit and couldn't find him. His room was cleared and empty. All his copies of National Geographic were gone. I was told at the nurses' station that he'd been moved out of NPI. I'd find him in the Medical Center building, up the block, on the fifth floor, in Cardiology.

Cardiology? The heart? What was he doing in Cardiology?

No one explained anything to me; no one even left word for me at NPI; no one phoned me at home and told me what was going on. They just moved Kevin, and he told me what had happened.

That morning, an intern, brand new on the floor, had come in to do a workup—testing blood pressure, pulse, vital signs, etc. The intern was left-handed, and that, combined with the particular arrangement of reading materials and other junk that Kevin had lying on the bed, made it clumsy for him to take a pulse the usual way, at the wrist. So he reached to take it in the neck.

But when he pressed his fingers against the carotid artery in the neck in the usual fashion, there was no pulse. Suddenly, the whole floor was in the room. And it was clear. There was no pulse.

The next thing they did was an angiogram, the procedure in which doctors insert a needle and shoot a dye into the arteries so they can get a good X-ray picture. They wanted, of course, to X-ray the artery in the neck that had no pulse. But the artery was so clogged that the angiogram created an incident in itself. Kevin passed out and convulsed during the procedure. When I found him in Cardiology, his whole left side had gone numb and he couldn't control his left hand.

The clogged carotid artery was cutting off blood, and thus oxygen, to the brain, which was causing neurological symptoms. The original seizure was probably caused by a tiny bit of plaque breaking away from the arterial wall and lodging in the brain.

It never occurred to anybody at NPI that there might be an arterial problem. Kevin was too young. You don't get clogged arteries when you're thirty-three years old. Besides, the omnipresent "no cholesterol" that we see today on margarine packages and cooking-oil labels was years away. The study of coronary artery disease was just beginning to break new ground.

Or, indeed, was the whole situation at NPI an embarrassing oversight? Is that why NPI moved him out of there so quickly? Is that why there was no one around for me to talk with? And did they compound the embarrassment by almost losing Kevin when they did the angiogram?

Twenty-five years later, all I can do is wonder. I wonder how they could have missed an artery clogged so badly. Was NPI so immersed in its own discipline—the brain—that they never did a complete physical? Wouldn't an electrocardiogram or a stress test have indicated the *problem? I think there's a very simple test that would have. All doctors do it when they give you a routine physical. They shine a pinlight flashlight into your eye and simply look at the arteries exposed there. Inside the eye is the one place in your body where arteries are out in the open and subject to visual inspection. You can actually see evidence of coronary artery disease.*

At the time it all happened, I was young and shy. I was, as most of us are, in awe of doctors. I never questioned. I tended to be grateful to NPI for hanging in there for two-and-a-half months until they found out what was wrong.

Today, I tend to think they missed it, and they got Kevin the hell out of there before somebody created a problem. I think they missed it because they weren't considering the whole person. And because diagnosis is really, really tricky.

That's why people should never hesitate to question a doctor. To get the facts. To get an understanding of a situation. To get second and third opinions. Medicine is not in any way a hard-and-fast science. It's not math or calculus, with answers governed by rules. No two doctors are going to handle a situation that's out of the routine in exactly the same way. Patients need to realize that doctors are fallible and diagnosis is tricky. Patients need to get past the "doctor as god" syndrome and rely more on themselves.

In a flash, that summer of 1963, Kevin went from NPI at UCLA to Cardiology at UCLA. About sixty days later, the surgeons in Cardiology performed the twelve-hour operation that was an attempt to clear the artery—the operation that failed; the operation where they didn't bother to cosmetically close the incision; the operation that caused Dr. Bracco to call us over to UCLA and sort of tell us that Kevin was going to die. ❧

Twenty-four years later, on Saturday, September 20, 1986, Ed and I found ourselves in the middle of a diagnostic disagreement between the doctors at the City of Hope, who wanted to remove the malignant tumor in the colon, and the doctors at Cedars-Sinai, who were advising against it.

To help find his way out of the dilemma, Ed decided to break the tie by getting a third opinion. He phoned Dr. Beckman, the rumpled young man from UCLA. I don't know how he got Dr. Beckman's home phone on a Saturday. But he got it.

I could hear a baby crying in the background as Ed talked with Dr. Beckman. I could picture him in his Saturday clothes. I wondered if his wife was mad because he got phoned at home. I remembered one time when Kevin, desperate over something I can no longer remember, was equally resourceful at getting a doctor's home phone number but when he phoned he was told, "how dare you," "you have no right," "don't you ever interfere with my personal life," etc.

Dr. Beckman, however, was terrific. He said, "Ed, phone me anytime. Don't feel because you aren't going into our program, you can't call."

He then gave Ed his opinions about the surgery. "Surgeons always want to cut," he said. "But there's no medical reason to remove the tumor. It's housekeeping. There might be a reason if it was fast-growing, but this kind is typically slow-growing." He said a lot more. But that was the gist of it.

The medical opinions tilted two to one against surgery. When Ed hung up, I asked, "Are you going to cancel?"

"Not yet," he answered. "There's one more thing I want to do."

September 22

ED DID THE ONE MORE THING. He phoned Dr. Ewen's superior at the City of Hope, Dr. Stanislaski. Ed wanted to talk with him not only because he was the boss but also because his first contact with the City of Hope, over the phone, had been with Dr. Stanislaski. Ed got him on the phone and explained the situation. He asked if not doing the surgery would jeopardize his participation in the experimental programs.

"Of course not," Dr. Stanislaski said. "It's certainly okay if you don't do the surgery. You don't have to."

"But should I?" Ed asked.

"It's a judgment call," Dr. Stanislaski said. "I can't make it for you."

Ed hung up. He sat by the phone still and silent for about thirty seconds. Then he dialed the phone again, asked for Dr. Marcos' office, and cancelled the surgery. Then he phoned Dr. Ewen's office and set the date—October 1—to begin the experimental program.

September 27

ED WAS A MORNING PERSON. I was a night person. When we got married, we worked the conflict out in a way any man would understand—I became a morning person.

I couldn't believe it happened to me. I hadn't seen the sunrise in forty years—maybe ever, I don't know. I hadn't had breakfast in twenty. It made me sick to eat before ten o'clock. I drank about four cups of coffee every morning, while I staggered around getting dressed, and I always took another mugful in the car. Even so, I'd yawn all the way to work.

Ed would bound out of the bed, trot onto the deck, beat his chest, drink in big gulps of air, then turn on the "Today" show. I couldn't believe it. Who were all those people talking about world events at seven A.M.? Jane Pauley drove me nuts.

Ed made a production every day out of breakfast. At first, I'd just stare at the trays he brought me. Pigs in a blanket, sausage-eggs, apple pancakes, corned-beef hash, crepes with blueberries, mushroom omelets. Occasionally, in desperation, I'd nibble on the toast and sip the juice until he'd go downstairs for more coffee. Then I'd throw everything over the deck into the Bougainvillea and pretend I'd eaten it while he was gone.

But after a time, I began to come around. He made me listen in the mornings, especially to mockingbirds. He showed me how sunrises streak the sky in a special way that's different from sunsets. He brought me roses from my garden with dew on them. (I had never actually seen dew.)

After about a year, my world turned upside down. I was getting up at six and going to bed at ten. I quit starting things—like baking cakes and writing TV commercials—after the eleven-o'clock news. I lost track of Johnny Carson. I started to like Jane Pauley.

This Saturday, however, I was suffering a relapse. I sensed Ed getting out of bed at six A.M., but it didn't faze me. Neither did the smell of coffee half an hour later. It wasn't until nine o'clock that I heard the sound of boomer-sized waves hitting the beach, along with the sound of Ed's hammer booming on the deck.

"What are you doing?" I called down to him.

"I'm starting the greenhouse," he called up at me.

We'd talked about the greenhouse for months. "We ought to build a greenhouse for the Plumeria," Ed would say.

"You're right," I'd say.

"We can put in an herb garden," he'd say.

"I can grow bromileads," I'd say.

"One of these days we should do that."

But this Saturday morning, there he was, with that macho look on his face men get when they work with tools. He'd moved an entire hardware store onto the deck. Hammer, saw, bags of nails, retractable tape, level, brackets, electric drill, electric saw, plane, lumber, chalk-line. He had on his "you-Jane-me-carpenter" outfit—corduroy shorts and no shirt. The portable radio was tuned to KLAC, the construction-guys' station. With Waylon Jennings wailing in the background, he was wailing in the foreground.

The reason for the greenhouse, of course, was the Plumeria. Plumeria is the bush that grows in places like Hawaii and produces a fragrant white flower with a yellow center used abundantly in leis. You find Plumeria all over the South Pacific. Once, when we came back from Tahiti, Ed decided he wanted a Plumeria on the deck. "They don't grow in Southern California. Too cold," he was told in nursery after nursery after nursery.

"They do grow here," he kept saying. "I've seen them."

He finally found a nursery that stocked Plumeria by phoning one in Hawaii and asking where they shipped. We went there and brought home a big bush, about six feet high, and two smaller ones in containers the size of coffee cans.

We left them in their pots, and all three thrived on our lower deck. They punched out their little white flowers for Ed to put on trays when he brought me breakfast. They thrived, that is, until the first winter. There was a sleet storm right before Christmas. And the day after, without a word of explanation, the Plumeria moved into the house. They spent that winter in the living room, fighting with the Christmas tree and the Dracena Magenta for attention. But they weren't meant to live in the house and when we put them back outside in the warming days of springtime, we first began to talk about the greenhouse.

"I think I can finish it in a week," Ed said as he bent over his plans. "I'll get all the glass pre-cut and hang ready-made sliding doors. Would you get me a beer?"

This is not a man dying of cancer, I thought to myself. This is a man building a greenhouse so his Plumeria won't have to spend another winter in the living room.

Being fairly adept with a hammer, I joined him. It was a great day. Normalcy.

October 1

THE ADVERTISING AGENCY.
The first thing you see when you walk in is Canary. She's six feet tall, give or take, with a great sense of style in the way she dresses and the

honey-coated voice of a southern Black as she answers the phone, "Kresser/Craig."

The eclectic, I think electric, nature of the people takes off from there and never stops. At one end of the office you see jeans, wild ties, no ties, men in pony tails, women in boots, levis, and 400-dollar blazers. You see posters on the walls and in the halls, Macs, printers, lines and lines and lines of type, storyboards, mechanicals, logos, discarded layout tissues all over the floor, and walls papered with ideas stuck there with masking tape, ready to be ripped off and added to the heap on the floor or ripped off and put into the hands of a renderer.

You hear the squeak of magic markers, the whirrr of the stat machine, the click-click-click of a writer putting a page of headlines into a Mac. And underneath everything the noise of creation. The copywriter/art-director teams lying on the floor, sitting on the couches, their feet on the desk, on the chair, on the windowsill— anyplace but on the ground—as they think up ideas for advertising.

My office anchors that end of the building. I'm a writer. The creative director. An owner of the company. I never dreamed, when I started as a copywriter in 1961, writing ads for Dormans Men Clothiers and radio commercials for Standard Shoes, that I'd ever be a creative director, much less have my own company. I just wanted to be a writer. I still do. I got there, I think, because I'm a master of short-term goals. "Get the TV spot written by noon. Get the meeting over by three. Get the kid to the doctor by four." I never really planned my career, but always concentrated on doing well whatever I was doing at the moment. I'd be great in a Nike ad. I "just do it."

At the other end of the building, you see suits, suspenders, and bow ties. You see women in heels and silk shirts. Women who wouldn't dream of wearing slacks to a client. On the men, you see a few wing tips. A lot of near-Gucci. You see maps with dots indicating TV markets, miles and miles and miles of overheads. You see charts that follow sales, that follow broadcast buys, that follow expansion, that follow advertising-to-sales ratios, that follow profits, that follow research, that follow follow-ups.

You hear the constant whirr of computers accessing data banks, the din of presentations escaping under the door of the conference room, the high-tech sound of new phone technology, the constant hum of voices conducting business by way of GTE. It's the noise of marketing. Selling products through advertising campaigns.

Bob's office anchors that end of the building. Bob Kresser. Head account hump, he calls himself. My partner. I'm the president. He's the CEO.

Everybody has locked into his or her brain a stereotypical picture of an "adman." Somebody who's slick and smooth, with a lot of moves. Dressed just right. Talks just right. On the glamorous side. And facile. Very facile. A person who could sell refrigerators to Eskimos (or hamburgers in am/pm mini markets). Whatever the perception, you may as well erase it, because Bob Kresser blows it to hell. To begin with, there's the way Bob dresses. He knows what he's supposed to wear, but he just can't bring himself to do it. He has perfectly decent suits, but then he'll ruin a natty look with the shoes.

He has this whitish pair with thick, crepelike soles. Or he'll put on his tan loafers with his gray suit. Nikes have even shown up from time to time as a complement to Bob's best CEO suit.

"My heel hurts, Craig," he'll say sheepishly. "There's a bone spur. One of these days, I've got to get it fixed."

Bob carries a 15-dollar nylon zip-top bag instead of a brief case.

"I always lose brief cases, Craig."

His socks are always the wrong color.

"Do you suppose I'm colorblind?"

He has a propensity for pink shirts.

"Bob, pink was the '60s."

"Oh? Well,...I guess I'm just a '60s guy."

When Bob isn't wearing his suits, he tends toward cotton khakis that are too short. Bob is a loose-limbed six-feet-five, about six feet of which is leg, but apparently he's never noticed.

"I don't know why everybody's always saying my pants are too short, Craig. They look fine to me."

Bob wears his khakis to the office on days he thinks he won't have to go to the client. He wears plaid shirts with them and solid-color knit ties, the kind you haven't been able to buy since 1964. Invariably, on these days, he does end up at the client with Paul Anton, our executive vice-president, nodding sadly as Bob pulls his papers from the nylon brief case.

Once, Bob had his feet on the desk of Joe Tebo, our client at ARCO, and Joe noticed a hole in Bob's shoe. So he pulled the shoe off his foot and threw it in the trash can. Paul was mortified, but Bob was undaunted.

"Those are my favorite shoes, Craig. One of these days, I'll get them fixed."

Another non-adman trait is that Bob stammers sometimes when he talks. He doesn't stutter, he just loses his place, rambles along for a while, then backs up and starts over. He's also disorganized. His desk has phone messages on it from 1973.

But Bob is blindingly bright. And a genuine entrepreneur. He innovates. He thinks new thoughts. He tries new things. He's an inspirational leader and relentless in his pursuit not only of success but of excellence. If I had a company and wanted to succeed as a marketer, I'd give my business to Bob in a heartbeat.

As a human being, he's a touchingly sensitive man, funny and warm. Kindhearted. He's the person everyone wants to sit next to on the plane. The person everyone wants to dance with at the Christmas party.

Bob and I each had an agency of our own that preceded Kresser/ Craig. We'd each been in business on our own about ten years when we merged. Ed had a hand in putting the two companies together, and it had proven to be magic. In less than two years, we'd doubled the size of our company and had picked up one of the most prestigious advertising accounts on the West Coast—ARCO.

On this particular day, however, we were in turmoil. Hamburgers were in a tailspin at ARCO's am/pm mini markets and we were rushing a new commercial to finish. The account people were nervous; the creative people were grumbling. You could feel the tension in the halls. It's an exciting business, but there's a lot of pressure. I was also horribly worried about Ed.

Bob knew about Ed, because I talked to him about everything in my life, both business and personal, and I told him about Dr. Bornstein and the doctor's prognosis as soon as Ed and I got back from Hawaii.

Like my daughter Sug, Bob yelled out loud in disbelief.

That afternoon, at an ARCO meeting, he reached under the conference table and took my hand. With our client explaining something about the pricing of gasoline, he and I sat there, holding hands under the table, and I knew that this sweet, sensitive man I was so lucky to have as my partner was holding back tears.

On this day, I was horribly worried because Ed had left for the City of Hope early in the morning. To begin chemo. And I hadn't heard from him. I expected him to call by ten. By noon, I still hadn't heard, so I cancelled my lunch and waited. But nothing. Around two-thirty, I went into a meeting in our conference room, and finally Kimi interrupted it with a message. Ed was calling me from his car phone. I bolted from the meeting and took the call in my office.

"I need to talk to you," Ed said. "I don't want to do it on the phone."

"What is it? Where have you been? Are you okay?"

"I'll pick you up in about fifteen minutes. I really don't want to do it on the phone."

I was downstairs in front of our building in Century City when the Porsche came into the carriage area. Ed had the top down and the car and the man both turned your head. Ed had an ever-present tan and incredible blue eyes. The wrinkles and creases of time had outdone themselves on him as they do with some men, adding character, not age. But what dominated his face was the moustache. It had been white since he was twenty-nine years old and stood against his tan and his eyes like a white forelock on the face of a roan stallion. He took my hand as I got into the car and started at the end of his story, not the beginning.

"I didn't have chemo."

"Why?" I asked.

"The surgery is on again," he said.

"What?" I couldn't believe it. "Ed, you were so sure last week you didn't want to do it."

"I need to tell you about my meeting with Dr. Ewen."

It had been testy. "You ask seven people, you get seven opinions," the doctor said. He then went back over his logic, item by item. He didn't care that three doctors at Cedars and one at UCLA disagreed with him. He didn't care that his boss, Dr. Stanislaski, didn't have a strong opinion. He repeated his belief in the Goldman hypothesis. He said that the tumor was bleeding and could rupture. He said that it would undoubtedly grow and eventually cause an obstruction. "You see," he said to Ed, "the others don't expect you to live long enough for those problems to develop. But I do."

Ed took off the driving cap with the Cobra insignia on the front that he wore when he drove with the top down. The soft pink light of late afternoon diffused reality. The traffic speeding by on Century Park East, the people crowding through the revolving doors into the twin towers, and the motorcycle from ABC Messenger revving its engine all faded into the background. His face was foreground. What I saw was the tilt of the chin, the sparkle in the blue eyes, the crinkles at the corners of the moustache—the signs I'd learned to read on his face. The signs of strength. I knew at that moment that Dr. Ewen had engaged his spirit, and given him hope and courage. And that was far more important than the medical efficacy one way or another regarding the tumor in the colon.

"The surgery's set for next Monday," said Ed.

"Can we get the greenhouse finished before then?" I asked.

"You bet," he smiled.

I wished Dr. Ewen had been there.

October 3

THE PEOPLE WHO LIVE IN MALIBU
have a few secrets they try not to let out. Like where you can see good fireworks on the Fourth of July. Where you can find public access to seemingly private beaches. How to cheat the traffic when the coast highway is jammed.

Another little secret was the restaurant that sat right on the sand near Zuma Beach. It had been a hot-dog-and-hamburger joint for the beach crowd. But the owner turned it into a fine restaurant. They served trendy California dishes like Ahi tuna in cilantro sauce or Santa Barbara shrimp in tarragon butter. Despite the chic menu, it was a comfortable place. A lot of the famous people who live in Malibu made it a watering hole. So did a lot of the nonfamous people who live in Malibu —like Ed and me.

We went there for dinner because it was time to go, once again, onto the clear-liquid diet. And we decided to eat, drink, and be merry until midnight—the fasting hour.

We spent most of the evening, however, fascinated by two other couples who were also having dinner in the small upstairs dining room.

The first couple caught my attention when the man got up and went to the phone. I couldn't help but overhear snippets of his conversation.

"Stop rattling your glass," I said to Ed. "I can't hear."

The man was a doctor and was being phoned from his hospital. I heard him say, "Where the hell is the resident?" Then he said, "Oh Christ, not again." Then he said, "Well, give her 500 cc's more."

When he went back to his table, the young woman he was with was irritated. I couldn't hear, no matter how hard I tried, but her face was deep into sullen, about to turn the corner into surly.

"It's their anniversary," I said to Ed. "This is the first time they've had dinner alone in months, and he keeps getting called to the phone."

"Bullshit," said Ed. "You can tell by looking that he's divorced, and hot to trot. So's she." Ed occasionally used '50s terms like "hot to trot," which always amused me.

"If they were dating," I countered, "she'd be more tolerant. You don't get that mad unless you're married."

"She's not married," he said. "I can tell."

The doctor got called to the phone again. I couldn't hear much this time, but he was obviously very irritated. There was one "oh, shit" and one "is she conscious?"

Ed and I turned our attention to dinner. We talked about going someplace as soon as he recovered from surgery. We talked about finishing the greenhouse and whether or not we should try to grow orchids. We were talking about Tahiti when the doctor's voice came flying through the air. He was on the phone again. He was half shouting. His words formed a spear that sliced through the air and landed on our table.

"What do you mean she died?"

Ed and I just looked at each other. Life and death are going on around you all the time. You just don't know it.

The second couple we eavesdropped on that evening was Johnny Carson having dinner with a lady friend. "She's about a third his age," I said glaringly at Ed as if there was fault and it was his.

I was delighted that they didn't seem to be having a good time either.

October 4

ANNIE.

Ed got the glass onto the roof of the greenhouse, but it was a bitch to make it fit and he was going like a buzz saw to get it all finished. About noon, he got the glass in place on the sides. About four in the afternoon, he told me I could start my job—painting—while he went to work hanging the sliding glass doors. It wasn't a big greenhouse—3 feet by 8 feet by 10 feet high. But there was suddenly a lot to paint. We skipped dinner and kept on working. Ed couldn't eat anyway—he was on the clear liquid diet. The sun went down. But it was one of those balmy October evenings. So we kept on working, and we were painting by the lights from the deck when Annie just barged in.

Annie and I had been friends for twenty years. Her children and mine were all in elementary school when we first met. Trevor was the same age as Chris and Sug. Laura was a little older. Trevor played endless games of Marco Polo in our backyard pool, invited Chris to all of his birthday parties, and was Sug's date to her senior prom.

The friendship began a bit tentatively when Annie became part of my creative group at Foote, Cone & Belding, the worldwide advertising agency where my career took hold and took off. Tall and blonde, with a directness and an earthiness that were a bit unsettling because they made her so attractive, she was recently divorced and had, at age thirty-something, gone back to school at the Art Center College of Design in Pasadena. She had studied for a couple of years, got her portfolio together, and joined our group at FCB as a collateral designer, specifically to work on the Sunkist account. But she was very good and quickly became a full-out art director.

It was 1969 and while I was into backyard barbecues, trips in the Ford Ranch Wagon, baking cookies at Christmas, and pride over the moon landing, Annie was deep into the underside of the times. Shrinks. Divorce. Relationships. Men. Getting in touch with your feelings. Letting go of guilt. Perhaps we've always been opposite sides of the same coin and I see in her that part of myself I find hard to let out. I greatly admire her candor about life, her independence. Since I've known her, she's lived as a single woman and has done it better than anyone I know—with poise, grace, and never an ounce of self-pity. She reminds me, in that sense, of the screen heroines played by women like Katharine Hepburn and Bette Davis.

You wouldn't pick Annie out of a crowd as a rebel. She has classic taste. In her personal style. Her clothes. Her home. Her demeanor is gracious, her conversation cultivated. If you want to know where to put the fish fork (Annie actually has fish forks) when you set a table, Annie will know. Yet she has a rebellious streak that belies her country-club upbringing as a doctor's daughter in Battle Creek. The paradox of Annie is that she can be a little shocked if a friend wears an inappropriate dress to a social event, yet she can dare to be shocking herself in far more substantive matters. Attitudes about life. Relationships. Taking risks.

Reticent at times in business situations, another paradox of Annie is that she can breezily take off on her own and gallivant around the world. She took a month once and went by herself to Paris. She's traveled alone in Mexico, Australia, and the Caribbean. She swapped houses with a family from Nice and spent a summer in their home in the south of France.

We shared a lot of her love affairs and heartaches over the years, and when Kevin died she helped ease me into the world of dating and I got to share a heartache or two of my own with her.

And, we shared the threads that make up the everyday fabric of life—recipes, shopping, decorators, doctors, adolescent behavior, too much to drink at office parties, children with poison ivy, which car to buy, should I color my hair, do I dare paint the dining room red? (I did.) Neither of us had family, other than our children, in California, so we shared Thanksgiving, Christmas, and the Fourth of July. We even shared Ed for a time. She went out with him before I did. And she was one of two or three people, other than my family, to whom I'd told the story of Ed's illness.

She knew he was going to surgery the next day, and she barged in unannounced.

I remembered another time she did the same thing. Another October evening, shortly after Kevin died.

&. *Kevin died October 17, 1977. There wasn't any particular warning, although in retrospect, I should have known. He was getting so thin. He was having so many problems with his eyes and his memory. He was working, but most days I dropped him off and picked him up, because he'd slowed to the point where he was better off not driving.*

His father was visiting us. Sir John Craig. Kevin's family had been wealthy and prominent in Oklahoma/Arkansas during the 1930s and '40s. They owned lead and zinc mines, and while the rest of the world struggled through the Depression, they lived a Kennedyesque kind of life. Ten children, Mama's chauffeur, Daddy's chauffeur. Trips to Atlanta in the Dusenberg to see the opera, Little Lord Fauntleroy suits. There was a summer compound in Eureka Springs, Arkansas, and the family home in Tulsa took up a square city block.

In 1939, Kevin's father was "knighted" by the Catholic Church. Knights of the Holy Scepulcher date back to the eleventh century, but the honor is given today to lay people who contribute a lot to the Church. John Craig's pride was such that he took his knighthood literally and let himself be known as "Sir John."

Kevin's relationship with Sir John and his mother, Mary Holland, had a lot to do with why a man with his brains and background was running a window at the post office in Beverly Hills. Kevin was sandwiched between John, who was one year older and the out-and-out favorite of his father, and Ricky, who was one year younger, and the out-and-out favorite of his mother. Kevin spent a lifetime looking for approval from his parents, especially his father, but never got it. As a little boy, he retreated to the company of the cooks and the chauffeurs, because he felt more comfortable with the servants. In their company he was another of Sir John's sons, on equal footing, and wouldn't be criticized. By the time he was a young man, bravado, intelligence, and a charming eccentricity well obscured the low self-image. Even I didn't figure it out until well into our marriage. But it was there, and it was at the core of Kevin's inability to accomplish in terms that today's world understands.

Sir John was visiting along with Father Paul Brown, a priest from Tulsa. Over Sunday dinner, we made bets with the two old men on the World Series. The next morning, Kevin got out of bed and ran to the bathroom. When he came back, I fussed that he shouldn't run around naked with Father Brown in the house, then rolled over for another forty winks. Seconds later, Kevin had a heart attack.

I wasn't sure what it was at first. I thought he was convulsing again. Then, suddenly, he wasn't breathing. I ran to the phone to call the paramedics, then out the front door to call the children back. They caught a seven-ten bus to school and had already started down the street. Chris and Sug were fifteen. Erin was thirteen. Maureen was twelve.

I brought Erin with me into the bedroom. She'd taken a lifeguard course that summer, which included CPR, and gave her father mouth-to-mouth resuscitation while my heart wrenched at the scene. Then the paramedics came. The minute they saw Kevin, they were on their radio phones to UCLA Emergency. They restarted the heart with electric shock, but I could tell from their faces it was all over.

Chris and Sug came with me to UCLA, and after about fifteen minutes Alan Fogelman came into the waiting room. He'd been Kevin's doctor for seven years. It was Alan who had concluded there was a hereditary problem surrounding Kevin's atherosclerosis. It was Alan who had put our children into the Coronary Pediatric Center at UCLA. It was Alan who humanized for Kevin and me our entire relationship with UCLA.

It was Alan who came to tell us that Kevin was dead.

Sug called his name and bolted from the room. I grieved to Alan that I should have phoned the paramedics faster. He took my hand and said, "Jeanie, his situation was so tenuous."

We had the funeral two days later. Kevin's family and mine poured in from all over. Tulsa. St. Louis. Kansas City. Oklahoma City. Dallas. Longview. Some of them were still there a day later when Sir John, who was still there as well, went into cardiac arrest. The paramedics came again. Again we went to UCLA Emergency. Alan Fogelman took care of him. But he died at UCLA a week later. Kevin was forty-seven. Sir John was eighty-two.

October 31—Halloween—was Kevin's birthday. Everyone was gone by then. I was sitting in the living room of our house on Benecia wrapped in a red terry-cloth robe of Kevin's. I hadn't cried very much.

But the delayed reaction was starting to happen, and I was crying at that moment. Suddenly, there was a knock at the door and Annie just barged in. She knew it was Kevin's birthday, and she didn't call, she didn't ask, she just came.

When she noticed the red bathrobe, which she'd seen so often on Kevin as we whiled away Sundays around our pool, her eyes welled up. And the two of us sat there and talked about him until the children came home.

I told her I was angry at Sir John for dying too and stealing from me and the children our time for grief. It was a difficult thought for me to express, but she understood. ❧

Now, a decade, a lifetime, a million moments of feeling later, she was here, barging in again. She had a casserole with her and a bottle of wine. She kissed my cheek and said softly, "I'm so sorry this is happening to you."

But to Ed, she said aloud, "Where's the corkscrew?" And we sat on the deck, eating her famous chicken with artichokes and speaking of ships and shoes and sealing wax and my friend, Ann King.

October 6

THE SURGERY.

They took Ed from his room at six-thirty in the morning. Erin came down from Santa Barbara to be with me for the day, and she and I barely made it into the hospital and down the pea-green corridor to his room before they wheeled him away. In fact, we ran through the lobby, past the vending machines and the nurses' lounge, past the trolleys trundling through the halls with breakfast. The gurney with Ed on it was already being pushed toward the elevator.

"Wait a minute!" I yelled.

They stopped. Ed was groggy from the pre-op injection, but he squeezed my hand. "I made a deal with Dr. Marcos," he said. I didn't know what he was talking about.

He smiled at Erin. "How's your guy?" Then they pushed him on toward the elevator.

Erin and I walked to the cafeteria and had breakfast. We smiled at how everything at the City of Hope is endowed. Every chair in every lounge, every X-ray machine, every table, every bed, every scope, every gurney, every trolley—everything has a dymo label on the back that says: "A gift to the City of Hope from George and Iris Reiner." Or whomever. You come to expect the plastic spoons and paper napkins in the cafeteria to be inscribed.

We had a second cup of coffee. We waited. We talked. We went to the lounge where Dr. Marcos had asked us to wait. Erin brought along a bunch of graduate-school catalogs. She was getting ready to go back for a Master's and was thinking of MIT, so we talked about that and about her boyfriend, Rich.

Erin was only twenty-two years old, but she had already graduated from Stanford with a degree in geophysics and had been working for two years as an environmental planner for the County of Santa Barbara. She had one of the most beautiful faces I'd ever seen. Incredible brown eyes with lashes so long they'd brush my cheek when she kissed me goodnight as a child. Dark-brown, thick, naturally curly hair like her father's. A smile that could light up a room. A laugh that filled our home all the years she was growing up.

She'd always been an amazing child. She accidentally learned to read when she was three years old, sitting on my lap, while I read Dr. Seuss out loud. By the time she started school, she'd already read all of the Hardy Boys and Nancy Drews. When she was in the first grade she was identified as gifted and caused all of the other children to be tested as well, because brightness often runs in families. All four of the children were identified as such and went to the special classes for gifted children at Westwood School, but it always seemed to show the most in Erin.

She skipped the third grade and graduated from high school at sixteen. When she got accepted at Stanford, I was a little reluctant to let her go and I didn't know if I could afford it, as advertising was paying me well—but not wonderfully—at that time. Besides, I already had two kids in college and was anticipating all four being there at once before we were through, a strain on the budget of anyone, perhaps, save J. Paul Getty. But I talked to her high-school counselor.

"She's still a little kid," I told him.

"I've never had a student more qualified for Stanford," he told me back.

So she went. She worked to help, and she got a scholarship in her junior year. Together, we afforded it.

Ed and I were married when Erin was a junior. She became very independent and a stubborn feminist during her years at Stanford. She never lived with us, but she was around a lot. She dubbed our home

"Club Med Malibu" and would drop in with bands of friends from hither and yon. She had a certain reserve with Ed. She wasn't chagrined by him, like Chris. But neither did she let herself flat-out adore him, like Sug and Maureen. Still, she loved his margaritas and had his same kind of gusto when it came to having a good time. The sound of the two of them laughing together is in my mind forever.

Erin had no memory of her Dad's surgeries. She was a baby when he had the first one and only three or four when he had the second. But she'd spent her share of time in hospitals. She and Sug inherited his atherosclerosis, which was eventually identified more formally as familial hypocholesteremia, and went into pediatric coronary care at the UCLA Medical Center when Erin was about three. We talked about her health a little as we waited. She was taking Questran, a cholesterol-reducing drug, and her count was reasonable, in the low 200s. There was a new drug called Lovostatin that everyone was talking about. It was supposed to be even better.

The time dragged by. The candy-stripers came and offered us coffee. (The candy-stripers at the City of Hope are not the teenagers you're used to seeing in the role, but wonderful sprightly women in their sixties, seventies, and eighties.) Another volunteer came by and told us the hospital was very short of blood and that if either of us could give, we should come up to the second floor. "People are not giving blood as much," Erin told me, "because they think they can get AIDS from the needles." You can't, of course. I didn't want to leave the waiting area for fear of missing the doctor, but Erin went up and donated.

It was only ten-thirty when Dr. Marcos, still in his blue surgical cottons, walked into the lounge, but I felt like we'd been waiting a year.

Dr. Marcos was an Argentinian, and there was something about the way he took my hand that caused me to know him as a compassionate and giving person, although I had only met him the day before.

He smiled as he handed me a folded piece of paper. "Your husband gave this to me right before he went under."

It was a note to the doctor. It said, "No colostomy. If you have to choose between leaving the tumor in and giving me a colostomy, leave the tumor in."

"Ed is fine," said the doctor. "He came through the surgery very well, but I had to put in a colostomy. It's temporary. Three or four months. It's a compromise."

I knew Ed had a fear of colostomies that went beyond, I think, his fear of death. "The tumor was bigger than we thought," continued Dr. Marcos, "and lower. It's a good thing we got it out."

I asked how it could be bigger. They had taken so many X-rays. How could it be bigger? How could it be lower?

Dr. Marcos explained that much of it was embedded in the wall of the colon and didn't show up on the X-rays. "We were expecting something the size of a quarter," he said. "What I took out was the size of a lemon."

They'd removed a six-inch section of the colon that was dangerously close to the lower part that becomes the bowel. They'd put in the colostomy to give the area a chance to heal.

Dr. Marcos spent a comforting five minutes with us, answering questions, easing minds, then he directed Erin and me to the Intensive Care Unit where we waited another hour or so. Then they let us in to see Ed.

It's a real shocker to see someone right after surgery. The body is full of tubes and suction cups. Monitors are beeping. Bags are hanging from metal trees. IVs are dripping fluids. The skin in the surgical area has been shaved. The face is sallow.

Ed was drugged, unconscious. The first thing I did was pull back the covers and look at the colostomy. I decided that I couldn't be afraid of it. That marriage is intimate and you share everything. That my attitude toward it would have a lot to do with his attitude toward it. If I was repulsed, he would be ashamed. So I pulled back the covers and the dressings, and took a good look.

"That's not so bad," I said to Erin. She had the guts and the composure to look at it, too.

"It's not bad at all, Mom," she said.

At that moment, Ed woke up for one brief instant. He saw us. He saw it. He said, "Oh, shit."

A colostomy is a new anal opening. You get one because your bowel has been removed. Or because, as in Ed's case, your bowel needs to heal and can't be used for a time. Your anal opening is between your legs. If you get a colostomy, it's in front, usually about halfway between your belly button and your pubic area, but toward the right or the left. The surgeons make a slit in the abdomen, pull the colon through to the outside of the body, then open the colon so that fecal matter can pass. At this stage of the body's processing of fecal matter, however, it's semiliquid and you can't control the flow. There's no "I have to go" feeling. So, the stuff just drains out of the new opening whenever it gets there, and people wear a bag around the opening to catch it. Hundreds of thousands of people have colostomies, yet they are the most taboo subject among all the body's physical problems.

I stood there looking at it with Erin and said to myself, "This will be okay." Of course, I wasn't the one who had it.

Erin and I sat with Ed all the rest of the day and into the night. Every now and then, a stab of pain would shoot open his eyes. Erin said, "There are no words for pain. You can't really describe it."

Dr. Ewen came by. Ed was semi-awake. The doctor took him by the hand and said, "You and I have some fighting to do."

Dr. Marcos came by. Ed tried to talk about Fangio, the Argentinian race-car driver who was almost as famous as Eva Peron in the '50s. Dr. Marcos also took his hand. "Yes. I know Fangio." He turned to me. "He is going to be fine."

Erin and I left about nine o'clock at night. We were mostly silent as she drove the long fifty miles from the City of Hope to Malibu—the 210 Freeway to the 605 to the Pomona Freeway to the Santa Monica Freeway to the Coast Highway to our own little street.

We'd come a long way, but we had just begun the fight.

October 7

THE INTENSIVE CARE UNIT AT THE CITY OF HOPE looks like the Manned Space Center at NASA. In the middle of the room is "Mission Control," a ring of beeping, flashing monitors, computer screens, and electronic sensors. In command of Mission Control is a scurry of nurses—you assume the best and the brightest—and a parade of doctors, technicians, orderlies, aides, and specialists. Around the perimeter are the patients, each one in a curtained cubicle, lying in a bed that looks like the cockpit of a jumbo jet, with its dials, gauges, switches, and flashing lights.

There is constant noise in ICU, not just the whirring, beeping, buzzing cacophony of the high-tech equipment, but the human noise of telephones, conversation, people bustling, patients coughing, doctors going in and out. You have to push a buzzer to get in, identify yourself, then wait a few minutes until they're ready for you. A regular human being, like myself, looks strangely out of place—like an Earthling among Martians. As I walked through to Ed's cubicle, I felt I mustn't touch or say anything lest I disrupt the whole mechanism. I also wondered how anybody can get well there. It's not exactly peaceful and serene.

Ed recognized me through the haze of morphine and said "hi" and "I love you" before he drifted back under. I was frightened by how bad he looked. His nurse, Josie, told me he was fine, that I could swab his mouth from time to time with peppermint-flavored sponges on a stick and that I could put cold compresses on his forehead, but other than that there was nothing to do but wait. I was alone. Erin had gone back to her job in Santa Barbara. So I sat in the darkened cubicle, hearing Ed breathe, hearing the monitors beep, becoming immobilized and frozen by the icy thoughts collecting in my brain.

I didn't know if Ed was going to live or die. I didn't know if the surgery had been right or wrong. I doubted Ed's decision to opt for privacy. I felt so alone and so lacking in support. Then, slowly, like water freezing in a pond, I began to doubt my whole life. What would there be for me without Ed? My children were grown and gone, immersed in their own lives. And I suddenly hated my work. It was superficial and shallow. What did it mean? What was it for? What was there of worth for me without Ed? Some lines from T.S Eliot's "The Love Song of J. Alfred Prufrock" kept repeating themselves over and over in my mind.

I grow old ... I grow old.
I shall wear the bottom of my trousers rolled.
Shall I part my hair behind? Do I dare to eat a peach?
I shall wear white flannel trousers and walk upon the beach.
I have heard mermaids singing, each to each.

I do not think that they will sing to me.

Fear. Depression. Stress. Isolation. I could feel them physically present in the room pulling me under the ice, in a slow downward spiral. I know now, but I didn't know then, that Fatigue was also present in the room, confusing my shaky hold on reality. I began to feel desperate. I knew I had to get away, so I mustered all the tiny snippets of energy I could find and made my legs walk away from ICU, to the elevator, to reception, outside to the warm air of the afternoon. I walked around the rose garden for a while, chasing away the demons by trying to identify all the beautiful hybrid roses—Mr. Lincoln, Chrysler Imperial, Bing Crosby, Sterling Silver. Then I walked to sit down by the fountain, and that's where I met Tom Coughlin, a man I had never seen before and will never see again but who saved my life that afternoon.

He was sitting by the fountain, too, and started up our chat with something like "nice day." We made small talk for a while, about the roses and the weather. He was an older man, in his late sixties. He had a friendly, accessible face, like the guy who runs your neighborhood drugstore or a spry grandfather in a McDonald's commercial. I found myself telling him about my husband in Intensive Care. I told him we were going into an experimental program as soon as Ed recovered from surgery and that I was scared.

"Most everybody here is in an experimental program," Tom Coughlin said. "I've been in one myself for twenty-two years."

"Twenty-two years?"

He thumped his chest. "I was one of the first people," he said, "to ever get a pacemaker. It was a real big experiment when they put mine in. They didn't know if it would work at all, or for how long. I was ready for it to give out in a few weeks or a few months." He thumped his chest again. "It's still there."

I asked him if he'd ever had problems with it.

"Just one," he said.

"What's that?"

"It's only one speed."

"I don't understand."

"It means I have a one-speed heart," he grinned. "It always goes at 72 beats a minute, no matter what. If I need it to go faster—to walk up a hill, for instance—it won't go faster. If I need it to go slower, it won't do that either. It's a real problem when I need to get mad."

I laughed out loud and thought to myself, "or when you need to have sex." The problems of a one-speed pacemaker began to unfold in my mind.

Tom Coughlin was continuing to chat. "Newer models have two speeds," he said. "You can turn it up whenever you like. They're getting more sophisticated all the time."

I talked with Tom for another twenty minutes or so. He brought me back to reality and put a calming perspective on my fears. Perhaps the most important thing he did, without even knowing it, was remove me from isolation. There is nothing more helpful on earth to people than people.

Thank you, Tom Coughlin, wherever you are.

October 8

THEY MOVED ED OUT OF INTENSIVE CARE and into a private room, but I thought he looked awful. Just awful. I thought he looked worse than forty-eight hours before, when he came back from surgery. He was still full of tubes; the colon was still "in shock." They were pumping this ugly green stuff out of his stomach. He had continuing nausea, intense pain in the surgical area, and a frightening disorientation.

Dr. Marcos told me these things are "very common after surgery." I didn't believe him.

The atmosphere at the hospital was like a Fellini movie, with people walking in and out of scenes, creating strange images and forming eerie tableaux. Nursing specialists walked into the scene every few minutes to do a procedure, take a pulse, give a shot, read a monitor, or scan a meter. People passed by in the hallway. The tall, thin man with one side of his face completely gone. The short, fat lady in the yellow bathrobe who paced the hall and talked aloud to herself. The coveys of doctors, interns, and residents walking in groups, talking in their confidential tones and using their secret codes. The constant crashing and banging of gurneys, trolleys, beds, equipment, and people.

To pass the time, I took notes on the nurses. There was "Vampira," the one who took blood. She took enough blood from Ed, it seemed, to transfuse an army. Then there was "The Thumper," a big black man whose job it was to roll surgical patients over on their sides—no simple task a lot of the time—and thump their backs with a rubber mallet, in order to loosen phlegm so it could be coughed up. There was "The Pin Lady," a nurse whose inexplicable job it was to stick needles into various parts of the body, especially the feet. But my favorite was "The Bag Lady."

Her name was Betty. Her job was to help people deal with colostomies. "What did she do wrong to get that job?" I asked one of her compatriots.

"She volunteered," I was told.

Betty had had a colostomy herself, for a time. Now she taught people the things they needed to know. How to keep the area clean, how to attach the bags, where to get supplies, how much time to allow to take care of it every day, what kind of clothes to wear. She was dropping in on Ed to see if his colostomy was working. Through the haze of his disorientation and morphine, Ed managed a feeble wisecrack. "Are you an old bag?" he asked.

She flashed an enormous grin. "That's terrific," she smiled at me. "People don't usually joke about colostomies until about a year."

Late in the day, Dr. Marcos ordered an X-ray. Ed had been throwing up for too long and he wanted to see if there was an obstruction somewhere in the stomach. I shrank with fear. "An obstruction," I concluded to myself, "means the cancer has spread to the stomach."

But Ed came back from X-ray with clear pictures, and nobody had an answer for why the vomiting continued.

I tried to bond with the three-to-eleven-P.M. nurse, Renee. She was forty-five-ish, a tall, thin woman with short blonde hair. She reminded me of Shirley MacLaine when she plays a character like a waitress whose life has been closer to a bowl of soup du jour than a bowl of cherries. I struck up a conversation and Renee told me about her three grown daughters. How she was tired of supporting them. How she was tired of nursing. How she'd been a widow for two years.

One of the amazing things about nursing is the matter-of-factness with which nurses handle the intimate body mechanics of perfect strangers. Ed had a colostomy, he was throwing up bile, his incision was oozing, and he was being forced to cough up phlegm. Renee would wash him up, sponge him up, dry him off, and pat on baby powder, as if she was dusting and cleaning a living room. Once, when she had to pull hip-high rubber stockings onto his legs to help circulation, she climbed into his bed, got on her knees between his legs, and with her fanny to his face, forced the stockings on.

Toward evening, she told me she was going to get Ed out of bed. I was shocked. "He needs to walk," she said. "Things will work better if he gets on his feet."

I was fascinated by the time and attention it took to accomplish a simple thing like walking. Renee rearranged all of his tubes and bags. She checked his colostomy, the IVs, and the catheter. She got down on her hands and knees and put slippers on his feet. She rigged two hospital gowns so that his fanny wouldn't hang out the back. She got him to his feet. Then she put her arm around his waist and his arm around her shoulders, and they walked about twenty-five steps down the hall and back. He was absolutely dependent on her as they walked, leaning on her, physically and mentally. I wondered if I could ever be that intimate with someone I didn't know.

It is a very giving thing to be a nurse, even if, like Renee, your compassion has cooled and the warmth of human touch has become the pat of matter-of-factness.

I went home that evening and thought about quitting advertising and becoming a nurse. I wonder if Renee went home and thought about how she had got stuck in nursing and how I was in a glamour profession like advertising.

October 9

ED CALLED ME AT HOME AT SIX A.M. The ringing telephone pulled me from a dream I was having about fear. I was on an island, with bad guys of some sort about to converge. I knew I had to run, but I couldn't. I was paralyzed by fear. I shook off the dream and talked to Ed, who was cuckoo. He told me he spent the night in an airplane. He told me to look through the kitchen drawers for the nasty letter he'd written to Chris. "I didn't mean it," he said. "Tear the letter up." He also apologized for whatever he had said to Erin that made her leave. I told him that he wasn't on a plane. That there was no letter. That Erin left because she had to go back to work.

I went to work myself and ran into a buzz saw. Hamburger sales at am/pm still had us in a turmoil. I was trying to get a commercial through the process of legal approval, production-company bids, pre-production meetings, and the rest of it. One of the copywriter/art-director teams was pissed about something and acting truculent. Another writer's work wasn't getting sold at the client and he was getting moodier and moodier. I had a shouting confrontation with an account guy over storyboards.

"Shit," I thought to myself.

I whizzed through the mine fields of the advertising agency and got to the City of Hope around one P.M. Renee gave me the news that the colostomy was beginning to work. The colon was beginning to empty the stomach. The nausea had eased. The vomiting had all but stopped. But Ed was still disoriented. Dr. Marcos came by and tried to ease my mind. "It's the drugs," he said, "the IVs, the pain, the day-into-night atmosphere, the people taking blood, taking urine, taking blood pressure, taking temperature every five minutes. Also, nobody wants to be here. It scrambles the brain," he smiled.

"What can I do?" I asked.

"Conversation is the best medicine," he said. "It helps reconnect with reality."

I read to Ed from *Advertising Age* and the *Los Angeles Times.* I told him that the Plumeria seemed happy in the greenhouse. I told him that his grandson, Matthew, had left a message on the phone machine. His squeaky little two-year-old voice had been taught to say "Por-sche. Por-sche."

Ed asked me again about the letter to Chris and if I'd phoned Beverly about the tickets to London. I didn't say "What tickets?" I said, "I'll phone her on Monday." It's not a bad idea, I thought, London.

October 10

ED WAS SITTING UP IN A CHAIR WHEN I ARRIVED. "I shaved this morning," he said proudly. "They took the catheter out. I also pissed."

But he was still disoriented and had developed a fixation about food. He offered a nurse 100 dollars to go out and get him a hamburger. "Call Chris," he said to me. "Tell him I want some Jimmy's chicken."

"You can't eat yet," I said, repeating what Dr. Marcos had told me. "Your system isn't ready for it." They were barely letting him have water.

He got on the phone and called Dr. Marcos. Then he called Dr. Marcos' assistant, Dr. Unger. Then he phoned Dr. Ewen. He wanted to know when he was going to eat and when he was going to be released. He phoned the head nurse because his room was hot. The nurse couldn't help. So he phoned Maintenance and got a fan.

"Ed's back," I said to myself. Then I went down the hall to the john, locked myself in a cubicle, and had a good cry.

October 11

SUG AND ERIN HAD COME FOR THE WEEKEND, to be there and to help. On Saturday morning, Sug brought me coffee— as Ed would have done—then crawled into bed with me.

She was twenty-four years old that Saturday morning, my first child, having beaten her twin brother into the world by ten minutes.

"I'm naming her Deirdre," Kevin had pronounced, shortly after he'd met her for the first time. "I'll name the girls, you name the boys," he'd said, as if we'd discussed this deal before, which we had not.

"That's okay," I had thought to myself. A proprietary interest in daughters is a fine trait in a father. So he'd named her Deirdre, after the brooding Irish queen and because he loved all things Irish. I named the boy Christopher Kevin, partly after his father and partly because I thought that Christopher Kevin Craig was one of the world's all-time beautiful names. To separate him from his father, we called him Chris.

But as soon as we got Deirdre home, Kevin began calling her "Sugar." "My little Princess Sugar," he'd coo into her crib. Obviously the name stuck, because here she was, a twenty-four-year-old graduate student at Hastings College of the Law in San Francisco, still being called Sug by the entire world. I'm not the sort of person who likes nicknames, but I can't seem to call her anything else.

Sug deals with most things and all people, including me, on an emotional level. And most of our conversations, even when she was a child, took that tone.

"Are you angry, Mama?" she asked, as she crawled into my bed.

"I don't know, Sug. I was angry when Kevin died. I was very angry when I first found out about Ed. But right now... it takes so much energy to be angry. I feel I have to save my energy for Ed."

"Sometimes anger is good, Mama."

"I know. You can get so mad, it gives you an edge and pulls you through. I don't think it's bad. I don't know. I guess I just don't have time for it right now."

"Well, I'm angry. It's so unfair, Mama."

"I know." I could never think of a comment when faced with the unfairness. It so obviously was unfair. But there was no comfort in that and no way to change it.

"I worry about you as much as I worry about Ed."

"I know you do. You all do. And I worry about each of you. It gets all mixed up. I know as much as you love Ed, you're more angry because of me."

"What are you going to do?" she asked.

"I don't know, Sug. I really don't know. In my whole life, I've never had a plan. I'm keeping a sense of humor. That's really important. I'm not thinking too far ahead. He's strong, you know. I don't want to ruin whatever days we have by thinking too far ahead."

"But aren't you afraid?"

"Yes."

"Were you afraid when Daddy was sick?"

And a memory seeped out of the back of my mind and filled the sunlit room in Malibu.

🐚 *I was in our bedroom on a Sunday afternoon, sitting at the home-made desk Kevin and I had fashioned—an oak-stained plywood door from the Akron sitting across two filing cabinets. I was making enough money at Foote, Cone & Belding to buy the house, but not enough to furnish it. I didn't really care. At this stage of the game, the kids just tromped in muddy shoes on top of furniture anyway.*

As I sat at the desk paying bills, I could hear the voice of Benjamino Gigli, the Italian tenor, mingling with the name of his Italian ancestor—"Mar...co...Po...lo"—being chanted incessantly by a gaggle of neighborhood children in our pool.

Kevin was in the living room, playing his Gigli records. They were reproductions from Angel Records of Gigli's recordings made during the '20s. They had the hollow sound of monaural, but Kevin thought that no other tenor had ever equaled Gigli. He would play the sextet from Lucia de Lammermoor over and over and over again.

I looked up from the gas bill as Sug ran into the room. Some twelve-year-olds are physically on their way to becoming women. Some are still little girls. Sug was a little girl, in a little girl's silly swimsuit with ruffles on the fanny. She stood in the doorway, dripping water without regard for my hardwood floors.

"What's the matter, Sug?" I asked.

"Mama, I'm afraid there's something the matter with Daddy."

The fear that napped at the back of my brain came awake. I never knew when Kevin's clogged arteries would cause a problem. He'd pass out once in awhile. He'd have convulsions. His eyesight would go out. He'd become confused. His knees would buckle. He couldn't use his left arm. He couldn't walk because his legs would turn to jelly. Every time he coughed too loud, I'd turn my head to check.

"Where is he?" I said to Sug. She grabbed my hand and pulled me to the living room.

Kevin was lying on the couch, his hands behind his head, his eyes transfixed on the ceiling. Benjamino Gigli was reaching an "A" over high "C." The music was so loud it almost drove you from the room.

"He's crying, Mama. Is he sick?"

My fear melted along with my heart and I took her hand. "Daddy's crying," I said, "because he loves the music so."

And so fear came and went, like it did that afternoon. Or sometimes came and stayed, like when he passed out in a motel in Barstow on our way home from a trip, starting a chain of events that didn't end until he was hospitalized again at UCLA.

But if I look back on those thirteen years with Kevin, it isn't fear I remember, or UCLA, or convulsions, or failed surgery. I remember children laughing and cookies baking. I remember Erin's seventh-grade band concert when Kevin leaned over to me in the darkened Emerson Junior High auditorium and asked quizzically, "What are they playing?" and I said, "God Bless America."

It was not a family life tainted by ill health. It was normal. I'm proud of that for Kevin. And I'm proud of that for me.

October 12

ERIN, SUG, AND I SPENT SUNDAY
with Ed at the City of Hope. My daughters filled his room with silly
things. Halloween pumpkins made from crêpe paper, some car toys, a
paper rainbow. They brought wax Halloween moustaches for each of us
to wear.

Eric and Mary Davison came by and spent some time. When Ed
joined Della Femina in Los Angeles to start up the Isuzu account, Eric
was the first person he had hired. They'd become colleagues, compatriots, car buddies, and confidants, and Eric and Mary were the people he
had taken into his confidence when he had learned he had cancer. But
Ed frightened them a little that day.

"Look out for the spider on the wall," he shouted at Eric.

There wasn't any spider.

Later on, Erin, Sug, and I took him outside in the sun after scroung-
ing a bed table and some chairs from an empty room. We listened to the
World Series on the radio and we talked and talked. "Conversation is the
best medicine," Dr. Marcos had said. Slowly we saw him coming back to
reality. He began negotiating with Dr. Marcos about his release.
Dr. Marcos said Wednesday. Ed said Monday. Dr. Marcos said Tuesday
afternoon. Ed said Tuesday morning.

Around noon they let him eat. He had strawberry jello and apple
juice, and the look on his face when he ate it was one of near rapture.
His colostomy gurgled a little. We told all the "shit" jokes we could
think of.

It was going to be okay.

October 13

ALICIA PHONED ME AT WORK.
She'd come to clean the house, as usual, and Ed wasn't there. That
wasn't out of the ordinary, but Ed's mess wasn't there either. The clutter
he made when he worked at home, the shoes in the middle of the
bedroom floor, the wine glasses all over the kitchen, the scrap-of-paper
trail he left all over the house.

Alicia phoned me in panic and in tears.

"Yean"...she pronounced her "J's" like "Y's"..."Yean," she shouted into the phone...she always shouted over the phone..."Yean, where is Ed?"

I decided it was time to tell her. She practically lived with us. She was part of the family. "He's in the hospital," I said. "He had surgery." I blurted the rest of it. "Alicia, he has cancer."

"Oh, my God, Yean, I thought he was dead."

She told me she'd been noticing things for a couple of months. Little things. A doctor's name scribbled on a note pad. A brochure from the City of Hope. Long-distance phone calls from my family. She'd begun assuming the worst.

Indeed, she'd been so sure he was dead, cancer was a relief.

"Thank God," she said, which made me burst out laughing not only because of the irony of the comment but also because almost everything that had to do with Alicia and Ed made me burst out laughing.

Their relationship had all the stuff of a TV sitcom. She'd taken care of my house on Benecia and stayed on to make the long trek to Malibu, when Ed and I were married. But when Ed left Della Femina and started being home once in a while during the day, they sort of...well...took each other on. Big, massive, bellowing, commanding Ed, who'd gotten his way in conference rooms all over the world, being pushed around by a five-foot-tall woman with a dustpan in her hand. She felt the house was her territory, of course, and he felt it was his.

"Jean, you've got to speak to that woman," he'd roar. "She's a terror, Jean. She tears through the house. You wouldn't believe it. She does it all in two hours. You ought to see her iron, Jean. She does a shirt in thirty seconds."

"I don't care if she's fast, Ed, so long as she does it. What difference does it make?"

"She breaks things. When she dusts, Jean, she could break a piano."

Alicia, in turn, had no compunction when it came to complaining about Ed. "Ed doesn't pick his clothes up, Yean. I don't mind. I'll pick his clothes up. But he ought to pick his clothes up."

She also tattled on him.

"I'm sorry to bother you at work, Yean," she'd shout into the phone, "but I wanted to tell you I need Tide. And by the way, Ed's supposed to be on a diet, but he went out for lunch and had pizza."

They battled constantly over who was in charge when they were both in the house at the same time.

"Ed, get out of the living room. I have to vacuum."

"Damn it, Alicia. Vacuum someplace else. I'm busy here."

"I gotta do the living room now, Ed, while the clothes are in the dryer. You better move, Ed." It was clear who won when she started sending him on errands.

"I need bleach, Ed. Can you go to Hughes and get me bleach?"

"Yeah, sure, . . . we'll have it for you next week."

"I need it now, Ed."

"And you know what?" Ed said to me later, looking perplexed, "I went."

All the while they battled: "You can't have lunch now, Ed, I just cleaned the kitchen."

"Do not let Alicia and Brasso near my antique telescope, Jean. Nowhere near it. I'll kill her, Jean."

No one could have guessed the role Alicia Lopez was eventually going to play in the life of Ed McNeilly.

October 14

ED WON.

Dr. Marcos released him at ten o'clock Tuesday morning. I was an hour-and-a-half late to pick him up because of an eight A.M. client meeting that wouldn't end. He was sitting by himself in the patio area when I got to the City of Hope. The morning was sweet and warm, with the scent from the rose garden drifting by on wispy breezes. Despite his size, Ed looked small and forlorn. He was edgy because I was late. He had a bag of colostomy supplies in his lap and his little suitcase at his feet.

"I thought you'd never get here," he said.

"I'm sorry."

"I want to go home so bad. I can't get well until I get my feet on my own turf."

We went straight to Malibu, and the first thing he did was go to the kitchen and look in the tea-towel drawers for the letter to Chris.

"There isn't any letter," I said.

"I know. You've told me. But it was so real."

He was a little wobbly, but he was too nervous to get into bed, so we went to Alice's Restaurant for lunch. He'd lost about fifteen pounds and the Hawaiian sport shirt that was covering his colostomy hung loose, which it never had before.

While we were picking at our lunch and trying to calm down, the head of one of the West Coast's largest advertising agencies walked in with a pretty young woman on his arm. He saw us. I waved. He pretended he didn't see us and walked out. "People always come to Malibu when they're messing around," I said.

Ed's colostomy gurgled. A look of apprehension flashed through his eyes. "He has his secrets, I have mine," he said.

October 15

I CHAIRED THE ANNUAL GENERAL MEETING of the Western States Advertising Agencies Association. On my way home at eleven at night, I decided to resign from that board and pull back from every other industry activity in which I was involved. Every hour chairing a meeting was an hour away from Ed.

October 16

IT'S DIFFICULT HAVING A SICK PERSON at home in bed. Every meal, every glass of water, every pill, every cold cloth, every cup of tea, every slipper, every sock, every pajama top, every pencil and paper, every book—every everything has to be fetched.

Then there are the trips. To the drugstore for prescriptions. To the grocery store for soft foods. To the video store, bookstore, and newsstand for things to occupy the patient.

Then there is the laundry. The sheets, towels, washcloths, bed pads, and clothes heap into mediciney mountains at an alarming rate.

There there is the "help." Help me to the bathroom. Help me to my feet. Help me into the chair. Help me reach the phone. Help me handle my colostomy. Help me clean up the mess I made.

Then there is the cooking. He can have this. He can't have that. Nothing that will make gas. Nothing hard to digest. Nothing with too much sugar or fat. Then there's nothing left that he wants to eat.

Then there is the nursing. Take his temperature. Write it down. Call the doctor. Mete out the pills. Take his blood pressure. Check his incision. Change his dressings.

Then there is the patient. Who isn't. Sick people tend to be self-absorbed. They get bitchy. They want their way. They want attention. They want to complain. They become childish.

I'm a very calm person. I seldom lose my cool, but I lost it from time to time with Ed. He was more demanding than I could bear and uncharacteristically inconsiderate.

"Damn it, Ed, don't ask me for another glass of water," I shouted one afternoon. "I brought you water five minutes ago."

"I know what I need, Jean. I'm burning up in here. I need water."

I got it for him, but when I walked into the bedroom it was everything I could do to keep from dumping it in his lap.

I also felt drained all the time. Like the way you feel a few hours after an automobile accident or some other crisis. I was working, or trying to work, in addition to caring for Ed—going to the office for an hour or so or handling things over the phone. Between the two, I just wanted to go away and sleep. But there was that voice all the time.

"Could you help me to the bathroom, Jean?"

It's very hard. It simply is, that's all. Any time people have the chance to help with someone bedridden at home, they should. There are few times when help will mean as much. The best thing to do is come as a twosome, with one person staying with the sick person for an hour and the other taking the caretaker out for a drink or a meal. The caretaker needs attention too, and understanding, someone to listen. It's also good to bring food for the people who aren't sick. Sometimes, if you know them well enough, it's possible to do their grocery shopping or run some of their errands. Or to walk in, gather up all the laundry, and bring it back clean. Little things help, too. Bring a movie on tape, especially a funny one. Joh (her unique way of shortening Josephine) Koppel, at my office, made us about thirty tapes from her home-movie library, and they saved many an evening. Or just drop a card and give moral support.

Remember. It's very hard. When you ask "Is there anything I can do?" you put the onus on the beleaguered caretaker to find a way to let you help. Instead, find a way yourself. Like Annie did.

She brought me a meat loaf. And three hours of her company on a Saturday night.

October 17

WE LEFT THE HOUSE TOGETHER AT SEVEN A.M. to be at the City of Hope by eight forty-five. Ed was a little pale, but steady. In fact, he wanted to drive. In fact, he wanted to go in the Porsche with the top down.

"Ed," I said, "don't be such a goose." And we drove in my car down the Coast Highway to the Santa Monica Freeway through the thick of the morning commuter traffic, onto the Pomona Freeway to the 605, past the gravel pits, into the Valley of Smog to Duarte. I felt now that I could do it in my sleep.

There was a lot to do at the City of Hope. See Dr. Marcos for a post-op exam. (Ed had been having a lot of pain. He kept thinking they didn't get all of the tumor.) See Betty to check the colostomy. (The area around the opening, which is called the stoma, looked like it might be getting infected.) But the big thing—the really big thing—was to see Dr. Ewen and start chemotherapy. Finally, we'd go to work on the doozies in the lungs.

I waited on one of the S-shaped vinyl couches in the out-patient reception area, while Ed went for lab work. There is always lab work. The decor in the area, from the blond tables that the S-shaped couches curled around to the plastic flower arrangement on the reception desk, reminded me of the 1950s. I thought about myself in 1954 or '55, with my pony tail streaming in the wind, riding my bike with Judy McCarthy out to the lake at the Branding Iron Country Club in Oklahoma City. We'd lie on the raft all day, oblivious to the 105-degree Oklahoma heat, and talk about Ava Gardner's love life with Frank Sinatra, that new record "Rock Around the Clock" from this wild group called Bill Haley and the Comets, and whether Sally Dill was ever going to break up with George McCaffrey and give Martha Tuttle a chance at him. Ed came striding toward me and pulled me from my reverie.

"Come wait with me," he said. "Dr. Ewen has gone to get me randomized." He was speaking of the computer process that would put him into the experimental program's test group or into the control group. The test group got the new drug; the control group got 5FU.

"Dr. Ewen was chary," he said, as we settled down in the examining room.

"What's the matter?"

"I think he's irritated with me because I got so many other opinions. Then I didn't want to sign the chemo release."

"Why not?"

"It absolves everybody here of any responsibility. Nobody wants to take responsibility," he said. "Somebody's got to. In business, I'm responsible for my clients."

"They don't want to get sued."

"It has nothing to do with getting sued." He was very upset. His eyes were red-rimmed either from anger or from the welling of tears, I couldn't tell which. "If you take responsibility it doesn't mean you make guarantees or promises. It means you acknowledge your role. Shit. Nobody wants to be responsible for me but me."

"Did you sign it?"

"Of course I signed it. What am I going to do? Walk out of the program? But it's bullshit. How can the medical profession not take responsibility for what it does? I've signed fifty papers so far, absolving everybody of everything. It's bullshit." At that moment, Dr. Ewen walked into the room.

"You're in the control group," he said. Ed's name had gone into a computer, which randomly placed him in the control group—the group being treated with 5FU, the accepted, standard drug for colon cancer—rather than into the experimental group, being treated with the new drug Leucovoran. Since the control group was getting a specific treatment, not a placebo, it wasn't a "blind" control group, and everybody in the program knew which group they were in and which drug they were getting.

I wanted to scream. When were we going to get some luck? I saw absolute devastation flash through Ed's eyes, but he blinked it back. I grabbed his hand. He forced a smile at the doctor.

"You said earlier that if I got the control group, I could get the test group's protocol, if my treatment wasn't working. Is that still the deal?"

"Yes. We can do that," said Dr. Ewen. I could see in the doctor's eyes that he understood how deeply Ed wanted to be in the experimental program. There was a lot of tension in the room. I tried to crack a joke.

"The best thing about 5FU," I said, "is the name."

Ed and I left Dr. Ewen and followed the color-coded lines to the yellow corridor, the area where patients receive their chemotherapy. Ed was going to get 5FU. We knew it didn't work very well—it shrank tumors in about 10 percent of the people treated with it—but nothing in general usage had ever worked better. Ed's program was simple enough. He was to get an injection every day for five days in a row. And to follow that pattern once every twenty-eight days. The injection took about two minutes, once the nurse found a vein. We picked up a prescription for nausea, some literature on side effects, and went home.

It had been two-and-a-half months since Dr. Kraft first discovered the tumor in the colon, but it seemed a century ago. The colon tumor was gone. Ed had a colostomy. He was on chemotherapy, but not in the experimental program that had brought us to the City of Hope to begin with.

On the way home, he was extremely hyper. He talked in random spurts, stopping one thought and starting another. "I think all the second opinions offended Ewen. Did you say your brother Carl's coming? My testicles hurt all the time, Jean. No matter what, Ewen's a fighter. Remind me to phone Robin. I'll get the test program one way or another. I don't feel a thing from the shot. Jean, did you know that Hubert Humphrey had a colostomy?"

"No, I didn't, Ed."

"I never voted for him."

Underneath that poignant comment and the sputtering of disjointed thoughts, I could sense fear sending out tendrils, trying to root in Ed's brain. The fear was very real. It appeared quite often. But it never turned to panic. Panic is what brings people down.

"Jean, let's call Eric and Mary when we get home."

"Okay."

"I want to debut my colostomy in front of friends. Can we all go out to dinner?"

And so, Ed fought off fear and conquered panic.

October 19

ONE OF THE BEST THINGS ABOUT LIVING on the ocean is the parade passing by out on the water. "It's out there for our personal amusement and amazement," Ed always said. He saw more than I did. "Look," he'd grab my arm, "there's a school of fish feeding." I wouldn't see a thing. "It's where the water is all stirred up."

"Oh, yeah," I'd say. Sometimes I'd really see it. Sometimes I wouldn't. We loved to sit on the deck and just watch what paraded past.

The man who paddled the kayak. The day-boat leaving the Malibu pier. The half-day-boat leaving the Malibu pier. The man on the jet ski. The Sunday-morning distance swimmer, always out about half a mile. The porpoise, always in twos, arcing in and out of the water. The spray, if you knew how to see it, from the gray whales. Pelicans doing the pelican smash as they went for fish. Sailboat regattas. Fishing boats when the halibut are running. Wind surfers all the time. Board surfers on the Malibu point. Freighters and tankers out in the shipping lanes. Spinnakers. Airplanes pulling signs that say "Catch the Wave—KTWV," a local radio station. Kites. The Fuji blimp. Army helicopters, on their way, I always thought, to the President's compound in Santa Barbara.

It's hard to leave it all, especially on the weekends. But we began a series of weekends where we drove to Duarte and back on Saturday and Sunday for the shot of 5FU.

On the way home, that first Sunday, we had a talk. I was driving. The Porsche. Ed wanted me to get comfortable with it, but it was not an easy car to drive. "Let the clutch out all the way," he'd tell me a hundred times, "before you accelerate." I was getting it, but it took practice and a driver's sense of timing. I felt superior in the knowledge that I didn't really like Porsches. Besides being hard to drive, they aren't especially comfortable, the air-conditioning stinks, and there's no place to put a bag of groceries. I thought I looked good in it, though.

As we turned onto the Pomona Freeway, Ed asked me, "Do you think we should change anything?"

"You mean about the way we're living?"

"Yes."

"I've thought about it some. I thought about it when Kevin was sick, too, but we never did anything."

"You had a house full of kids then. You don't now."

"That's true."

"We could go someplace for a couple of months. We could take a whole year."

"But you have chemotherapy."

He shrugged his shoulders. "I'm sure they have 5FU in other parts of the world. It's just a shot."

"What do you want?"

"I'm not sure," he said. "I don't want any regrets."

"We could travel more. I know you love it. But I wouldn't want to leave Malibu."

His Santa Claus eyes twinkled, because he loved the way I loved our home. Ed had bought the house a few months before we were married, gutted it, and remodeled it. It was the fifth or sixth house he'd built in his lifetime, and it caused me to know that he could have been a great architect if he hadn't been a great advertising man. The house was small, but it was perfect. The master bedroom opened out to the sea. There were decks on three levels, a small pool, ocean views and ocean sounds in every room. And the details were so lovely. A pelican etched into the glass on the kitchen door. Ceiling fans in the living room.

"So you want to go on with things just as they are?"

"I love our life," I said. "And I don't want to start a series of rituals," I added, remembering the dinner with Beef Wellington.

"But our life is different now. Our life is cancer. I see your kids looking at you. Deep in their bowels they must see their mother as a tragic figure."

"That's awful," I said. "That's an awful way to be thought of. I don't think they look at it that way."

"Do you look at it that way?"

"I'm driving a Porsche," I said, "on a Sunday afternoon with a terribly attractive man who's crazy about me. Is that tragic?"

There was a long silence as the Porsche roared past the gravel pits. Finally Ed smiled at me. "Don't brake so much; you ought to down shift."

And one more time, we decided on normalcy.

October 20

I GOT A LETTER FROM MAUREEN, written on the computer at Wesleyan where she was starting her senior year.

Dear Mom,
I'm pretty much planning on coming home over Thanksgiving. About Ed: Of course I'm worried, and also just really angry at this situation. I think he's really going to work toward a recovery, and he is certainly no wimp. If anyone can kick a tumor on its ass, Ed can. Mom, I'm also a little scared about how he's feeling in relation to us kids, or at least me. I know he could never openly ask for any support, and I don't want to hurt his pride, but I would do anything —absolutely anything—to help him out. I hope he knows how much I love him and want him to be healthy. I never dreamed six years ago that I would have ever gotten so attached to him. Lucky for me, I have.
You know, it's funny. This year when October 17 rolled around I was thinking about Daddy a lot. I guess I do every year, but this year, it seemed different. Our lives really have changed since Daddy died. It's remarkable. In a weird way, it's comforting to know that even when things get really screwed up, you just end up undergoing a lot of changes, and with a bit of luck, things get better. I don't think it's random, either. I mean, our family getting "back on track" wasn't just a freak event. Anyway, that was all the stuff I was thinking about. I love you. And Ed too.
Mo.
A collage of memories began to take shape in my mind. Of Maureen and her Daddy.

❧ Maureen came into the world angry. I remember the first time I changed her diaper, the day she came home from the hospital. Her four-day-old body turned purplish-red all over and she screamed and shook her fists. It's funny how you can hear different emotions in a baby's cry.

"She's mad," I said to Kevin.

"Well, I don't blame her," he came to her defense. "The womb is warm and the world is cold."

Kevin had a gift with children. He gave each of them attention that was very personal. Despite the closeness in age among the four of them —there were only three years and three days between the twins and Maureen, with Erin in the middle—he never treated them as a group and found a way to spend a kind of time with each child that was particular to him or to her. Only Erin got to sip out of his brandy glass. Only Sug played rubbie-nose-and-kissie-face. Only Chris got to go with him to the post office on Saturday. With Maureen, he sensed that she wasn't really mad, but shy and intimidated. So he looked for ways to make her feel important.

"C'mon, Maureen," he'd say to a groggy four-year-old at six A.M. when he was coming in from the night shift at the post office, "let's go get a waffle." And the two of them would troop off to Junior's and the little girl would hang out with her Dad, the truckers, and the Jewish businessmen who came into Junior's for breakfast. She felt like the Queen of Sheba.

Once when she was about eight, he went over to Westwood School on her birthday and took her right out of the third grade to go have lunch with him.

At about that same time, he started taking her to the library. "C'mon, Maureen," he'd say, "it's book time." Every Monday night they'd go together to the West LA branch of the public library. He got her her own library card and in time she read every book on the kiddie shelves.

By the time she was nine or ten, Kevin's eyes were getting bad. The clogged arteries affected his vision, and every now and again his eyes "would go," as he put it. First he'd see pinpoints of light. Then just black. Sometimes it would last ten or fifteen seconds. Sometimes it would last two or three minutes. He got into the habit of taking Maureen with him everywhere.

"C'mon, Maureen," he'd say, "be my eyes." And she'd grab his hand and watch the traffic lights and the curbs on their way to Duke's for Kevin's one-millionth waffle. She was a tomboyish little girl with bobbed hair and thick-lensed horn-rimmed glasses correcting slightly crossed eyes. Unlike her fastidious sister Sug and her neat sister Erin, Maureen had a lot of trouble staying kempt. There was always a shoe untied, a knee sticking through torn jeans, peanut butter on her glasses.

Kevin was a mess, too. He was one of those men who'd put on a plaid shirt with checked pants and then look at me strangely when I'd comment.

"These don't go together?" he'd say ingenuously.

The two of them walking hand in hand into the library were like refugees from an Andy Hardy movie.

I always knew that Kevin and Maureen had a lot of "don't-tell-your-mothers." "Don't tell your mother I let you order pie for breakfast. Don't tell your mother I got you to school late again. Don't tell your mother about the stray cat we're sneaking bowls of milk to."

He had them with the other children, too. The conspiracies between father and child created not only a bond but a web of household intrigue that made them all feel clever and reckless. "Don't tell your mother I let you drive the car around the block. Don't tell your mother we went in the pool with no clothes on."

No wonder they all adored him.

Maureen was twelve when he died. She told me, "I always knew that Daddy was sick. But I never thought he'd die." I don't think children have a concept of death until they experience it firsthand. Besides, Kevin's illness wasn't a focal point in our family life and our home wasn't a sick person's home. His eyes would go, his knees would buckle, but that was part of Kevin's persona—another oddity, like his obsession with back issues of the National Geographic or his predilection for pickled pig's feet.

Maureen mourned her father more than I did, I think. More than any of us. "It's like a giant hole in my stomach," she told me, "and no matter how hard I try, I can't fill the hole up and make it go away." 🙰

Nine full years after her father's death, I got a letter from her telling me, in so many words, that she'd finally healed. Only to see a new gash moving toward her heart.

"There are no answers," I remember telling Sug. "Anger is futile," I remember telling Sug. Yet, when I read Maureen's letter I wanted to throw a chair through the picture window.

How can life...God...fate...be asking her to go through it again? Be asking me to go through it again? Be asking us to watch each other go through it again?

I kept reminding myself that there wasn't a sinister modus operandi behind our bad luck. Nobody was asking us to do anything. Not God. Not fate. Not life. There was no intelligence with a plan inflicting pain. Sometimes lightning does strike twice, that's all.

There was some temptation to sink into a state of brooding and depression. But in the end, it simply wasn't my nature. I couldn't be a Pollyanna and pretend there was no pain. There was pain. Sometimes I'd watch Ed do the simplest of things, like put on his shoes, and I'd be aware of how much I loved to tease him about the twenty-two pairs of deck shoes he always wore without socks, and I'd be aware that some-day I might have to figure out what to do with his twenty-two pairs of shoes. And the pain would deaden my senses. But brooding didn't make it go away.

What made it go away was getting my mind on something else. And trying, always trying, to be positive.

Kevin was so incredible about being positive. His positivity caused him to suck more out of life than anyone I've ever known. He could have an adventure doing something as unremarkable as walking to the drugstore. He could feel enough to cry when he heard music. Once, he came home with ten years' worth of pre-World War I *National Geographic* maps he'd found in a used bookstore in Santa Monica, and for the next two weeks as he lost himself in the euphoria of his life-long fascination with maps; he was happier, I think, than I've ever been happy.

I asked him once why he never got depressed over illness, and he said, "Jean, I'm just stupid enough that if I were shoveling shit in a fifty-mile-an-hour wind, I'd find something to like about it."

I picked some of that up from him, I think. Or perhaps it was more symbiotic. Maybe I was born with more of it myself than I know.

Ed, who was not the shit-shoveler that Kevin was but who was the do-er that Kevin was not, expressed the same attitude in his own way.

Two weeks after major surgery, in the midst of adjusting to a dreaded and dreadful colostomy, under heavy pain medication, having just started chemotherapy with all its side effects for a cancer problem that had been diagnosed as terminal, he turned to me with a twinkle in his eye and said, "Well, are we going to London or not?"

And off we went.

November 6

ED AND I HAD GOTTEN INTO THE HABIT of trying to turn airplane flights into parties. He didn't like to fly, because he was such a large man and it was uncomfortable. But I said to him once, "Look at it this way, Ed, it's three or four hours alone together with no distractions and we can talk about the things we never get to talk about."

He liked that thought—especially the part about being alone together—and from that time on did things to make plane flights seem like romantic interludes. Once, he brought a bottle of chilled Perrier Jouet on the plane, the champagne we served at our wedding, along with a little basket filled with black bread, sour cream, and Russian caviar. By the time we got to Oklahoma City to visit my mother, I felt like I'd just come from a cocktail party with the Romanovs.

For the plane flight to London we brought guidebooks and maps to plan our time there, some copies of *English Country Life* to get in the mood, a small food packet with orange marmalade, toast squares, and Earl Grey tea bags, and two paperback copies of Norman Cousins' *Anatomy of an Illness.* We didn't intend to get deeply into Cousins' book—we wanted to think about England, not illness—but we each glanced at our copy and then couldn't put it down.

First published in 1979, it tells the story of how Cousins was afflicted with a crippling illness diagnosed as incurable but took his treatment into his own hands, fought for recovery, and won. The book talks about emotions such as panic, fear, and rage and how they contribute to disease. It talks about other emotions such as hope, faith, love, and laughter and how they can preserve our health.

Ed and I devoured the book and only nibbled on our toast and marmalade as we flew over the Atlantic. Cousins is an amazing man. The author of eighteen books and editor of *Saturday Review* magazine for twenty-five years, he made a dramatic shift in careers in his sixties and is now on the faculty at the UCLA School of Medicine. His job there is to bring a more holistic approach to the medical-school curriculum.

"I didn't like anybody at UCLA except Dr. Fogelman when Kevin was there," I said to Ed, "but this time, they seemed different." I was remembering young Dr. Beckman. "I wonder if Cousins is already having an influence."

"Listen to this, Jean," Ed said as we traded another insight, "he says here that 'the principal contribution made by my doctor...was that he encouraged me to believe I was a respected partner with him in the total undertaking.' That's what I'm looking for from the doctors, Jean. A partnership."

The book became a touchstone for me and Ed. We found in it an affirmation of the positive attitudes that Ed was mustering and that Kevin had mustered before him. We found an attitude that applauded the patient for taking responsibility for his own recovery, and we found thoughtful discussions about holistic versus traditional medicine and treating patients versus treating diseases. We found in it what we were looking for: heart, hope, and strength. And in that way, Norman Cousins turned our twelve-hour plane ride to London into a party.

November 7–14

THE WEEK IN LONDON.
It was unseasonably warm in London, allowing us to walk without the encumbrances of overcoats and mufflers. Through the stalls at Gray's Market and on Portobello Road, looking for antique pewter and brass. Down Oxford Street, already bejeweled for Christmas. To a pub called The Guinea down a mews off Berkeley Square. To a pub called The Grenadier, near the "Upstairs-Downstairs" kinds of homes in Belgravia. We bought chocolates at Selfridge's and an umbrella at Harrods. We walked across Hyde Park—where schoolchildren were breaking line to chase falling leaves—to Buckingham Palace to watch the gilded carriages, embassy cars, and the Queen's mounted Palace Guard as they paraded to the Opening of Parliament.

Near the end of the week, we took a cab to the British Museum, which, after half a dozen trips to London over the years, I'd never seen.

I was thunderstruck by the museum. The facade of an Egyptian temple, so tall you have to crane your neck to see it all, sits inside with the same nonchalance of a David Hockney painting sitting in the Los Angeles County Museum of Art.

But there was a sweet, soft moment as well as we wandered through the rooms that depict daily life in ancient Greece and Rome and looked at artifacts that have managed to survive two or three thousand years. Many of them were much the same as the items that got us through the business of our own daily life. Pots and pans. Dishes. Kitchen tools. Implements for sewing and working fabric. Hand tools. Things that might have been toys. (No civilization could remain sane without toys.)

I watched Ed looking at an artist's sketch of a floor plan of a typical Roman villa. He was looking at it with the eye of a builder and commenting on how the design allowed for good air circulation and how the layout of the kitchen was the same as ours in Malibu.

The comparison to our own life touched me very deeply.

I wondered about medicine two or three thousand years before. I remembered that in Greece, in the fourth century B.C., Hippocrates was born. Was he capable of diagnosing an incurable disease? Did he know about tumors?

I remembered a wonderful quotation from Thomas Wolfe's novel *Look Homeward Angel*. I had memorized it years before, when I left FCB and my boss, Jack Foster, quoted it in a letter telling me good-bye.

Each of us is all the sums he has not counted.
Subtract us into nakedness and night again,
and you shall see begin in Crete four thousand years ago
the love that ended yesterday in Texas.

As I watched Ed looking at the floor plan of the Roman house, I felt akin to that time and to the love that began in Crete and ended in Texas. I felt I was part of a continuum and Ed was too. The soul really is immortal. A thought never dies. An idea never dies. A love never dies. It isn't life and death that mark the boundaries of a human spirit.

There are no boundaries.

November 15

WE GOT HOME FROM LONDON feeling a sense of sharing deeper than we ever had before. Every little thing about Ed made me smile. I felt a oneness that was quite extraordinary. But we paid the price.

As the week had worn on in London, he'd had increasing difficulty with pain. It became hard to walk. He'd overused the area around his groin that was still healing from surgery. His stamina had also begun to ebb, and home in Malibu, he was exhausted. I said, "We shouldn't have gone."

He said, "Bullshit."

He'd done a remarkable job of handling his colostomy. It's not easy to service one in the lavatory of a 747. You need a little space and a little time to detach the bags, put on new ones, dispose of the bags, clean the skin around the area, apply the powdered deodorant. You also need to gain a little confidence. There's fear at first that the bags will leak, overflow, or come loose. There were a couple of times when we had to duck into a pub on the streets of London so he could find a bathroom because he was afraid there was a problem. But the problems, when there were any, were minor. He wore a sleeveless pullover sweater to hide the slight bulge below his belt. He carried the supplies he always needed with him, in a camera bag.

We'd been lucky with the side effects from chemotherapy. It looked like 5FU wasn't going to give Ed a hard time. He had some nausea on the days he got the shots, but it didn't persist. There were oddities. Things tasted strange. The skin broke out around his nose. He had some hot flashes. (Better him than me.) He lost some hair, but not too much. More noticeable was the fact that it changed color and texture. His hair was graying, pewter-colored. Under chemo, it went back to brown. We were both afraid he might lose the white moustache that had been under his nose for almost forty years. But it stayed where it belonged.

I'm downplaying Ed's problems with chemotherapy, his problems with pain, and his problems with the colostomy. But I downplay them because he did. He didn't wish to be perceived as a sick man by me, by himself, or by the world. If you expect chemotherapy to lay you out, maybe it will. If you don't have time because you've planned a trip to London, maybe it won't.

Kevin had been the same. Alan Fogelman said to me once, "Kevin denies his symptoms."

I said that wasn't quite right. Kevin ignores his symptoms.

Both men, Kevin and Ed, worked from the positive emotions of hope, faith, love, and laughter.

November 16

BACK AT WORK, I'D BEEN STARING all week at a phone message from Madeline. It said: "I heard Ed is ill. Hope it isn't so. Please call."

Madeline was Director of Marketing at ABC-TV in New York. But she grew up where I did, at Foote, Cone & Belding in Los Angeles. She was rising in the media department at the West's largest advertising agency while I was rising in the creative department.

When I joined FCB, in 1965, Madeline was already there. I was a copywriter; she was a media planner. After a time, she was an associate media director and I was a creative group head. We both became fixtures on the Sunkist account. Indeed, we both got reputations outside our own agency because of our work on Sunkist. She did a media plan in 1972 for Sunkist lemons that was extraordinarily innovative. And I worked on the ads, which attracted a lot of attention. So did our television work for Sunkist oranges. I wrote a campaign using Sunkist growers on camera and thought up their theme line, "You have our word on it."

We worked together on a lot of other things, too. Hughes Airwest. Mazda. Schick. United California Bank. Ore-Ida. Albertsons. We were part of a team and became good friends, as did Jack and I. But what was different about me and Madeline was that we had nothing in common. Nothing.

Well, . . . we were both women. But even on that score, we were about as alike as Madonna and Debbie Boone.

Madeline was from the Los Angeles-Jewish-wealthy-connected intelligentsia. I was from Oklahoma City—for pity's sake, as they say there—and wasn't connected to anything except a family legend about my grandfather making "The Run" in 1889. I grew up playing "Kick the Can" in the backyard and swimming on summer afternoons with 300 other kids in the public pool at Memorial Park. She grew up with ballroom-dancing lessons and summers away at camp. She joined a top sorority and went to Berkeley. I never joined anything and went to a Catholic college in Tulsa so small even people in Tulsa had never heard of it. When she was buying clothes at I. Magnin, I was tromping around in The May Company's basement. I had a husband and four kids. She never married. I had this peacefulness that irritated the hell out of her. She had this take-charge ability that drove me nuts. How come she always got her way? Yet, strangely, and this perhaps was the key, we never really competed. (Well, . . . maybe just a little.) We were such opposites, there was no common ground on which to put each other down, as women in business were wont to do in those days when there weren't many women in business and each of us secretly enjoyed having the territory to ourselves.

Madeline was close to me through the years with Kevin. She was involved with my children, my life, and my problems. She helped me from time to time, because she had a way of stripping off all the non-essentials and focusing on the simple reality.

"Madeline," I told her once in the late '60s when I was feeling overwhelmed by four kids and a demanding job, "I don't know what to do. I can't handle all of it anymore."

"Sit down," she said. "And be specific. What can't you handle? What is all of it?"

I talked and she listened. Then she told me to do three things. "For God's sake," she said, "get a dishwasher. Don't tell me you can't afford it. Then you need to make Kevin quit working nights. Then you need to get out of that house. You're cramped. You don't have conveniences. And that house is weird."

By the time a couple of years rolled around, we'd done all three of those things and our life was better. They'd probably have been done anyway, but Madeline brought them into focus.

Ed's wish for privacy regarding his illness had given me an excuse not to tell people like Madeline. I hated telling people. Without exception, they'd look like they'd just been kicked in the stomach. The word *cancer* puts both dread and discomfort into people's faces. Their eyes blink as thoughts flash past of being hit with cancer themselves some-day, then flit as they try to think of something to say. Some human way to react. But the double whammy of cancer and my having had another husband with another dire illness was enough to make people turn white, and that would make me as uncomfortable as they were. I often felt that both of us—the teller and the tellee—wanted to just run away.

So I hadn't told Madeline, but somehow, she'd heard about it any-way. The news was getting around. There were too many people at my office who either knew or sensed that something was the matter.

I didn't know what to do. I stared at the phone all week and never returned her call.

November 18

ED WENT TO THE CITY OF HOPE TO SEE Dr. Marcos. The pain around his rectum and in his groin was getting worse, not better. Dr. Marcos wasn't there.

Dr. Unger, his assistant, explained that the bowel is usually re-moved when there's a colostomy, but Ed's wasn't. So it was trying to work. Seizing. Contracting. Aching. He was going to have to grit through the pain until the colostomy was taken down and his body started to function normally again.

Neither of us quite believed her. There was a lingering fear that there was still cancer in the colon and that's what was causing the pain.

Sometimes I dreamed about the cancer in the colon. I thought I could see it there. I felt I could watch it growing. The dreams were as if I'd been miniaturized and was traveling through the organic chambers and arterial passages of the body. I could hear voices shouting, "Look out to your left" or "Danger ahead." Then, suddenly, the cancer loomed in the distance, as if a mountain of rock had fallen across the passage. I was startled awake one night when I couldn't tell whether the drama was happening in my body or Ed's.

Indeed, that's how I felt much of the time. "We" had cancer. "We" were getting chemotherapy. It had the same stranglehold on me that it had on Ed. As much as I loved him, I hated that feeling. I didn't like being trapped in the net of someone else's affliction, even Ed's.

November 19

A MAN NAMED ACE PHONED. He was with The American Colostomy Association. "Mrs. McNeilly," he said, "our group is to help people adjust, but we do other things, too. We have picnics and barbecues."

"Let me put my husband on the phone," I said.

"I'm happy to talk to you. We often find that the family needs more help with colostomies than the people who have them. Would you like me and my wife to come by?"

He offered to come all the way to Malibu, then extended an invitation to their next meeting. I told him we were adjusting well. "Besides," I said, "Ed's colostomy is temporary. They're supposed to take it down in January."

"That's okay," said Ace. "If you ever had a colostomy it counts for membership. We have a real good time, Mrs. McNeilly, and we'd be glad to have you with us."

I thanked him, and I hung up feeling touched by the sweetness of the man's outreach to me and Ed. It was another of those situations where I didn't know whether to laugh or cry. Ace was terrific. But the fact that his organization even existed, you have to admit, is . . . well . . . amusing. There's an organization for everything on earth. Absolutely everything.

November 21

IT WAS ELEVEN-THIRTY A.M. I WAS AT THE OFFICE, on the phone, when Kimi stuck a note under my nose. "Ed is calling from a phone booth," it said. I hung up on the other call and got on the line.

Ed didn't say my name. He didn't say hello. He just shouted in my ear. "The chemotherapy is working. Jean, the chemotherapy is working."

I choked and tried to talk through a strangling throat. I felt hot tears blinding my eyes. I couldn't get my breath. I couldn't see. I couldn't talk.

He told me about his morning at the City of Hope. Dr. Ewen had kept him waiting a long time. "I got edgy," he said, "because I feel the relationship with Ewen is tenuous. I wanted to ask him today if I could get my 5FU shots in Santa Monica because of the drive. But I didn't want to add to the perception of problem patient." Ed never hurried a story. "I also wanted to ask him about the doctor in Tennessee." (There was a physician in Nashville who would replicate any experimental protocol used in the treatment of cancer, because he felt people should have available the treatment they want. Ed thought he might be able to get the Leucovoran program through this doctor.)

He continued, "I was considering all this when he ran into the room waving X-rays."

"It's working," Dr. Ewen had shouted. "It only works on one in ten. You're one of them, Ed."

"He showed me the X-rays," Ed went on. "You can actually see how some of the tumors in the lungs are smaller."

I was still getting my breath. I couldn't believe it. I was afraid to let myself believe it.

Dr. Ewen didn't want to draw any long-term conclusions. His attitude was wait and see. "But," he said, "cancer cells by nature are rapidly growing. We have definitely stalled it for now."

"He noticed my hair is thinning," Ed was continuing to shout. "I don't care."

I hung up and ran down the hall of my office looking for Bob. I had to find him so I could tell someone, and I also decided to phone Madeline. I could tell her now. I had something good to say.

November 22

WE WERE SO HAPPY. Thanksgiving was coming. The children were coming. We spent the whole weekend grinning and bustling. Poaching pears. Cleaning silver. Doing up beds. White linen tablecloths. Turkey. Yellow chrysanthemums and navel oranges. Clean sheets. Clean rooms. Good images when they all arrive. We interrupted it for two trips to Duarte for 5FU.

5FU wasn't supposed to work. But Ed was making it work. Ed was making it work.

November 25

ED'S DAUGHTER ROBIN ALSO CAME for Thanksgiving. She left her husband, Michael, and her son, Matthew, in Florida and arrived looking pale and nervous. The three of them had just finished a year in Boston, where Michael was studying to become a "pump tech"—a profusionist. That's the medical technician who runs the heart-lung machine during open-heart surgery. Robin was an intensive-care nurse, and she'd put Michael through his year of training by nursing at Massachusetts General Hospital.

It had been a tough year. Boston wasn't home. They were scrunched into a tiny, temporary apartment. They were living on Robin's nursing salary. Matthew was a toddler and in between her job, her husband's erratic schedule, and the limitations of day care, Robin had had her hands full caring for him. And now, just as the difficult days in Boston were ending, she had to handle the fact that her father had cancer. To make matters worse, he didn't want her mother to know about it.

At twenty-six, Robin was still in the blush of young womanhood. I stared at her from time to time, not because she was Ed's daughter rather than my own, but because she was so pretty. Dark-brown hair, high cheekbones, skin the color you find at the base of rose petals. And blue eyes, deeper even than her father's, like two alien moons floating above a rosy sea. I was grateful to Robin because of her acceptance of me after Ed's divorce and because of her attention to him since he'd been ill. She phoned every week and there was an open, easy relationship between her and me, which had been heightened by sharing Ed's illness. When she got off the plane, I noticed she was terribly thin from the strain of her year, and her voice was reedy and sharp from the strain of her father's illness.

"Dad, we have to talk," she said, almost the first minute she saw him.

"Later," he said, knowing full well what was on her mind and wishing like hell to avoid it.

I felt for Robin. She had to fit herself in among my four children in a home that was mine and Ed's. She had to watch her father as titular head of a family that was not her own. I asked my children to be sensitive and not be preemptive of Ed. But it was hard. He was so clearly the "man of the house" and this house was so clearly "home" to my four children and to me.

Later in the day, Robin talked to me about talking to Ed. "I think there should be a family meeting," she said, "between Dad, me, Mom, and Kim."

"Uh-oh," I said. "I don't think he'll do that."

Ed had been married to Robin's mother, Donna, for twenty-seven years. He was married to her when I met him. She was living in Florida at the time and he had come to Los Angeles, but although they were living apart, the separation was for business reasons. There was no real thought of divorce. I think their time apart would have caused disruption, however, if not divorce, with or without me. But perhaps that's only what I like to think. Ed had been living for years in an emotional cocoon, shutting down his feelings, cloaking his needs, and using silence as a way to cope. When he moved to California, he came back to life and in a short time was a renewed person in a marriage that was passive and wanted to remain that way. But whatever the underlying problems, Donna was extremely angry about the divorce and her feelings were easy to understand.

Even with the passage of time, there were problems. After the divorce, Ed felt their encounters became opportunities to make him feel guilty, which he already did in buckets, and also to make him feel at fault for whatever of life's problems were now cropping up. It was a human reaction, but it caused Ed to back off even farther.

Finally, he just began staying away completely. He even got the alimony payments handled by the bank. One of the fallouts was that Ed also "lost" his younger daughter, Kim. It's difficult for children living with one parent or another not to take sides and feel pressure, and Kim was living with her mother during the time things were most difficult. So now, there was almost no communication between Ed and Donna and none at all between Ed and Kim, even though they both lived in Los Angeles.

There are a lot of questions that could be asked about Ed and Donna and about me and Ed. Or about any long-term marriage that ends in divorce. Is there a responsibility after twenty-seven years? Of course there is. But do you answer to it at the cost of your own happiness, perhaps for the rest of your life? That's the whopper, and there's no one answer. Usually, people work their way through the situation, things start to assume their own momentum, and the choice becomes inevitable. Either you just can't leave. Or you just can't stay. Ed couldn't stay.

"Mom and Kim have a right to know," Robin went on.

"Part of me agrees with you. But Ed has his reasons. He's very protective of his privacy. He doesn't want people to know. But you should talk to him about it, Robin. It's between you and him, really. I should stay out of it."

"It's so hard to make him talk."

"I know you think that." To me, Ed was an emotional teddy bear, yet Robin often saw him as stern and remote. "But if you choose the moment, he'll talk. He'll talk your arm off. Right now though, he's having such a good time with Thanksgiving."

"I'll wait until after," she said. But her voice was full of strain. From her tough year, her father's illness, her family's disarray. All of the above.

Thanksgiving 1986

WE USED MY MOTHER'S CRYSTAL, which she got when she married Papa in 1927. And my own wedding china, which I got when I married Kevin in 1960. Ed and I had our annual "stuffing-off." We always baked two small turkeys instead of one big one. He stuffed his with cornbread stuffing, the kind his mother used to make. And I stuffed mine with bread-crumb stuffing, the kind my mother used to make. Then everybody had to vote.

I lost, six to nothing, but I thought Ed cheated, because he monopolized all the tools in the kitchen and laced his stuffing with two cups of Grand Marnier. As I watched it all, I remembered my first Thanksgiving in California, in 1961.

❧ *First of all, it felt wrong because it was hot. One of those fall days in southern California when the Santa Ana winds blow and the desert air heats up the whole basin. It was in the '80s. And the swaying palm trees and white and pink ivy geraniums spilling all over the front yard of our apartment building did little to ease my ache for autumn in Oklahoma. I wanted to be where chrysanthemums were getting spindly because Mama had forgotten to cut them back, where wind sweeping down the plains carried the scent of baked apples and yellow leaves were falling from the cottonwood trees in the front yard.*

Second of all, I was pregnant. By that time we knew it was twins, because I'd gotten so big. The babies weren't due till March, but I already looked like I was two weeks late.

Third of all, I cooked a huge turkey, because that's what Mama and I always did on Thanksgiving. When it was done, Kevin and I sat down alone at a kitchen table in our tiny apartment to eat it. It was absurd. The turkey could have served twenty. It took all day to cook it and we couldn't go anywhere, which irritated Kevin.

"Let's go to the beach," he'd said.

"It's Thanksgiving," I said.

"So what?"

"You can't go to the beach on Thanksgiving."

"Why not?"

"It doesn't feel right. Besides I have to cook the turkey."

"Screw the turkey."

My feelings got hurt. I cried. Then, of course, the turkey was dry and the stuffing didn't taste a thing like my Mother's. She called me about four in the afternoon and the whole family was there in Oklahoma City. My oldest brother, Father Bob, who was a priest. Howard and his wife Jane, with their kids, Howard, Mark, Paul, Celeste, and Robert. Carl and his wife, Jacque, with Dawnie and Michelle. My sister, Marta, had run off to Europe, so she wasn't there.

And I wasn't there.

When Bob got on the phone and couldn't talk because his mouth was full of Mama's pumpkin pie, I cried again.

Kevin tried to make it better by running across the street and getting a bottle of three-dollar champagne.

We drank the champagne and got a little silly. We stayed up until two in the morning and went out for breakfast, at a dumpy little café we'd found tucked in among the pylons that support the Santa Monica pier. Sitting among the fishermen telling salty stories to the short-order cook, I felt reckless, grown-up, and glad finally that I was there at two in the morning on the edge of the continent rather than snug in my bed in the house where I grew up in Oklahoma City.

The next morning, when Kevin fainted coming out of the shower, neither of us paid much attention to it. It scared me when he fell, but he was only out for about thirty seconds. We attributed it to too much cheap champagne, not enough sleep, and no air in the cramped little bathroom.

Three years later, when he was going into surgery at UCLA, I remembered the fainting incident. It was the only precursor we ever had that there was a massive problem building inside his body. ❧

Since then, I'd had exactly twenty-five Thanksgivings in California. Kevin and I never went "home" for the holidays because of time, distance, two people working, and the cost of plane tickets. I ached for my family, but half a continent away we began to build our own traditions around the children and ourselves. After that first Thanksgiving, only one other was sad: the one right after Kevin died. We didn't know what to do with ourselves that year. Mercifully, Annie came to the rescue. She invited us all to her condo in Pacific Palisades and cooked a Thanksgiving feast so elegant we still talk about it.

It's easy to understand, however, how holidays can be sad for many people. When you're alone or unhappy and all the world around you is celebrating, it only intensifies the loneliness and unhappiness. We had reason to be sad Thanksgiving 1986. But we declined the invitation. We sat around the table, instead, with beaming faces and when we looked at Ed, we thought about champagne for breakfast. When he looked at us, he thought about who had snitched his chocolate cookies from the freezer.

Normalcy.

November 28

THIS IS HOW THE CONVERSATION WENT between Ed and Robin.

ED: "I don't want my days ruined by being regarded as less than a whole person. I may be crazy, but I may be able to reenter the business world. I want to keep that option."

ROBIN: "Kim has a right to know. Mom has a right to know. You were married for twenty-seven years. Whether you like it or not, there are emotional and financial ties that remain."

ED: "I would tell Kim, but she will tell her mother, and her mother might tell my business friends, like Jack Reilly. She sees more of Jack and Ellie now than I do."

ROBIN: "Trust her. Maybe she won't."

ED: "You're right. *Maybe* she won't. I can't take that risk. Robin, I do not want to share my cancer with the world. And I don't want to share it with Donna. I have a right to my privacy. I have a right to do this in the way that's best for me."

So they didn't have the family meeting. Maybe they should have, but Ed wanted his illness private. I told Robin that after all was said and done, it was Ed's call. "He has the right to do it his own way," I said, "including doing it wrong. No one else can decide for him what's best."

And no one can. Nobody has the right to *go around* a patient. No doctor. No family member. No friend. How a patient wants to live or die, whether or not he wants to be treated, should be respected. It's the ultimate nullification of human dignity to take away a person's rights in the matter of his own life or death.

December 1

ED GOT AN IMPORTANT LONG-DISTANCE phone call during the week. From Ed Russell.

Edward T. Russell (Eddie) and Edward R. McNeilly (Ed) worked together for almost twenty years on the Volkswagen account at Doyle Dane Bernbach in New York. Their careers were parallel in that both were meteoric.

"I screamed through that company," Ed told me once, speaking of his early years at DDB.

And the company itself screamed, as no other advertising agency ever has. Their brilliant campaigns for VW, American Airlines, and Avis set a style and an attitude that advertising has been emulating ever since. The company was catapulting from one peak on the growth chart to another, and the most celebrated of all its work was Volkswagen.

Eddie was the first account guy on Volkswagen. He carried the "Think small" ad to the client—who understandably didn't understand it, because nobody had ever done advertising that way—and sold it. A short while later, Ed joined Eddie on the account. Eddie was the account supervisor and Ed the account executive. For the next decade, they were the centerpiece of the business side of the account.

And what a time they had! They rode the crest of VW's success in the United States and then took the car and the advertising all over the world. They brought Porsche and Audi into the country and Porsche and Audi's advertising into DDB. They both ultimately controlled huge chunks of business along with VW. Ed had Lever Brothers, for example, and Eddie had Seagrams. They both made a lot of money when the company went public. They both made it through the labyrinthine corporate structure that grew along with the company, to be among the first select few to sit on the Board of Directors.

Eddie and Ed were both larger-than-life people. Daring, bold— at times, reckless. Eddie was the person who introduced me to Ed in Los Angeles in 1980. The two of them spent the evening seeing who could order the most bottles of Dom Perignon at ninety-five dollars a cork.

Their careers were also parallel because the advertising business and DDB ultimately broke both their hearts.

They were pushed out of the company in the early seventies, a short time apart. I don't know exactly why, although I've heard a hundred different stories, asked umpteen different people, and talked to Ed endlessly about it. It's all "Roshomon." The stories tell about the same incidents, but they don't match. The perceptions of what really happened are all different. Joe Daly, the CEO of DDB for many years and the man who fired Ed, has told a number of people that he never did it. "It was the client," he says.

In a nutshell, I think the top got too crowded at DDB, factions formed, and Eddie spoke his mind on an important issue that caused him to lose favor with top management. As for Ed, he was also on the wrong rim of a small inner circle. And he didn't politic enough. He didn't worry enough about how he was perceived. "I was never any good at that sort of thing," he told me. "I was good at running accounts."

After DDB, Eddie opened his own agency and Ed, nursing the deep wound of rejection, left the advertising business and moved to Florida. Later on, Eddie helped the startup effort to bring Isuzu into the United States and called on Ed. That's what brought him back into the agency business, out to California. And to me.

Now, on this day in early December, Eddie phoned from New York to invite us to Pound Ridge to help him and Mary Jane celebrate their fortieth wedding anniversary. They were going to open some wine Eddie had been holding in preparation for this occasion for more than three decades. "We're only inviting three couples," he said. "Could you come?"

Ed was so touched by the invitation, and so moved by Eddie wanting to share the occasion with me as well as with him, that he responded by sharing as well. He told Eddie he had cancer.

"I wanted to sound positive," he said to me later, "but I couldn't keep the fear out of my voice. I wanted to sound like I'm beating it because I am. But then my voice broke."

His eyes were misting up as he talked to me, and there was nothing I could do to comfort him but listen.

"I care about him so much," he went on. "His reaction makes me feel so loved. I guess that's why I cry."

December 9

WE WALKED TOGETHER INTO THE CITY OF HOPE, and as I waved to the volunteer at the reception desk, I said to Ed, "I feel like a regular."

He said, "I was a regular once at the 21 Club in New York. I prefer that."

We were there to have blood tests, X-rays, and a meeting with Dr. Ewen for the second report on the effects of chemotherapy. We were anticipatory and a little scared. If the news was good, what a great Christmas present! If the news was bad—well, that's why I came along. We'd find a way to give it some perspective. We didn't want depression or anxiety with Christmas coming up.

We'd been bustling, the two of us, over Christmas. All of the children were coming again, including Robin, with Michael and Matthew this time, and we weren't going to give this Christmas to cancer. We were going to look cancer in the eye and say, "You can't have it, you bastard. We want to laugh this Christmas and no aedinocarcinoma of the seigmoid colon is good enough to take that from us."

We'd also decided to take a trip in February to the Grand Cayman Islands in the Caribbean. Ed was absolutely radiant about the trip. He was charged up, energetic, full of vitality. Not that there weren't bad moments. Moments of weakness and fear. For me and for him. One night, he came out of the bathroom after caring for his colostomy, struggling with frustration and anger.

"I feel like I'm wallowing in shit," he said. "I dream about it. I can't get away from it."

I dreamed about it too. There was a distinctive odor left behind in the bathroom. I sensed that odor in my dreams. And sometimes, after he had chemotherapy, I'd dream that the chemical was rushing through my own veins and I'd wake up feeling it sear as it did its work.

I sat at the City of Hope, waiting while Ed had lab work, and watched the people. There were a lot of women wearing turbans, babushkas, and snoods on their heads to cover up their hair loss. Other people had fuzzy, wispy hair—an indicator they'd had chemo too. Some people on chemo lose a lot of weight, because the drugs do something to kill the desire to eat. They end up looking very frail and thin and move with a wobbly walk.

There was a lady across the room whose whole face was disfigured. I guessed she had no nose, because there was a plastic cuplike device where the nose should have been. All of the shape of her face was gone. No forehead. No eye sockets. The bones had been removed, I thought to myself. But looking at her in this setting was not at all discomforting. And no one stared. We were all here with a problem, and we all understood. No one had to hide his or her problem or be ashamed.

There's a brotherhood among the sick. But it also extends among the well at the City of Hope. A remarkable attitude permeates the very walls of that institution. It's as if the staff has been told, day by day, person by person, year by year: "No matter what your problems are as people, the problems of the patients here are worse. Be positive. Be giving. Be on their side. Put them first." There was involvement at the City of Hope. Camaraderie. The doctors, nurses, technicians, volunteers, patients, and families were all in it together. Things were a little dog-eared. Some screens needed patching. Some walls needed painting. Some furniture looked like it was from 1950. But the City of Hope had heart. And it did, indeed, have hope.

Ed came striding toward me across the waiting room. I thought he looked better than he'd looked since I'd known him and now, at 225 pounds, he appeared fit and healthy. He was wearing khakis and one of the white, 100-percent-cotton shirts he loved, with topsiders and no socks. He looked like a Portuguese fisherman ready to go for marlin off Majorca. I could tell by the tilt of his chin and the swing of his stride that the news was good.

"Your condition is stable," Dr. Ewen had said. Since the first set of X-rays, there had been no change. The tumors hadn't gotten any smaller. But they hadn't gotten any larger, either.

"No growth is good news," the doctor smiled. Dr. Ewen had been cheery and solicitous. He thought we should do a liver scan soon as a routine precaution, since the liver was the next likely place for the cancer to spread. "Not that we need another place," he grinned. Part of the brotherhood at Hope was humor.

Before we left, Ed started another round of chemotherapy. He'd get his fifth shot of 5FU in Christmas Eve.

Christmas 1986

THERE WERE TEN OF US TOGETHER in the house—a small house—for eleven days. It was a triumph of good will that we managed. There were Ed and I. Robin, Michael, and Matthew. Chris, Sug, and Maureen. Erin and Rich.

The images are still vivid. Tomato pizzas, crab bisque, and spinach salad (red, white, and green) on Christmas Eve. Ed's floor-to-ceiling display of white elm holding dozens of red ornaments. The blue spruce from Malibu Feed with hundreds of twinkly white lights. Christmas music chosen by Chris. The Beach Boys. Reggae. Pete Fountain, in honor of Ed. Chris baking traditional Christmas breads. Maureen spiking the punch. Painted eggs hanging from a mesquite branch as the Christmas

Day centerpiece. Quiche. Kumquats. Preserved oranges. Smoked salmon. Ham. Champagne. Many toasts. Walks on the beach and volleyball. Watching the high tide on Christmas Eve. Singing carols. Playing Pictionary. Family pictures taken by our friend Patrice. Ed showing Matthew the sunset. Ed showing Matthew how to work the juicer.

There was one bad moment. Robin asked Ed to leave his Porsche on the street overnight so when he took it at six in the morning to go to The City of Hope, the opening of the garage door wouldn't awaken Matthew.

Maureen, who can sometimes be cold, suggested in front of everyone that Ed could put his Porsche wherever he wanted and that Matthew, at two-and-a-half, was old enough to manage. Robin retorted angrily and left the room on the verge of tears. Michael followed after her, commenting on his wife's stress and fatigue.

There were tensions simmering beneath the surface of that one outburst. Maureen protecting Ed and Robin protecting Matthew were a microcosm, perhaps, of the deep-rooted feelings of both sets of children.

Robin, feeling the sting of being a visitor in her own father's home, was establishing new territory with her son. Maureen, so incredibly loyal to her father, now having given her love to Ed, was giving it with an intensity as charged as lightning. Maybe she was trying to say, "I love him more than you do." Maybe Robin was trying to say, "It's my father's house, I'm his daughter, and I have rights."

Any family in which there's been divorce knows how emotionally charged it can be when the children are mingled. It's a new unit and nobody knows exactly where they fit. "Is the oldest in charge even though he's not *my* older brother?" Loyalties get confused. "If I like Dad's new spouse, is it an affront to my Mom?" Styles clash. "At our house, we never got away with that." It takes a long time for personalities to rub against each other and wear down the rough edges.

Our two families didn't have a long time. We had now. And in a superb showing of love for Ed, and each other, we eased our way through the eleven days with only one negative incident.

If cancer couldn't rob Ed of Christmas, a quarrel wasn't going to. The matter was put to bed along with Matthew. Ed didn't leave his Porsche on the street. Matthew was awakened, but it was okay. He made the orange juice.

When Christmas was over, and everyone was gone, Chris said to Ed, "Everybody forgot you were sick."

Ed chuckled and said, "I know."

Cancer lost.

January 11, 1987

ED'S COLOSTOMY WAS SUCCESSFULLY taken down. Neither of us thought it would be, until it was actually done. Dr. Marcos performed the surgery. All of the children were scattered by then into their own parts of the family puzzle, except for Chris. Robin, Michael, and Matthew had gone home to Florida, where Michael was beginning his new job as the pump tech. Sug was back in San Francisco, in law school at Hastings. Erin was in Santa Barbara, as was Rich, who worked for Exxon there. And Maureen was back in Connecticut, finishing her senior year at Wes.

So Chris and I held the fort. Chris. The most paradoxical of my children. The quietest. The hardest, perhaps, to understand. At twenty-four, he'd become a good-looking young man, brushing six feet, lean and taut, with my almond eyes and a tough-set chin. But his looks were shrouded by a killer shyness only other shy people can ever understand. Fear of picking up the phone. Fear of approaching someone and asking directions. Fear of being called on in class. People that shy hate being that way. Chris hated it. But it's like being left-handed. You just are that way and you don't know where it came from or quite how to change it. I was the same way until I was well into my twenties.

But the paradox about Chris is that underneath the shyness, he's also tough. And so very, very sure of himself. He was the first of my children to ever look me in the eye and refuse to do something he'd been asked to do. He was about eleven. I asked him to apologize to one of his sisters for slugging her or saying something nasty; I can't remember the details. He looked at me with a piercing gaze and said simply, "No. I won't."

I was taken aback by the sureness of his answer and the steely look in his eye that told me he was willing to take whatever the consequences. I don't remember exactly how I handled the situation, but I do remember that I admired his stance.

Chris is a person who knows who he is and is true to himself. And while his feelings are cloaked by shyness, they are deeply held.

With the heart and schooling of a naturalist, he was working as a hydrology specialist for the U.S. Army Corps of Engineers in Los

Angeles. He'd always wanted a job that had to do with weather or the environment. When he was seven years old, he began keeping weather statistics—on the amount of rainfall in LA, the amount of snowfall at Mammoth. He went to UCLA for a while but got his degree in Watershed Management at Colorado State University, which had a great school in that discipline.

His job took him around Los Angeles County doing things like checking dams, putting in weather stations, and monitoring rainfall runoff into the Los Angeles Basin. He installed a small weather station on our upper deck and gave us reports from time to time on precipitation. (I think he did it so Ed wouldn't overwater.) Of all my children, he had the least in common with Ed and was the most disapproving of him. "He drinks too much," Chris said to me once, "and he causes you to drink too much. Someday he's going to fall asleep at the wheel and you're both going to get killed."

Chris was fifteen when Kevin died and became my buddy when it came to dealing with "things." "Chris, could you help me light the pool heater? Chris, my car won't start. Chris, would you climb up on the roof and figure out where it's leaking? Chris, can you fix the toilet?"

Every Sunday night for years, Chris took my car out, without being asked, and put gas in it for me. When Ed moved into the house on Benecia with Chris, me, and Maureen, Chris asked if he would still be the one to pick me up at the airport when I traveled on business trips. It was such a poignant little question, but underneath it was the whole story. "What is my role now?"

I tried to let Chris know I still depended on him, because indeed I did. I'd ask his advice on family matters and made a particular point to look for help from time to time, without turning to Ed as well. Ed did become the one, however, to pick me up at the airport. It was time for that. He'd become my "main man."

The relationship between Ed and Chris was complicated by the fact that Ed was everything Chris was not, and vice versa. Chris was like a young gazelle—frightened by the noises of life, conservative, content to be alone in the forest. Ed was like a moose, thundering through the woods. Reckless, dominant, commanding the herd.

Yet, in time, they found some ways they could communicate and a friendship and a fondness grew that played at the edges of love. Chris let Ed educate him about cars; Ed let Chris make him knowledgeable about the Los Angeles Lakers. And of course, there was me. Ed and Chris shared a love—an extraordinary one, I think, for one lucky woman. And that was a bond of its own.

Chris' job at the Corps of Engineers ended every day at three in the afternoon. By four, he would join me at the City of Hope. He always wanted to know the minute details of Ed's progress. "Has he had a bowel movement yet? Is he off morphine? Have they let him walk?" And he always stayed and had dinner with me at the hospital cafeteria. He didn't put many of his feelings into words, but there was a quiet sweetness to his actions that was as endearing to Ed as it was to me.

I don't know if they talked about it among themselves or if it just happened, but all during the time of Ed's illness, one of my children was always at my side. And I loved the hell out of them for it.

January 12

I WAS JUGGLING NOTEBOOKS AT THE LINE of public telephones behind the receptionist's desk at the hospital, trying to find where I'd written down my charge-card number so I could phone Robin, my brother Carl, and the handful of people who knew Ed was in the hospital and let them know he was okay.

Suddenly, a voice slashed through the fog of my own confusion. "This is Mario Zamparelli," I heard. It was the man in the phone stall next to mine.

Mario Zamparelli was a designer who worked for Hughes Airwest during the time FCB did their advertising. The year was 1969, I believe. Howard Hughes had just bought the airline and Mario was given carte blanche to make it look different from anything else in the sky. He painted the entire fleet a fluorescent yellow and did the windows with mirrored glass. I was the copywriter at FCB who wrote the advertising campaign. "Flying Hughes Airwest," my radio commercials said, "is like riding in a streak of sunlight." We built the campaign around the theme line "Come Fly the Sun," and we named the flight attendants the "sundance kids." I worked on Hughes Airwest for five years and sat in a few meetings with Mario. Once he had me out to his design studio to do some writing on a special project of his own. But that had been a long time ago.

I listened for a moment or two to Mario's end of the phone call he was making. It was apparent someone he loved was at the City of Hope gravely ill. But I decided not to turn around. He might remember me. He might not. He probably would. But somehow I didn't want to share the realization with him that we'd both ended up at the bottom of an unfortunate barrel. There was a poignancy to it that made me shy and uncomfortable.

So I watched Mario go without speaking to him. My shyness has caused me to do that a lot in my life and I usually regret it. As I do now with Mario.

I hope his story had a happy ending.

January 15

THERE WERE A LOT OF TIMES, especially when Ed was in the hospital, that stress reared its nasty tentacles. Life at Kresser/Craig hadn't stopped. Indeed, it followed me. I sat at the City of Hope one afternoon, writing a new business presentation to the California Egg Commission. It was murder trying to handle my working life and lead a second stressful existence at the City of Hope. One morning, I ran through the kitchen on my way out the door to work and spotted a dirty cereal bowl, milk on the counter, and an open box of Grape Nuts. I'd eaten breakfast but didn't remember having done it. I also found myself losing track of things, like whether or not I'd made the house payment, watered my plants, or called my daughter back. I got a speeding ticket on the 210 Freeway, not because I was in a hurry, but because I got lost in my thoughts and didn't notice how fast I was going. Stress did all those things.

I have my own ways of handling stress, and I don't do things you're supposed to, like go to the gym and work out. Or take some time off. Or get out and go to a movie. Usually, you can't do those things. If you could, you'd be leading a life that wasn't stressful to start with.

I do bad, untidy things instead. I drink. I unload on my children. On Bob. On whoever's handy. And I follow a "leave-it-out" philosophy.

One of the most stressful times in my life was when the children were small and I was trying to run both a home and a job. I left things out with reckless abandon. Things that are supposed to be important to women: hairdressers, manicures, shopping. I got my hair cut for years at the Yellow Balloon, where I took the kids, so I could leave out trips to the beauty salon. I swore the kids to secrecy, of course.

To this day, people find it strange to go shopping with me. "She buys one of everything," they comment.

What they don't know is I learned to shop for a whole season while on a single lunch hour, and it's a habit I can't seem to break. I still sneak my purchases from Robinson's into the house, because I don't want the kids to see how much I bought at once.

I left complete categories of things out of my life to avoid stress. Most of them are still out.

- Taking things back. Nine on the stress meter. In my entire adult life I have never taken anything back, though I must admit others have done the task for me.
- Arguing with the housekeeper. However Alicia wants to do it, she can do it. I have learned not to care whether she uses Pledge or Endust.
- Balancing my checkbook. A flat ten on the stress meter. I take the bank's word and while it may have cost me two or three hundred dollars over the years, I figure it's added ten to my life.
- Reading women's magazines. They are designed to make a person feel guilty for not being perfect.
- Washing woodwork. I found it easier, when the children were little, to paint it. How's that for killing two birds with one cleanup.
- Ironing. My rule was—if it needs ironing, don't buy it.
- Saving and filing bills. I pay the electric bill, the phone bill, the gas bill, and throw the stubs and everything else away.

Once my mother came to visit and soon after she arrived, she discovered one of my "leave-it-outs" and came to me, perplexed.

"Jeanie, I wanted to do your laundry and change the children's beds, but I can't find your linen closet."

"I don't have one, Mama."

"Well, where do you keep your extra sheets?"

"I don't have any extra sheets."

"You don't have extra sheets?"

"Well, . . . what we do is wash the sheets and put them right back on the beds."

"Why do you do that?"

"It saves steps. I don't have to fold them up and put them away."

"Jeanie, you can't run a house without extra sheets."

"Mama, you can't have more than one set of sheets on a bed at once. The only thing extra sheets do is sit in the closet."

"I never heard of such a thing."

Mama never got over the sheets. Every year or so she'd ask me if I had a linen closet yet. Actually, I never did until the children were gone and Ed and I moved to Malibu. I should ask them someday if it warped them.

A sense of humor is also a great stress reliever. And that's what that little story is all about. Handling the advertising agency, the illness, and the solitude caused by Ed's wish for privacy all caused a great deal of stress. My left eye developed a tic from anxiety. I was half ill myself from exhaustion some of the time. Night after night, driving home from the City of Hope at ten or eleven o'clock, I'd open the windows and turn the radio up so I wouldn't fall asleep at the wheel. I was scared. I wasn't ready for another operation so soon. Ed's incision had gotten infected. His restored plumbing hadn't started to work the way it should. He had to stay in the hospital longer. I was so sick of sickness.

What got me through it was a sense of humor. Ed's. The staff's at the City of Hope. They all knew about a sense of humor. And my own. When you think you can't make it, crack a joke. And the best joke to crack is about whatever's causing the stress.

Ed finally did that. He put together a pool on the surgery floor about when he'd have his first bowel movement. Everybody on the floor—nurses, residents, other patients, and me—picked a date and a time and put in a dollar. It buzzed all over the halls when he came through.

"Ed had a bowel movement. Ed had a bowel movement."

Dr. Marcos came onto the floor and Ed called out to tell him. But the good doctor stopped him. "I heard," he smiled.

Laughter is, indeed, the best medicine.

January 24

ED FINALLY CAME HOME FROM the City of Hope with his colostomy gone forever and the incision healed and closed. But inside his body, there was rebellion. His plumbing was working, but it was like an out-of-control fire hose—starting and stopping, coughing, sputtering, then gushing, only to go dead with no warning.

"I'm shitting bricks," he'd say at seven in the morning, only to have uncontrollable diarrhea by noon. One day, he was in the bathroom every twenty minutes for seven hours. He'd get exhausted, dehydrated, and demoralized. "It makes me so angry," he said, "to be holding off cancer, but to be brought to my knees by bowel movements."

There was pain in the rectum, pain from uncontrollable urges, pain around the incision, and pain in the lower back. He used codeine to control it. "I'm not going to get into morphine," he said. "Once you start morphine, you don't stop."

And for the first time since he'd been ill, Ed became self-absorbed and focused on his problems. There was no normalcy.

We'd made plans to visit friends in Florida. But we had to cancel because Ed's insides were going haywire. Then I got demoralized. I wanted to go so badly. I wanted to have some fun. And to laugh.

"I have to get away from being sick," I said to Ed. "I feel like I'm mired in sick." Then I lectured him. "You're negative," I preached, "and self-absorbed. You've got to get your mind off yourself. I can't listen twenty-four hours a day about being sick."

There weren't many moments like that with Ed. Moments when sickness won. Moments that made me feel trapped. But there were some.

And there had been some with Kevin, as well.

᠗ *We were beach freaks when the children were little, spending Sunday after Sunday after Sunday with our collective bare feet leaving footprints on one or another of southern California's great public beaches.*

We got to know them all, from San Clemente to Santa Barbara, but Kevin dubbed Will Rogers State Beach in Santa Monica "bikini alley" and it became our favorite haunt. We'd pile into the Ford Ranch Wagon on Sunday morning with lunch in the cooler and set up camp. Kevin-at-the-beach was a phenomenon. It took him about twenty minutes to get organized. First, he'd unfold the full-size lounge chair he'd found at Thrifty Drug that collapsed so you could carry it in the back of a car. Every Sunday, it would collapse into itself and onto Kevin a dozen times before he got it sitting on the sand. Then he'd attach to the arm of the chair a clamp-on beach umbrella and hang from its back a canvas tote bag containing back issues of National Geographic, Car & Driver, Motor Trend, English Country Life, Playboy, Popular Mechanics, *and yellowed* Sunday New York Times Magazines. *"Kevin," I'd say, "you always bring those and you never read them."*

"I do too read them," he'd lie.

Then he'd put on one side of the chair a huge black vinyl suitcase, about the size of a giant economy box of Tide. Indeed, he had shoved an empty giant economy box of Tide into the bag to make it rigid. In this bag-around-a-box, Kevin had his "stuff": a small Sony tape recorder, jumper cables, a stapler, dental floss, a hand-held calculator, a Thomas Brothers map book, a wooden ruler, a steel pica ruler, a T-square, plastic bags, pliers, a notebook, an alarm clock, a Timex with no band, a stop-watch, a fly swatter, a compass, a tire gauge, a collapsible drinking cup from the Sierra Club, birdseed, four John F. Kennedy half-dollars he was saving for some day when the kids were good, Band-aids, a paring knife, a church key, a wine opener, three bungi cords, duct tape, black shoe polish, Cutter's insect repellent, and half a roll of toilet paper.

Kevin seldom took anything out of the bag, but he always wanted it with him. Indeed, he took it to work every day.

On the other side of the chair, he'd dig a hole in the sand and parti-ally bury a cooler that had his beer in it. You aren't supposed to drink beer on the Santa Monica beach and he thought that nobody could see it, which flew in the face of the fact that a quart-sized bottle of Coors was always in his lap.

He'd sit in the chair wearing a straw Mexican sombrero, mirrored sunglasses, paisley swim trunks, and Mexican huaraches. He kept a pair of binoculars handy to use for looking at girls and sat there all day and read—I never understood it—the huge classified section from the Los Angeles Sunday Times. "Kevin, what in the world do you find to read in the classifieds?" I'd ask. He wouldn't even look up. "You either under-stand it, girl, or you don't."

I liked to lie on the sand on those Sunday afternoons after I was tired of reading, shut my eyes, and listen to the sounds. The chatter-laughter-swelling-ebbing-talking sounds of grown-ups. The shouting-yelling-joyous-crying-piercing sounds of children. The hawking of the vendors. The lifeguards on the bullhorn. Portable radios scattering the talk of DJs into the summer air.

Then there were the waves coming in. Five, six, seven, eight, crash. You could tell the size of the wave or whether the tide was coming in or going out by the sound. Some waves boomed. Some rolled. Some slapped. You could hear the birds. Gulls with their aching, lonely cry. Pelicans smashing into the water. Sandpipers skittering as people came near. You could lie on the sand and almost hear the earth heaving as it breathed in rhythm to the swell of the tide.

Our favorite wintertime beach was Leo Carillo, because there were lots of things to do there when the sun wasn't warm enough to darken a tan. There were dunes to climb and caves to search. There were rocks that jutted into the water and long rocky walls that dared you to take precarious walks. There were even fire pits, so you could end a winter Sunday sitting in the glow of a driftwood fire with hot dogs snapping on the end of a stick.

We went to Leo Carillo beach one January Sunday when the children were at the gangly, frenetic, runny-nosed ages of thirteen, thirteen, eleven, and ten. As we drove up the Coast Highway they were bouncing off each other in the cavernous back of the Ford Ranch Wagon like caged Dalmatians. We parked in the lot at Leo Carillo, and when we opened the car door you could feel the sharp salt spray hit your face. It was one of those blue-and-yellow winter days when the sun was so bright it made your eyes hurt and the snap of the wind made you want to run, just run.

"It's a blustery day," shouted Erin, who loved to quote from Winnie the Pooh, and off the four of them went, running up the hill to the crest and down toward the surf. I followed them, running as fast as I could, feeling like a kid myself, kicking rocks and stomping on leaves. Then I turned and saw Kevin, way behind me now, struggling to get up the hill. He wasn't in trouble, but he was laboring. The hill was steep and his clogged arteries were hard pressed to get him the oxygen he needed.

Out of nowhere, a gush of tears came to my eyes. Tears for myself, not him. "Don't run, don't jump, don't skip," I thought. "He can't keep up. Watch him every minute. He might lose it." I wanted him to be able to run on the beach with me. I wanted to be free myself. I wanted to shout, "Let me out of here."

But the wind blew my tears away, I waited for him, and we walked together to join the children. I wouldn't have changed my life or asked for a different one.

But, yes. There were moments like that. Moments of feeling trapped and wearied by it. 🙠

And, there were moments like that with Ed.

January 25

DON CUNNINGHAM PHONED TO TELL ME that Benjamin Root had died. Benjamin was Richard Root's son. Richard was a mentor of mine when I was at FCB, my first business partner when I left FCB, and a person I loved to pieces.

His family, like mine, got struck by lightning twice.

When I left Foote, Cone & Belding in 1977, I left it to go into business with Don Cunningham and Richard Root. But it was really Richard who got me out of there. There was no good reason for a thirty-nine-year-old woman with four children and a sick husband to leave the womb of a large corporation and become a partner in a fledgling advertising agency, when most fledgling advertising agencies go belly up in their first five years, but Richard talked me into it.

"I'm in a terrific position at FCB," I kept telling him. "I'll be Creative Director when Jack steps down. Why should I leave?"

"They won't give it to you because you're a woman, and their biggest client is Japanese. They'll say that your kids keep you from traveling and crap like that."

"But my kids have never kept me from traveling."

"I know that. Listen, they won't give it to you. Besides, this is more fun."

He and Don Cunningham had been together about a year and a half. Both of them had also worked at FCB; Don had even been head of the office. But they'd both stalled there, moved on, and eventually thrown in together.

They were doing advertising and media projects for a variety of smallish clients. Don had been persistent in staying in touch with a large client he'd worked with at FCB, AVCO Financial Services. When he went on his own, he did brochures for AVCO, direct-mail programs, neighborhood flyers—any little project they had. Eventually, they started giving him more important stuff. Then Richard joined him. And lo and behold, the two of them got the whole account. AVCO was a big national advertiser at the time with a big budget, and getting them was quite a coup.

But Cunningham & Root was an advertising agency that couldn't do an ad. They used freelancers to write and art direct, as many boutiques do, but real growth was going to require a partner on the creative side, and that's where I came in. Richard encouraged me to join them for about a year and then pounced when they won the AVCO business.

"They've never even given you a VP," he said. "You're second in the department and look at your salary. Craig, you deserve to be creative director, but you won't get it. They're too conservative. Besides, wouldn't you like to do your own thing?"

"I don't know if I would or not."

"We'll be rich, Craig."

"But what if it doesn't work? Then what'll I do?"

"Get a job. You can always get a job anywhere."

It was his confidence in me, more than my own, that did it. Cunningham & Root became Cunningham, Root & Craig, and the three of us were a terrific team.

Don was conservative, stable, and full of integrity. Richard was bold, brash, and full of ideas. I brought a good reputation as a creative person, and we took off. The first week after I joined them, we got the Hungry Tiger Restaurant account. A few months later, we got a big Southern California Savings and Loan. We got an automobile dealer association. And after about a year, we got another national advertiser. The California Iceberg Lettuce Commission.

During this time, when the business was growing, Kevin died. Richard was the one who steered me through the darkness after death. "I'm not going to let you feel sorry for yourself," he said. "We've got a meeting on Monday, and we need you there." He also helped me pick up some of the threads of my life. "Would you like me to teach Chris to drive? Come have dinner Saturday night with me and Parm. Do you realize you need new tires on your car? Let me take your kids skiing."

Then, on a Sunday afternoon eighteen months after Kevin's death, Richard was running on Broad Beach and had a heart attack. He died in a hospital in Thousand Oaks ten days later. He was only forty-seven years old. Kevin had also been forty-seven.

I was crushed. Don was crushed. Nobody who knew Richard could believe it.

I saw a lot of the Root family—his wife, Parmele, and the children, Cynthia, Ben, and Alexandra—right after Richard died. But I was still out of focus from my own husband's death, as well as reeling from Richard's, and I had to pull away from them. "You're taking on too many of their problems," my psychologist told me. "You have to work on your own life. Let them go and don't feel guilty." So I did. But I did.

Don and I continued in business together, but it was never the same. The company grew some for a while but eventually, without Richard's boldness, it stalled. When I wanted to merge with Bob Kresser, Don didn't. So we separated and I took my half of the company, which became Kresser/Craig.

I don't remember exactly when or from whom I learned that Richard's son Ben had cancer. But I grieved when I heard it. Out of sadness for the Roots. Out of shock at the parallel to my own life. Because by this time, Ed had cancer too.

Ben was thirty years old. He had testicular cancer and the doctors seemed to control it for a time. There was surgery, and I heard that Ben came out of it "clean." Then, a few months later, he was down again. The doctor said he'd never seen cancer return with such vengeance.

I didn't know it at the time, but Ben was at the City of Hope when Ed was there. Parmele and I could have passed each other in the rose garden or at the vending machines and, each deep in our own problems, never seen the other—as Mario Zamparelli never saw me.

When I went to Ben's funeral, Cynthia and I hugged each other and she said, with a sad irony in her voice, "What is this, a contest?" I spent only about two minutes with Parmele. Neither of us knew where to begin and small talk seemed gross under the circumstances, so we said very little. Sometimes, indeed, words are poor excuses for thoughts and feelings. Parmele and I knew what the other was feeling, but there was no way to put it into words.

Cynthia and I had a phone conversation some weeks later and we talked about lightning striking twice, for her family and mine. We talked about grieving, loss, and the futility of trying to find a meaning. We realized as we talked that we'd each, separately, reached an understanding that might not make sense to others. It was a point of view completely lacking in sentimentality and seemingly cold, but it was forged with the white heat of reality.

"I don't dwell on it, Cynthia."

"We don't either. We don't talk about it."

"You try to find reasons and there aren't any. If you think about it too much, it makes you crazy."

"I know," she said. "It's a waste of time."

February 2

ERIN PHONED.

She said, "Rich asked me to marry him."

I said, expectantly, "Well...?"

She said, "Well, what?"

I said, "Well, what did you say?"

She said, "I said 'yes.'"

I said, "Well!"

I was thrilled, actually. Rich was terrific. Smart, ambitious, and crazy about Erin. Ed had often said of him, "I like him. He's got a lot of integrity and a good heart." He was a chemical engineer, working for Exxon. He and Erin had met on opposite sides of an environmental issue. Exxon wanted to drill in the Santa Barbara channel. The county objected. It went to court. Rich was part of the team representing Exxon and Erin part of the team representing Santa Barbara County. They eyed each other for a while; then Erin asked to be taken off the project so they could start going out. They'd been seeing each other for only six months, but we all sort of knew from the start that they were permanent.

They weren't going to get married right away. Rich thought a lot about his future and decided to go back to school and get his MBA. Erin wanted a Master's degree, as well. So they were going to do that first, probably at Eastern schools, and then get married.

Erin's would be the first wedding in the family unless somebody else eloped, which wasn't likely. I cried when I hung up the phone, because I was a mother and one of my children would be leaving me. I was also wondering whether or not Ed would see the wedding. I tried to keep my thoughts in the present, but emotional moments often opened doors on the future. Good Lord, it would be a great wedding if Ed was there to throw it! He made everything so much fun.

Or would I be by myself?

I hated being by myself. I hated being a hostess without a host. I hated attending advertising functions by myself. I hated going to someone's house and walking up to the door by myself. I hated being Mom at events in the children's lives without a Dad around. When Ed and I got married, I thought I'd never have to do any of those things alone again. But now I didn't know. And the thought that Ed might not be at my side at Erin's wedding was almost more than I could bear.

February 14

WHEN I GOT HOME FROM WORK, Ed was waiting with a present for Valentine's Day. It was a red, heart-shaped plastic bucket to use when I did my gardening. He'd filled it with fresh-cut daisies and looked cow-eyed when he handed it to me. It was the most endearing thing. Where in the world do you find a heart-shaped bucket or a man who can see the tenderness in such a simple thing?

Ed had been feeling great. The problems in his colon and rectum hadn't gone away, but they'd eased, and his energy was amazing. He tore up our hillside to landscape, but instead of planting azaleas or

hydrangeas like a normal person, he trucked in three full-grown specimen palm trees and had them lowered into place with a crane. "It needs
to look more tropical," he said sheepishly when I gasped at the size of
the truck and the crane creeping to the top of our street.

He did a hundred little things. He carved a sign to hang over the
door to the greenhouse that said "Bora Bora Room." He searched
through nurseries for a yellow trumpetlike vine we'd seen in Tahiti.
Alamanda. He wanted an alamanda on the deck. He built shelves in the
garage. He started renewing contacts with his friends in the automotive
and advertising worlds. He started dropping in at the advertising
agency and got involved in upgrading the equipment in our audio-
visual room. And suddenly, he was talking again about buying a
business.

"It may be stupid," he said, "but I want to start looking at car washes
again. Do you have any problem with that? It's a lot of money."

Car washes are an interesting and strangely lucrative business in
southern California. Ed had looked into them for several months and
was on the verge of buying one when we found the tumor in his colon.
We'd canceled the deal right after the session with Dr. Bornstein. It'd
seemed insane, considering the prognosis, to even think about buying a
business.

But now, he was doing great. And I wanted him to know I thought
he was and that I had confidence in him.

"I think it's great," I said.

And he phoned his broker.

February 20

WE WENT TO SEE DR. EWEN
and got another favorable report. Ed's condition was still stable. Not
only that, the CAT-scan on his liver showed no evidence of involvement.

We started another round of chemo. On the fifth day, Ed was to get
his shot at eight-thirty in the morning, and then we were leaving for the
Grand Cayman Islands in the Caribbean.

Islands had a special place in our hearts. In fact, we had a goal to
visit all of them, all of the islands on earth. I don't know how many there
are but there are certainly thousands—more than any person could visit
in a lifetime. But still, it's a wonderful thought. Wherever you find islands, whether the Seychelles in the Indian Ocean, Fiji in the South

Pacific, or Catalina off the coast of California, you find a common mystique that links them together, as if they were once a string of pearls that came apart and skittered across the kitchen floor.

Islands have a pace, a peace, and a passion for natural beauty that sets them apart from any more common kind of land. They're peopled only with the extraordinary: adventurers, bums, expatriates, sailors, traders, tourists, Chinese merchants, pearl divers, treasure hunters, sportsmen, the wealthy, the wicked, the wild—and, always, the islanders themselves.

Islanders put this moat called the ocean between themselves and things like gang violence in Los Angeles.

Islanders go fishing all the time and put flowers in their hair. They think a motor scooter is a terrific way to get around. They know all there is to know about essential things like the tides, the stars, and the dolphin. They dance a lot.

You can go barefoot on islands, and finding places where you can go barefoot had become important to me and Ed. So we chose an island as our place to go away and be with each other.

February 26

TWO STORIES FROM THE TWO WEEKS in the Cayman Islands. The first is the snorkeling story.

Ed and I rented a house on Grand Cayman, on the Cayman Kai side of the island, away from the tourists and the big hotels on Seven Mile Beach. Cayman Kai is where serious divers hang out. If you rub zinc-coated noses with the subculture in this world that snorkels, dives, and scubas, you become aware of the most treasured underwater locales and you talk about them with the relentlessness of the tides coming in and going out—"reef-dropping," I call it. You hear men in tattered khaki shorts washing down the battered hulls of their Grand Banks 32s and talking about the reefs off Belize and Cancún. You hear them comparing Green Island to Dunk Island on the Great Barrier Reef. You listen to arguments over Tahiti versus Fiji. Truck versus Cook. Little Dick's Bay versus Montego Bay. Nobody ever brings up Hawaii. That's the sure sign of a novice, because there aren't any reefs there and reefs with their live coral are what makes diving glorious.

Grand Cayman is known as one of the great meccas for divers. The reefs around the island form a great underwater wall where live coral has spent a millennium creating a spectacle that takes your breath away. There's also black coral in the Caymans and several wrecked ships lying on the ocean floor, all of which add to the allure of diving.

"I dove the wall off Grand Cayman" is one of the lines you like to sneak into a reef-dropping conversation.

Ed and I had snorkeled together off Raitea, Fiji, Key West, Bermuda, Moorea, Bora Bora, and Grand Cayman. We'd ridden the swells through the opening in the reef off Rangiroa in the South Pacific and seen schools of fish—25,000 strong—riding the swells along with us. We'd seen brain coral, antler coral, fan coral, staghorn coral—all the bright blues, oranges, and purples. Ed had taught me to recognize many of the tropical fish. The omnipresent and charming angelfish and Sgt. Majors. Parrot fish. Groupers. Blowfish. Bluefish. Mullets. The spotted Triggerfish.

We'd snorkeled on this trip till we couldn't kick our flippers any-more. We could walk from the porch of our rented house down to the water and, in five minutes, swim right out to the reef. We'd rented an inflatable boat and putt-putted to a farther reef. We'd spent half a day on a tour boat that took you outside the reef where swells, coral heads, and fish were bigger. We'd gone to a secret spot told to us in confidence by Bill Wadds, our next-door neighbor. Ed had an underwater video cam-era and he looked like an oversized Jacques Cousteau as he jumped off the sides of boats and into the water, with his camera gear, his snorkel, his mask, and his flippers, paying no heed to the fact he was supposed to be sick and had just finished chemotherapy.

"You want to take scuba lessons?" Ed asked one morning.

What we hadn't done was scuba dive, because neither of us was certified.

"Well,…yeah,…sure," I sputtered, trying to cover up my astonish-ment. How in the world could a man with lung cancer be talking about taking scuba lessons?

But Ed walked down to the Cayman Kai resort about half a mile from our house to inquire about lessons. When he came back, he told me he'd changed his mind.

"Thank God," I thought to myself, "he's finally remembered his lungs and figured out that scuba diving is crazy." But I was wrong.

"It's my sinuses," he said. "I did a little diving in Florida and it hurt like hell. My ears, too. Do you mind if we skip it?"

"You're amazing," I said.

"Why?" he asked. And he wasn't being ingenuous.

"Never mind," I smiled.

The second story has to do with platelet counts.

Ever since he'd started chemotherapy in October, Ed had had a blood test every week to check his platelet count. He had the test done at a lab in Santa Monica and the lab sent the results to Dr. Ewen. The platelet count kept tabs on the number of red cells in his blood. If the count fell too low, it was a danger signal that the chemotherapy was wreaking havoc.

Dr. Ewen asked Ed to continue to get his blood tests while we were in the Caymans, so the first Friday we were there we went to a clinic near Seven Mile Beach and got the test done. It's pretty simple. You whirl the blood sample in a centrifuge to cause it to separate and take a count. I suppose you can get one anywhere in the world that has a lab. We took the test about nine in the morning, then hung around that side of the island to do some things we wanted to do. We shopped for black coral, rode the Atlantis—a submarine that takes tourists down sixty feet for a look at the wall, had fried conch fritters at The Lobster Pot, and then, while I double-parked, Ed ran into the clinic to get the lab report.

In his rush to get back to the car, he didn't even look at the report. He didn't look at it after he got in the car, either, because he was too busy back-seat driving all the way around the island. "Drive to the left, Jean. Slow down, Jean. I want to take a picture. Jean. Look at that boat out there. Jean. Don't pass. Jean. Pass. Jean." You know how it goes.

He finally took the lab report out of his shirt pocket as our rented Nissan pulled into the driveway of our rented house. "Jesus Christ, Jean, look at this," he bellowed.

The platelet count showed 7,000. The counts we had been getting regularly were 150,000 to 170,000.

"Oh, my God," I said. My mouth and throat go dry when I'm shocked or afraid and I can barely talk. "What does it mean?" I rasped. "What should we do?"

"I don't know what it means. And I don't know what we should do. This is frightening, Jean."

We tried to call Dr. Ewen, but we couldn't get a long-distance line. I grabbed the Cayman phone book and began searching frantically for a local doctor. We talked about driving immediately back to town and going to the Grand Cayman hospital. We talked about flying home. We talked about flying to Miami.

We tried again to get Dr. Ewen, but still no long-distance line. I knew we wouldn't get him anyway, at least not for hours. Doctors tend to call you back at the end of their day, and with the four-hour time difference, it was only noon in Los Angeles.

"Ed, there are several general practitioners in the phone book. And there's one guy who's a specialist on the colon. Let's go back into town and find one of them."

"They don't have any information on me," he said. "The first thing they'll do is slap me in the hospital for tests. And to protect their ass. Shit. I don't want to do that."

"Ed, we've got to do something." I was starting to panic. I felt stupid because I didn't fully understand the significance of a low count. I knew it meant danger. But danger of what?

Suddenly, I looked up and Ed was at the refrigerator getting out the mai-tai mix and the rum. "What are you doing?" I shrieked. "You shouldn't drink. You don't even know what's the matter. Your whole body may be haywire."

But he was smiling. "Look. Look at me," he said. "I'm fine. There's nothing the matter with me. I feel great. I'm not dizzy. I'm not weak. I'm not nauseous. I'm not running a fever. Maybe the problem isn't me. Maybe it's the lab. They could have made a mistake."

"What do you mean?"

"They made a mistake."

I sat down and took a sip of his mai tai. After all these years, it still didn't naturally occur to me that the medical profession could make a mistake.

"It's a little lab in a little clinic on an island," Ed went on. "This isn't Cedars-Sinai. I'm going to call them and we'll run the test again. And stop drinking my drink."

He called the lab and explained the situation while I mixed my own rum punch. The doctor, who had been educated in England and was one of those marvelous black men with an Oxford accent, was articulate and sure of himself. He didn't think they'd made a mistake but they'd be happy to run the test again.

We drove over the next morning, took the blood, and waited for the results. This time the count was 120,000. Lower than we were used to at home, but nowhere near the 7,000 from the previous day.

"Platelets deteriorate rapidly," the technician explained. "Perhaps the first time, we didn't run the test soon enough."

"Perhaps you didn't," said Ed.

We decided not to phone Dr. Ewen to make sure there was nothing wrong. We were sure. We also decided not to get a test on the second Friday.

"Good thinking," I said.

"Let's go snorkeling," Ed said.

March 9

AS SOON AS WE GOT HOME FROM the Cayman Islands, Ed got a blood test at the Santa Monica lab. The platelet count was 106,000—lower yet than in the Caymans. Ed phoned Dr. Ewen to tell him, but Dr. Ewen never called back.

"Actually," said Ed, "my message was 'please phone if there's a problem,' so he didn't *have* to phone. But I wish he had."

It seemed to me I'd spent a lot of my life wishing doctors had phoned.

March 11

MY BROTHER CARL DID PHONE. My poet-philosopher-oilman brother. The object of my adulation for most of my life, except for the time he chased me with a dead rat when I was five and he was ten. Or the time when I was eighteen that he told Mama I'd started smoking.

My brother Bob, the apple of everyone's eye when he entered the seminary as a junior in high school, was ten years older than I; Howard, the first one off to college, the first one in the army, the first married, and the first to have a child, was nine years older than I; and Carl was five. We also had a younger sister, Marta, born when Mama was thirty-seven and who was something of a golden child. Carl and I looked upon ourselves as the middle children with all that implies and had a bond as far back as I can remember.

If you took parts of James Garner, Burt Reynolds, Willie Nelson, and a smidgen of Richard Burton, that would be Carl. Witty, charming, brashly bright but not always dependable, with one foot over the line. As a kid, he was usually in trouble. He'd gotten kicked out of the parish school for rolling cherry bombs into the cafeteria at lunch. "They're just firecrackers," he'd said. But to stern, unsmiling Sister Mercedes, they were bombs. And away he went to boarding school—St. Gregory's in Shawnee. "Maybe the monks can handle him" was the drift of that decision.

But even there, it wasn't long before he found himself on the holy carpet. For dropping bowling balls down four flights of stairs in the middle of the night. For getting tipsy on sacramental wine. For driving the monk's John Deere into the frog pond.

Mama was at her wits' end a lot of the time, yet she never doubted him. "He got his first summer job when he was twelve years old," she liked to brag, "boxing groceries at Safeway, and when he came home with his first paycheck, he handed it to me."

Carl did a lot of things that made you love him. He played the guitar and sang Hank Williams songs. He stood in front of the bathroom mirror perfecting an imitation of Harry Belafonte: "Day-o, daaaayo. Daylight come and me wanna go home."

One hot, cricket-chirping August night, when I was eleven and he was sixteen, he took me into his room. That in itself was an event. For reasons only God and Carl will ever understand, he was an amateur taxidermist and his room went a considerable distance beyond belief. There was a stuffed squirrel in there and some sort of huge reptile, like an iguana. There were skins drying and macabre scalpel-like tools. Mail-order books from Northwest Taxidermy School were all over the floor, and there was a microscope with green stuff on a glass plate under the lens. I really didn't like to go in there, yet it was an honor.

He wanted to talk about sex.

"Don't ever neck," he said getting right to the point. "Nice girls don't neck. No matter what a guy says to you, don't do it."

He was very serious and big-brotherly. I knew the subject was important, but I didn't have the heart to let on that I didn't know what necking was. Well,... I was only eleven, and still on roller skates. I listened real hard, searching for clues. I knew it had to do with sex, but beyond that it was a mystery. You have to admit, it's a strange use of the language.

Along with sex education, Carl and I shared something else—poetry.

This reckless teenage kid who thought it was a prank to shoot a twelve-gauge shotgun blast into the dirt under Virginia Haig's front porch (that one brought the cops into Mama and Papa's living room) could quote from Thomas Gray's "Elegy Written in a Country Church Yard" or T.S. Eliot's "Love Song of J. Alfred Prufrock." He knew Dylan Thomas, W.H. Auden, and John Donne. He would walk into my room at night reading aloud: "I must go down to the seas again, to the lonely seas and the shore." He got me into it when I was eight or nine by betting me five bucks I couldn't memorize anything longer than two verses.

I showed him. I etched into the clay of my girlhood mind the epic poem about Alaska by Robert W. Service, "The Cremation of Sam McGee." It's the endless and ghastly story of a man who dies on the

Arctic trail and makes a deathbed request of his prospecting partner. "It ain't being dead, it's the awful dread of the icy grave that pains. And I want you to swear that foul means or fair, you'll cremate my last remains."

Forty-five years later, I can still recite the entire poem and only wish I'd chosen Dante. It's been hard to find a use for the lines of Robert W. Service, as they don't drop easily into cocktail-party conversations. "Sam McGee" started the habit, however, and the summer I was sixteen, I memorized a dozen or so of Shakespeare's sonnets, from which I do drop a line from time to time in an effort to prove literacy.

When we were in our twenties, Carl married Jacque (short for Jacqueline, pronounced Jackie), tiny, black-haired, a little sassy, but with a kind heart and the sunny warmth of an Oklahoma morning in July, when the corn is as high as an elephant's eye. They moved away to Texas and eventually to Longview; I married Kevin and moved to California, straight to Los Angeles. Years went by when we didn't see each other, but the closeness remained.

Carl was a successful independent oil operator working out of Longview by the time I married Ed. He had two grown daughters and a grandson, but he looked like a kid, drove a pickup truck, and still had at least one of his armadillo-boot-covered feet over the line.

He and Ed took to each other immediately. A man's man can always spot a man's man. Ed, who was an only child, said to me once in a classic bit of understatement, "If I had a brother, I wouldn't mind if it was Carl."

Carl was the first person, after the children, I phoned when Ed got sick, and Carl did what he could. He put Ed in touch with a man named Rusty Miller, who had inoperable lung cancer but who got treated at M.D. Anderson and was still around after five years. Jacque phoned once a week or so, and the two of them came to see us after Ed's first operation. They were an anchor, not just for me, but for him as well.

This particular evening, however, Carl didn't phone to talk about Ed. He wanted to talk about God.

His daughter wasn't going to church and it bothered him. "Let her be," I said. "I don't go to church either."

"I know you don't, but with you it's not a loss of spirituality."

"It's not with her either."

"I'm not so sure."

And there followed a forty-five minute free-form talk about spirituality, the Church, faith, God, and the cosmos. We went from Aristotle to Jacques Maritan, with a brief stop at Thomas Aquinas.

Ed kept shaking his head in disbelief. "What are you two talking about?"

"Shhhhhh. I can't hear. We're talking about God."

"How can you talk to your brother, for God's sake, on the phone, for God's sake, about God?"

"Why not?"

"I never heard anybody talk to their brother about God."

But a couple of days later he said out of nowhere, interrupting our reading in bed, "Do you really believe in life after death?"

"Yes."

"I don't."

"I know you don't."

We'd talked about our beliefs before. In fact, we'd had a long conversation shortly after we met. Ed told me he believed in God, but not in the immortal soul.

"I believe that when it ends, it ends," Ed went on. "Death is the end. There isn't anything after that."

My mind was racing to cope with the moment. How do you talk to a man who may be dying *about dying* without making it seem you're talking about him? I decided there wasn't any way. Shit. He knew we were talking about him and I knew that he knew. We might just as well spit it out in plain English.

"Don't you ever think about your mother?" I asked, "and sort of see her in a place?"

"Well, yes, but that's just the way the mind works. That doesn't mean she is in a place."

"I'm not so sure. I think after all this time, she's still alive in your heart and you actually feel her presence sometimes. And that's because she is in a place somewhere."

"I wish I believed that, Jean."

"You should believe it. When you die, whenever that is, you're going to join your mother."

"I've been dreaming about Mother, lately."

"Well, maybe that's because she's still a presence somewhere." And I paused for a moment. "Ed?"

"What?"

"I'm not afraid of dying. I think it's like taking a trip and when you get there, you find a lot of people you love."

He smiled at me. "I know you're trying to comfort me." And then he took the conversation into yet another sensitive area. "Remember my telling you once I wanted to be cremated?"

"Yes." I tried hard to pretend we were having a normal conversation. To act casual. But my heart jumped into my mouth. I'd wanted to talk to him for months about funerals and things. It was the one subject I was afraid to bring up, because it seemed to say I'd accepted the verdict.

"Well, I've changed my mind."

"Really?"

"I remember you telling me you could never be cremated because Catholicism teaches that bodies should turn to dust so they can be reunited with the soul at the end of time."

"It's something like that."

"Well, I don't know if I believe it, but I think I'd like to hedge my bets."

"What do you mean?"

"I'd rather not be cremated," he smiled, "just in case they're right."

I laughed and hugged him. He hugged me back. And I marveled at how a conversation on such a touchy, terrible subject could end in a laugh.

March 28

WE WERE IN THE PORSCHE AGAIN. We were driving to the City of Hope again. Down the Coast Highway to the Santa Monica Freeway past downtown Los Angeles to the Pomona Freeway to the 605 that goes past the gravel pits to the 210 to Highland Street in Duarte. Chemo always started on Friday and continued Saturday, Sunday, Monday, and Tuesday. I always went along on Saturday and Sunday, and the trips to Duarte became part of the rhythm of our lives. It reminded me of going to church when I was a child. I didn't really like sitting through the ten-o'clock High Mass on Sunday, but I didn't really mind it, either. Ed and I made a game out of finding acceptable places to eat in Duarte. Chili's was a winner. So was the Charlie Brown's near the aptly named City of Industry. But today, Ed was agitated.

"It took an hour yesterday to get a vein," he said. "They almost called it quits."

Getting a vein had become the worst part of chemo. Ed's veins were small to begin with, and he'd had so many shots that some of them had weakened and couldn't hold the needle if it did go in. After three or four unsuccessful stabs, a patient tends to get nervous and tighten up. So does the nurse. Some nurses have a knack for it. Ed had developed a special affinity for those with the knack and a horror for the ones without it.

"They finally had to get a supervisor," he continued, "but I can't stand it anymore. I'm going to ask for a Heparin lock."

"What's that?"

Ed described it as a shunt into the vein that you leave in place for a few days, taped to the inside of the arm. "If I had a Heparin lock," he said, "they'd only have to get a vein once during each round of chemo."

"Why didn't they start putting one in months ago?"

"I didn't ask."

"Why didn't you ask?"

"I didn't know about it."

"How'd you find out?"

"I saw a patient with one in his arm and asked him."

The practice of medicine makes you crazy. I couldn't believe no one had suggested this device, knowing what a problem he had with his veins. And once again, I saw the value of taking control of your own situation, finding out about things yourself, and making them happen yourself.

One of the nurses Ed really liked was on call. She got a vein on the first try and put in the Heparin lock, which didn't show at all under a long-sleeved shirt.

Ed got his sixth dose of 5FU. The tumors were still in check. The side effects were still mild.

April 30

I'M ALWAYS ASKING MY CHILDREN TO MAKE LISTS. "What are your ten favorite foods? What are your ten favorite all-time rock recordings? Name your favorite movies. Who are your best friends? What would you do for a million dollars?"

It comes, I think, from all those trips in the Ford Ranch Wagon and the effort to keep the four of them occupied. Wherever it came from, it's stuck with me and it's something I do for my own amusement—on airplanes, for example. I make lists of books I want to read. Or trips I want to take. Or plants I want to grow in the greenhouse.

Once, when Ed and I were driving from Monterey to Los Angeles we whiled away the time making a list of his all-time favorite cars. The list ended up 176 cars long. "Ed," I kept saying as the list kept mounting on the backs of envelopes and road maps, "you can't have this many favorites."

He was very thoughtful for a moment. "Well, I could leave out the 1938 Delahaye."

"But that's my favorite."

"I know," he smiled.

At least one of my children had picked up the habit. Erin keeps a "Book of Lists" in which she records her favorite things at given moments in time. I added to her list once with a list of "Things I Love About Erin," beginning with her minestrone soup.

I've used my lists from time to time to break the ice at events like client dinners. Once, at an epic nine-course extravaganza with a Japanese client, Bob and I started a list of all the meanings, in English, of the word *shit*. The list was astounding. First, there were all the connotations of the word in its purest form:

- bullshit
- horse shit
- dog shit
- chicken shit
- monkey shit
- ape shit
- pig shit

Which leads to the confounding: "Happy as a pig in shit." Especially when coupled with: "I feel like shit." Here's another interesting duo:

- Shit-faced.
- Shit head.

The list is endless:

- Shit out of luck.
- No shit!
- He doesn't know shit.
- Shitless.
- You're shitting me.
- He's got his shit together.

We must have listed a hundred different meanings to the word. Honest. I wouldn't shit you.

Once, Jack Foster and I sat at lunch and made a list of things we'd add to the Ten Commandments to update them for the modern world.

Like "Thou Shalt Not Cut Off Thy Neighbor in Traffic." Jack and I also exchanged correspondence for months on an all-time list of things without which modern civilization could not exist:

- jumper cables
- duct tape
- plastic trash bags
- charcoal lighter
- bungi cords
- Remy Martin

I've made several lists of the most beautiful words in the English language. They tend to change according to time and place in life, but I almost always include: peace, daffodil, music, champagne (I know it's not technically English, but I find it acceptable). And April.

April sounds like rain pitter-pattering. Or, if you drag out the last syllable, like wind blowing clouds across a springtime sky. The April rain is sweet and soft in California and while it may turn the day to lead-pencil gray, there are strokes of color that won't be denied. Rows of vivid pink azaleas slash across lawns, bluish-purple jacaranda trees make scalloped patterns against the sky; Fuchsia drip from hanging baskets in unlikely places like gas stations.

Ed and I flew to the East Coast to visit Eddie and Mary Jane in New York. We glowed from the warmth of their friendship. We saw beauty wherever we looked. A million daffodils near a church. The near-garish yellow of forsythia spilling over fences. And everywhere, the red and yellow of tulips. Every flower box, nook, cranny, clay pot, and footpath in Pound Ridge, New York bobbed with tulips. The giant magnolia tree at the side of Eddie's house was dressed in white, as if for Easter Sunday, and its huge white flowers dropped a carpet onto his lawn.

Before the trip, Ed buried himself in the work of the advertising agency. We were pitching Daihatsu, a Japanese car account, and he was our car guru. He put in a couple of exhilarating seventy-hour weeks, one of them with his Heparin lock taped to his arm, under his shirt. The few people who knew he had cancer, or who suspected, had forgotten. He was also keeping his eye out for a car wash to buy.

After the trip to the East, he started planning a birthday party for him and for me. He had just turned sixty on April 29. I would be fifty on June 1. We'd have a party at the mid-date between the two.

We spent time with Erin and Rich, who'd moved into Rich's apartment in Ventura. We began making plans for the two big graduations—

Sug's from law school in May and Maureen's from Wesleyan in June. We talked about going back to the Grand Cayman Islands at Christmas with the whole family. We talked about going to Florida to visit Robin, Michael, and Matthew. We planted ajuca on the hillside under the specimen palm trees and marveled at the creamy white flowers bursting from the Plumeria, obviously quite at home in the greenhouse.

April is a beautiful word. April was a beautiful month.

It was also a significant one, in that it marked six months since the controversy over surgery and removal of the tumor from the colon. I wondered what the circumstances would have been had we left the tumor alone. It was larger than anticipated and lower. Would it have ruptured by now? Obstructed the colon? Broadcast to the liver? Put Ed into the horrible pain so many cancer patients endure?

Removing it hadn't been easy. We'd gone through two difficult operations and their aftermath. Yet I felt we wouldn't have had this April— at least not in the peace, serenity, and normalcy we enjoyed—had we left the tumor alone.

Not everyone has Ed's courage. Not everyone has his stamina. And I say, humbly, not everyone has his me, because support from someone who loves you is of inestimable value; but people who are fighters like Ed, who have his will, his sense of self, his love of life, ought to be encouraged by their doctors to fight. But largely, they're not encouraged. They're advised, instead, to try to be comfortable and not become a Steve McQueen.

Isn't that sad? Isn't it truly, truly sad? Ed and I would have missed April.

May 3

ED WAS IN A LOT OF PAIN OVER THE WEEKEND. He ran out of the Empirin-with-codeine he'd been taking regularly since it all started. He couldn't get anyone at the City of Hope to okay the prescription until Monday morning, and the drugstore wouldn't give him the pills without the okay.

He also took a litmus test on his urine and found out that his blood sugar was up. He was a borderline diabetic and his blood sugar got out of control from time to time, usually from too much drinking.

He quit drinking, but he had a lot of pain every time he urinated. I could hear him yelling in the bathroom.

I felt the same frustration with the City of Hope I'd felt years before with UCLA—dealing with an institution, not a person; having nobody to talk to, unless your problem comes up between nine and five, Monday through Friday.

May 7

WE GOT A CALL FROM MAUREEN. After months of feeling she might, followed by months of feeling she couldn't possibly, she got the letter telling her she'd made Phi Beta Kappa. College was going to end on the ultimate high note, which was all the more thrilling for Mo because it certainly didn't start that way.

Unlike the older three children, who had specifically wanted to go to college in California, or at least in the West, Maureen had always wanted to go East to school. I wasn't surprised. She was always wandering off from the rest of the family. As a five-year-old, she would stray away on the Santa Monica Beach. It would be time to go home. Chris, Sug, and Erin would be all in a row, playing in the creek that emptied into Santa Monica Bay at Will Rogers State Beach, but Maureen would be off somewhere by herself.

"Don't worry about her," Kevin would say as I'd crane my neck, scan the faces of 400,000 tanners, and begin to panic. "She'll turn up." She would, of course. But I always panicked anyway.

As she got older, she was late to supper a lot, because she was outside wandering off somewhere, and late getting home from school, as well. She'd wander off from the rest of us at the supermarket, on picnics, at events in the school auditorium. She was often a no-show at family activities like "clean-your-room day," "let's all vacuum before we go out to the movies night," and "let's *all* help make cookies for the Girl Scout bake sale Saturday."

But what seemed like the harmless quirk of a tomboy little girl became something more than that when Kevin died. Erin had skipped a grade by then and was one year behind the twins, so the three of them were clustered at Uni High. Maureen was by herself at Emerson and felt left out.

"They all sit around at dinner and they all have the same friends and the same teachers and I don't have anything to say," Maureen would tell me.

In my own way, I felt left out too, because the balance shifted in everything we did as a family, even including Sunday dinner.

The kids took over.

When there are two parents at the dinner table, the family talks about what grown-ups talk about. When there is one parent at the dinner table and four kids, the family talks about what kids talk about. It made me feel awkward. Dinner-table conversation in the home should be the time when children learn from adults about Republicans and Democrats. Not when the adults learn from children about Twisted Sister and Moby Grape.

I didn't like Sunday dinners anymore. They didn't either, really. So we stopped having them. Indeed, we stopped doing a lot of things we'd done before. Sunday afternoons with Annie and others around the pool. Weekend jaunts to Idyllwild, Pearblossom, and Pt. Mugu. It could be that we would have stopped them anyway. The family was just about to change when Kevin died, to enter the stage when kids start to have their own activities and don't want to hang out with their parents anymore. And yet, it was different. They wanted change. Children instinctively want to move on as their way of handling grief. To put the sadness behind. To get back into the happenings of everyday life as soon as they can. Adults want to linger in the memories and rituals, to let it be known these things were treasured.

Children don't want grief to show. They don't like limelight shining onto raw emotions. They don't know how to handle the overwhelming nature of it. Adults very often want grief to show, to let it be known this person was loved.

Moving in opposite directions to a degree, the family changed. We became five people living together—and loving each other—but functioning less as a unit. And I was outnumbered, the only adult in a sea of term papers, acne creams, ghetto blasters, Pacman, proms, and those tiny little rubber bands that tightened up the braces on the children's teeth. I ached for adult companionship and I went out looking for it. Not men, at first. Just grown-ups. Indeed, right before I met Ed, I was so lonely and starved for friends I went to the extreme of starting an organization for copywriters and art directors called the Los Angeles Creative Club. The club is still around to this day and that surely isn't why I *said* I started it, but that's why I started it.

So Maureen, left at the dinner table by the older children, got left by me as well. She sank into herself; then, after a while, she got angry. Hostile at school. Surly with her brother and sisters. Just plain mad at me. When Ed came into my life, she countered with a relationship of her own. She was sixteen. He was twenty-nine. She wanted my attention and she got it. I told her she couldn't see him. She saw him anyway.

We went together to a counselor. He said the problem wasn't the boyfriend, it was our own relationship. There was a lot of tension. Feelings neither of us liked to admit were simmering under the surface. She resented my relationship with Ed. I resented that she resented it.

Sometimes there are troubled situations in life where both sides are right, and I think that's the way it was for me and Maureen.

Maureen was right. Her family dissolved before she was ready for it; and I spent too much time away from home at her expense. But I was right too. For twenty years, Kevin and I built a life around the family. Now he was gone and I needed friends. I also needed a man. And I had a right to pursue those needs. But being the adult, the onus was on me to strike a better balance and dispel the anger. I didn't do either of those very well. I regret that. But I don't feel guilty about it. I was doing the best I could at the time.

When Ed moved into our house on Benecia, it made things better. Ed and I came to Mo's track meets; Ed answered the door when Leonard Bailey came to pick her up for the Senior Prom. We were feeling like a family again. But Maureen was still unsettled and eager to be off on her own. She wanted to get far away, into an environment that was her own, not mine and Ed's, and not a copy of her brother's and sisters'.

So she decided to go to college in the East and applied to a great list of schools: Princeton, Yale, and Georgetown. She had the credentials to get into all of them—the grades, the activities, the IQ, the SAT scores— but she didn't get into any of them. It was a terrible blow. I think the reason she didn't get in is that she came across as a hostile and unhappy person. Her interviewers didn't bother to find out why she might be troubled; they just sensed a problem personality.

We got her into UC Santa Cruz at the last minute, and when she and I went up there to tour the campus, she came away crying, "It's beautiful, Mom, it's just not what I wanted." But she didn't give up, and midway through her freshman year, she made a short list of second-tier Eastern schools and applied again to Tufts and Wesleyan. She was accepted to both and went to Wes. But it was hard. Transferring as a sophomore. Making new friends. Trying to be accepted into already engrained social groups. But she hung in there and she made it. And somewhere along the line, while she was at Wes, the anger died.

Now, at twenty-one, she was a whole, healthy person. Bright as charged electricity. Articulate. Afraid of very little. Independent. Resourceful. And about to cap off her college career with Phi Beta Kappa.

It was a terrific comeback. I'd never been more proud of a person I loved.

Ed was as proud as I was.

He went out and got her a gold bracelet with a medallion hanging from it. On the medallion he had engraved: "Phi Beta Mo." We'd give it to her when we went East for graduation.

As Sug had said a long time before, "He's not my father, but he might just as well be."

May 8

ED SAT ME DOWN TO HAVE A TALK. "I loved working at the agency," he said.

"I know you did," I said. We'd made a great presentation to Daihatsu, but we didn't get the account. Advertising is like that.

"The best part," Ed continued, "was working on the creative." Ed had stepped out of his marketing role and into just about everything else, to the chagrin, I knew, of some of the people who worked for us.

I could imagine them mumbling amongst themselves about the boss's husband getting into things he had no business getting into.

But it was incredible therapy for him and I wasn't about to put a damper on it. Besides, he was doing great. He sat with Cameron Day and Joe Bui and helped them develop television commercials. Then the three of them went out and shot test spots, one in the parking lot of the Hughes Market and the other at Zuma Beach. We used both commercials in the presentation.

"I want to be a creative person," Ed went on.

"You are a creative person," I said, misunderstanding his meaning.

"No, no, no," he said. "I want to go back to work in an advertising agency as a creative person."

The way an advertising agency works is that there are creative people and account-management people. The creative people—copywriters, like myself, and art directors—think up the ads; and the account-management people and media people run the business. Once in a while, I'd seen a creative person switch over to account management. But I'd never seen an account-management person switch over to creative. It's the same in most other industries where creative people mix with business people. An actor, like Warren Beatty, can start producing movies. But a producer, like George Lucas, hardly ever becomes an actor.

"Are you serious, Ed?"

"I'm very serious."

"But you're sixty years old."

"So what?"

"You don't have a portfolio."

"I'll get one."

"I don't know, Ed."

"Would you work with me sometime?"

"We work together all the time now."

"You're not listening to me. You're not understanding my meaning. I don't want to work with you as the account man, I want to work with you as the art director."

"Oh." But what I was really thinking was "Oh, shit. Ed wants to come to the agency and work with me on a project and do storyboards."

It was one thing for Ed to contribute as a marketing person. He had no peer at that and everybody knew it, even if he was my husband. But to come into the creative department as my art-director partner? That was quite another thing.

But in the microsecond where the computer that is the mind weighs a thousand different possibilities and considers a hundred different conclusions, I arrived at a point of view.

He can draw as well as most art directors I know. God knows, he's conceptual. I give strangers a chance every day of the week. Should I rule out friends and husbands? So what if he's sixty years old? So what if it pisses off people in the company? I don't have to explain myself. It's my company. If any of the people here ever have their own company, they'll have the freedom to piss people off too. And they probably will.

"I'd love to work with you," I said. "We'll do it first chance we get."

"Don't patronize me," he said. "I'm not fooling."

"Neither am I."

May 15

ED MET AGAIN WITH DR. EWEN. Things seemed to be okay. He was on a program to bring his blood sugar down, which seemed to be working. But there were some tumors behind the heart that didn't show up on ordinary X-rays, so Dr. Ewen ordered a CAT-scan for the twelfth of June.

Ed was having some new pains in his back. "It's like somebody whacked me across the back with a board," he told me. The lungs are actually in the back of the body, not the front. When he told me about the pain, his eyes misted over.

"Don't worry, Ed," I said lamely, "you've had so many weird pains. It could be a million things."

"Of course, you're right," he said. "Besides, we have to get the party on."

May 16

IT WAS THE BIRTHDAY PARTY FOR the two of us. We called it the "Concours d'McNeilly" and everything about it had to do with cars. The birthday cake was in the shape of a car. Car magazines were stacked in the bathrooms. The Porsche was on display in the driveway. Ed's car memorabilia was scattered all over the house. We served Carroll Shelby's chili and had on display a picture of Ed in the AC-Shelby Cobra we'd sold to buy the Porsche.

Fifty or sixty people came. As Ed and I marched into the living room, each of us carrying a birthday cake, with the crowd singing, I caught a look in Bob Kresser's eye as he leaned against the fireplace. He wasn't singing and his look was very pained. I knew he was thinking about Ed. About me and Ed. About the cancer in Ed's lungs. About the poignancy of the moment. Bob was one of the few people in the room who knew for sure what Ed's condition was. Bob and his wife, Rosanne. They were holding hands. She wasn't singing either.

I looked away. I wanted the moment to be normal. I didn't want cancer in the room. I wanted my birthday with Ed and I was glad—so very, very glad—that people were sharing the moment with us as if it were just a silly birthday party for a couple of silly friends.

Had they all known, we couldn't have thrown the party. Too maudlin. Too touching. Too many smiles forced onto worried faces. Instead it was normal and filled with honest laughter.

Once again, cancer lost.

May 23

THE TWO BIG GRADUATIONS HAPPENED— Sug's from law school and Maureen's from Wesleyan—a week and a continent apart. I'd lived in mortal fear for three years that they'd happen on the same weekend, that we'd have to choose one over the other, and that the unchosen child would be warped for life.

As it turned out, we made them both, even though Ed had to sandwich in a round of chemo between the weekends.

Sug's graduation from Hastings was heightened by the fact that law school had been a struggle. She was just as gifted as her brother and sisters, but it didn't seem to help as she fought to stay afloat. She almost dropped out after her first year and again halfway through the second. I told her dropping out was okay.

"It's a left-brain profession, Sug, and you have a right-brain mind."

"I know, Mom, but I'm halfway through and I can't stand the thought of being a quitter." So she stayed in. And she made it.

Carl and Jacque and Howard and Jane joined me and Ed and the other kids in San Francisco to mark the event.

It was the same weekend that San Francisco was celebrating the anniversary of the opening of the Golden Gate Bridge, so the atmosphere was already heady. Ed was bounding onto cable cars, striding up hills, laughing with my brothers as if he hadn't a care in the world and this daughter was his.

I found things to weep about at every turn. Sug's beauty. Her perseverance. Ed's courage. My brother's coming halfway across the country. We stood on the roof of Sug's apartment building, all of us, to watch the lights turn on across the suspension cables of the bridge. You'd have thought it was my bridge, I was so moved to tears. Then I repeated the performance the following weekend in Middletown.

Maureen's graduation was like a medieval pageant. Trumpets blaring. Drums beating. Bells peeling. The graduates wore cardinal-colored caps and gowns and marched across the huge, grassy quad with banners flying proclaiming their schools. Professors in their caps, gowns, and capes marched too, looking like pilgrims on their way to the Cathedral at Bath. I expected Richard the Lion-Hearted to come riding in at any moment.

Bill Cosby was the commencement speaker. His daughter Erika was a graduate. "Get out on your own," he told the young people. "You're twenty-two years old and your parents are sick of you."

Maureen told me most of the graduates didn't think he was funny. Ed and I thought he was a riot.

As I watched Maureen accept her diploma, tears trickling into my sixty-seventh Kleenex, I couldn't help but wonder what Kevin would have felt had he been able to see his youngest child graduate, Phi Beta Kappa, from a fine Eastern University.

🐦 Kevin and I graduated from the same college a year apart, but it certainly wasn't a fine Eastern school and nobody there ever heard of Phi Beta Kappa.

He missed his own graduation ceremony, because he got there late. But they didn't give him a real diploma anyway. It was a fake because he got an "F" in Government, which was required for graduation.

"I learned all I need to know about Government in the Army," he told the Dean. So he never attended class. He passed the final exam, but because he was never in class, they gave him an "F." He wouldn't take the class over, because he had passed the exam. Kevin went through life creating those kinds of stalemates and never, that I can recall, gave in. (I would have to think about whether or not, on the other hand, he ever won, either.)

When he came home from Korea in 1953, Kevin dreamed of going to Georgetown University in Washington, D.C., to study law or political science and get into the Foreign Service. He was very gifted intellectually and had an uncommon feeling for languages. But his mother was ill and he never left Tulsa. In retrospect, I think he allowed the illness to become an excuse, because he feared failure. In addition, he never seemed able to get his life moving.

There is an engrained "idle" quality in some men raised in the gentility of the American South. Indeed, F. Scott Fitzgerald begins a short story with a definition of the verb "to idle" and comments that Southern men have it down pat by the time they reach puberty. Whether or not that was the reason, Kevin was never able to make his dreams reality.

To me, he was an older man, made worldly by Korea, more literate than anyone I'd ever known, iconoclastic, and challenging. He was always yelling at me to think. I was young and traditional, and he blew my mind open. "You're saying that because you've been taught to say it," he'd jab. "Think about it and then say it or not because you believe it."

I admired his brains and his cultivated background and was beguiled by his nonconformity. On our first date, he told me we were going to dinner at this place he knew that served the best fried chicken in the world. And we drove 400 miles to Rogers, Arkansas (the chicken capital of America) to the AQ Chicken House, where we had fried chicken, honey, and biscuits, then drove home at four in the morning. My mother was aghast. But I loved it. At that time, Kevin was living at home with Sir John, working nights at Andy's DX Service Station and going to school, when the spirit moved him, during the day.

The school was Benedictine Heights College, Tulsa, Oklahoma—the ill-founded and underfunded dream of a community of Benedictine Nuns in Tulsa. Their idea was to build a coed Catholic college (an innovation at the time) with a high percentage of lay faculty (another innovation) and an idea about learning they called an "integrated curriculum." If you were an English major, like myself, you studied science courses that were relevant to English majors. You might take astronomy, for example, instead of physics. If you were taking the Tragedies of Shakespeare in your English classes, you would be studying the European political history of the same era in your history classes. And because the purpose of a college education is to make you think, everybody—everybody—had to minor in philosophy.

The school was heady for a time and attracted an interesting, if offbeat, faculty. But it never really panned out. Small liberal-arts colleges didn't fit the profile in a part of the world that equated Bud Wilkinson, football, petroleum engineering, and other macho pursuits with college. Indeed, the school went bankrupt in the early '60s and its buildings became part of Monte Casino High School, a practical if inglorious end.

But I've always felt I got a good education. I understand, for example, the rhythm of an English sentence and did indeed learn, I think, how to think. But it's not the kind of credential that leaps off a résumé. What college? Where? Nuns?

I felt the irony of it all as 750 cardinal-colored caps were thrown at the sky by the graduating class. At its peak, Benedictine Heights had no more than 350 students, and that's if you counted the part-timers and young women in the Novitiate at the Convent. Kevin's graduating class had eight people in it. Mine, if I recall correctly, had fourteen.

Yet his children and mine graduated, in order, from UCLA, Colorado State, Stanford, and Wesleyan. He would have been very proud, of course, but more than that, he would have been amused.

Had he gotten there on time. ❧

May 30

WE MADE AN OFFER TO BUY ROBERTSON CAR WASH. Ed had begun looking at car washes as his stamina renewed in the early spring. Phoning his broker. Looking at sites. Bringing home pictures and lease agreements. But I didn't know if we'd actually ever buy one. It took a long time to find a good location and get a deal going. I decided to worry about it when the time came. Then, suddenly, it came.

"I found a deal on West Side, Jean," he hollered enthusiastically into the phone. "There aren't many on West Side. It's only been on the market a few days. I think we ought to move."

"Holy, shit," I thought to myself. "What're you going to do now?"

Looking is one thing. Buying is quite another. Buying now, another still.

Car washes are an interesting business phenomenon, especially in southern California, where people live in and semiworship their cars. A well-run car wash can make money. A lot of money. Ed began looking at them because they had to do with cars. He also thought they would provide a semiretired lifestyle that would be very accommodating for the two of us.

"It'll keep me busy," he said. "But not too busy."

Car washes have owners and they have managers. Managers are the ones who get the cars washed. Owners run the business. Owners can be away for days—even weeks—at a time. It all sounded good to me until Ed mentioned one morning how much money it took to get involved.

"About half a million dollars," he said casually.

"God, Almighty," I coughed, spitting my coffee halfway across the breakfast bar.

"Well, Jean," he went on as if any fool would know, "you can't get into a cash business without putting a lot of cash down."

"Oh, silly me," I said. "But Ed, it's so risky."

"We'll get it back in three years," he said confidently. "Maybe two. The only problem is people look at you funny when you say that's what you do."

But that had all been months before. We'd dropped the car-wash idea shortly after D-Day with Dr. Bornstein. I should have known that if Ed picked it up again he'd be successful in finding something and that he'd want to move fast. It was his nature. But at the moment, it certainly wasn't mine.

I felt like I was standing on a muddy hillside, starting to slide. I didn't want to go down the hill, but I couldn't stop sliding and I couldn't go back. What in the world would I do with a car wash if something happened to him? A *car wash*? I barely knew what to do with the advertising agency half the time. A retail business open seven days a week? I knew I ought to stop the whole thing. It was crazy to even think about it under the circumstances. I also knew that one word from me would stop it. But somehow I couldn't bring myself to say it.

Ed was going ahead with his life and defying the verdict. In treatment that was working and feeling good, he wanted to pick up where things had left off before cancer. How in the world could I stop him? I simply couldn't.

As the deal with Robertson Car Wash began to take shape, I hid from the reality. I didn't go to any of the meetings with Ed. I didn't want to hear about leases, liabilities, insurance, crew costs, debt—especially not the debt. It was horrible.

It would take 450,000 dollars down, with another 25,000 due in three months. An additional 50,000 dollars in cash would be needed to start up the business. Then, there would be a 915,000-dollar loan, to be taken back by the seller—10,700 dollars a month for fifteen years.

The cash came from the sale of 19,996 shares of Doyle Dane Bernbach stock. Ed's life in the advertising business was going into the car wash.

I felt like Scarlett O'Hara in *Gone With the Wind.* Whenever I thought about the enormity of the debt, or the fact that we were taking it on in the midst of lung cancer, I'd say to myself, "I'll think about it tomorrow." But now tomorrow was here.

Ed made the offer. It was accepted.

"Holy, shit," I kept saying to myself.

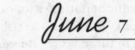

June 7

ED WAS WORKING ON THE DETAILS of the car-wash deal. In the meantime, he'd been coughing all week.

"I have a heaviness in my chest and trouble getting my breath," he told me, "but I think it's a cold."

"Ed, you never get colds."

"But, cancer doesn't make mucus."

"How do you know?"

"Look, my head's stuffed. I can't taste anything. It's a cold."

"Have you phoned Dr. Ewen?"

"Yes, but I couldn't get him."

"Did you leave a message?"

"I talked to his nurse. I asked her to ask Dr. Ewen if mucus would affect my CAT-scan. She called back and said, 'take the CAT-scan when you're feeling better.' What kind of an answer is that? Christ, I don't want to delay it. I just don't want it fucked up."

Ed almost never used that word.

"In business," he said angrily, "you deal with people. You work with them. You have answers. In medicine, they can't be bothered with people. They just want to deal with the disease. Now what the fuck is that all about?"

I didn't have an answer. But I frequently had the same question.

June 8

WHEN I GOT HOME FROM WORK about seven P.M., I found Ed in his car in the garage, asleep. He'd driven home from a meeting with Marty Reed about the car wash and had gotten himself down the Coast Highway, up our street, and into the garage, but he couldn't make it out of the car.

Chemo had caused fatigue from time to time, but this time it was devastating.

June 19

IT WAS THE DAY TO GO TO THE CITY OF HOPE, get the CAT-scan, find out what it said, meet with Dr. Ewen, and talk about the coughing, the mucus, and the heaviness in the chest. It was an important day, and the things that stick in your mind about important days are odd. Tiny details that otherwise would fade unremembered into the seamless backdrop of life etch themselves forever into the forefront of the brain.

What stuck in my mind about that morning was what I was wearing. I had on a khaki-colored cotton skirt and a white linen shirt. I'd added a Hopi Indian bracelet and necklace Ed had gotten for me in Sedona, Arizona. The bracelet was a solid silver cuff with a rain-dance design carved in bas-relief. The necklace was a fetish necklace—three strands of hand-carved birds and beasts intricately cut from onyx, coral, jade, turquoise, and other stones indigenous to Arizona. Both the necklace and bracelet were museum pieces. I wore them because Ed loved them. But that day, when we got to the City of Hope, they made me feel self-conscious. I thought they screamed "money" and I was sorry I had them on. My instincts told me Dr. Ewen resented money and that was one of the reasons he wasn't entirely comfortable with Ed. So, I decided to wait while Ed went in to see him. I thought he was more open with Ed, anyway, when I wasn't there. More one-on-one. More man-to-man.

I waited about an hour. The minute I saw Ed coming toward me across the waiting area, I knew the news was bad. His head was held high, his shoulders were thrown back, and he was marching toward me—not walking. When he got in front of me, he said, "Let's go."

"Are you all right?"

"I want to get out of here."

He was walking so fast I had to trot along behind, but he finally slowed down as we left the building, and I grabbed his hand.

"Was the news bad?"

"Yes."

He was struggling for control. There was anger in his face. There were also tears in his eyes. By the time we got to the car, I was feeling shaky and afraid. I saw a little plot of grass not far away, beside the hospital building.

"I don't want to get in the car," I said. "Let's go sit over there for a minute."

So the two of us sat down on the dewy, damp grass on this June morning with the scent from the rose garden drifting by on gusts. Ed cried. I put my head on his shoulder and held his hand.

"I don't like to appear weak in front of you," he said finally.

"Ed, it's not weak to cry. Just tell me what the doctor said."

He did a curious thing. He began focusing on his link with the forward momentum of life. "It looks like we won't be able to go ahead with the car wash."

"What did the doctor say, Ed?"

"He strongly advised against any investments or buying any businesses. The CAT-scan shows the tumors are growing again. He said there's no way to predict how much time I'll spend in the hospital during the next six months."

"But there's still the other program."

"That's right. Dr. Ewen said there are still cards to play. We can switch to the other program. But there wasn't a lot of confidence in his voice. He kept pointing out that the other program can't cure. It can only stall."

"We've known that all along. We've stalled it a long time already. I don't want to give up, Ed."

"I don't either, Jean. I was really looking forward to buying the car wash and making a go of it."

We were talking about life and death there on the grass. Affirmation or denial. Optimism or defeatism. I knew it was time to stop playing the ingenue about the car wash. I couldn't pretend it wasn't there any longer. I either had to support it and take the consequences. Or put an end to it.

I supported it. "Maybe we still can."

"What do you mean?"

"Well, there are ways it can be handled, I'll bet. We could get a partner. We could hire a general manager. And I'm not exactly a stranger to running a business, you know."

"Do you really think we might be able to go ahead with it?"

"I don't know, but we can talk about it." I didn't know. I had no idea.

"I love you," he said.

"I love you, too," I said.

We got up off the grass, went to the car, and drove back to Los Angeles. Onto the 210 to the 605, past the gravel pits, to the Pomona, past downtown LA, to the Santa Monica Freeway. All the way, we talked. We talked about the car wash and how we could go ahead. We talked about switching to the other program. We talked about Dr. Ewen and the City of Hope. Switching to the other program would take Ed out of Dr. Ewen's research group. Maybe it would make sense to get the other program through a private doctor in West Los Angeles or Santa Monica, someplace closer to home. We talked about all those things, and ever so slowly the sick feeling eased from my stomach. I could still see, however, the edges of terror in Ed's eyes.

That evening, we were due in Ventura for dinner with Erin and Rich at their apartment. It was the first time they'd had us to dinner, the first time for them to be grown-ups in a home they shared. We knew it was an important evening for them, but I thought we ought to call it off.

"No," said Ed. "Don't call it off and don't tell them what happened today, either. What does it accomplish? I won't feel any better and it just ruins their evening."

So we drove to Ventura, but the forty-five-minute drive took two and a half hours. Ed had to stop every few minutes and find a john. He couldn't stop throwing up.

June 20

WE GOT UP AT FIVE-THIRTY IN THE MORNING to catch an eight-o'clock plane to Albuquerque, on our way to Santa Fe. When we got home from the City of Hope, Ed said—as he'd said after the very first meeting with Dr. Bornstein, when we'd learned the "spots" were cancer—"Let's get out of here. Let's go someplace for the weekend."

We picked Santa Fe and somehow, in a couple of hours, Ed got us two plane tickets and a place to stay. I phoned my friend Gary Freund, who goes to Santa Fe every year for the Indian market, and found out which galleries to visit, which restaurants to try, and where the museums could be found.

As we wandered in and out of galleries and shops near the Plaza and behind the Cathedral, looking for paintings by R.C. Gorman, Ed's mind began to settle down and his voice was no longer tinged with fear. But that evening during dinner at Coyote Cafe, he started shaking and he couldn't stop. He couldn't walk, either, because his legs had turned to jelly. So we sat there in the southwestern-chic restaurant, crowded with the trendy people who live in Santa Fe and the trendy people who visit there, and held hands and looked at each other until the trembling stopped.

It made me wonder how many unknown dramas are happening around us all the time. Underneath the chatter about blue corn tortillas and banana salsa on the swordfish, how many people are holding back fears or struggling for control? It also made me feel that all the people around us were fools. They were sitting there eating dinner while Ed and I were dealing with life and death.

June 22

ED RETURNED TO THE CITY OF HOPE as soon as we got back from Santa Fe. By then, Dr. Ewen had a more detailed prognosis.

"The tumors are getting bigger," the doctor confirmed. "And there are more of them. We'll put you in the other program, but it will be three months before we can know if it's working."

The "other program"—the one Ed had wanted to get into in the first place—combined 5FU with massive doses of an experimental new drug called Leucovoran. The program required hospitalization for six days every month because of the amount of Leucovoran that got infused into the body. An IV needed to drip into a vein, twenty-four hours a day for six days, in order to get all of the drug into the system.

Because of the need to be hospitalized and the distance to the City of Hope, Ed worked it out with Dr. Ewen to transfer his case to a doctor in private practice in West Los Angeles. The doctor was familiar with the protocol for using 5FU with Leucovoran. His name was Sherman Moore.

By the time I got home from work that evening everything was done. Ed had personally gone from department to department at the City of Hope, collecting all his X-rays and records so they could be transferred to the new doctor.

"The only way I'm sure they'll get these is if I do it myself," he told me.

"I'm not sure I want to leave Hope," I said. "I feel at home there. I feel confident with them." I remembered Alan Fogelman and the difference he'd made for Kevin and me. "I like research doctors better than private physicians."

"Dr. Moore practices out of several hospitals in West LA. He's so much closer to home and to your office. When I'm in the hospital, you can visit at lunch time. It'll be so much easier on you, Jean. And so much better for me to have you near."

"I know," I said. "Of course, you're right." Nevertheless, I felt like an astronaut on a space walk whose umbilical cord had just been cut.

June 23

"EVERY TIME I MEET A NEW DOCTOR," Ed said as we stood in front of the elevator in the doctor's building, "I have to sell him. I sell him and then he works with me. He realizes he has a fighter, but first I have to sell 'em."

Dr. Moore's office was like a zillion other doctors' offices in a zillion other medical buildings. A cookie-cutter decor ordered, it looked to me, from a 1940 Sears catalog. The waiting room was very small and cramped. The receptionist was behind the sliding-glass window, as usual. The sliding-glass window in doctors' offices has become an important piece of symbolism to me. Not only is it very unfriendly, it also says "them" and "us." It makes a separation between the medical staff and the patients. It makes a boundary that says what any boundary says: "Stay out. Don't bother us. Speak when spoken to."

If I could wave a magic wand over the medical profession, the first thing I'd do is rip out all those glass windows and make all those receptionists sit out there with the people and answer the phone in front of them, like Canary does at Kresser/Craig.

Ed tapped on the sliding window and the receptionist opened it. Her name, I learned later, was Reba. He said, cheerily, "Good morning. I'm Ed McNeilly."

She, in a language called frozen-polite, said, "Take a seat, please."

Here we go again, I thought. You pick up vibes in a doctor's office the minute you walk in. You can sense it over the telephone, like you can sense whether or not you're going to like a TV sitcom within the first couple of minutes of dialogue.

Why couldn't she have talked to Ed like a person? "Good morning, Mr. McNeilly, we've been expecting you. Dr. Ewen has told us all about you. We're delighted we're going to be working together."

When Ed went in to see Dr. Moore, I waited. It was very important to Ed that he establish a rapport. That he get an understanding. I felt he could do that better one-on-one. Besides, there's an unwritten law in doctors' offices. "Try to keep family members out of the examining rooms. If they ask to come in, let them. But don't offer and try not to give them the opportunity to ask."

In my opinion, it's because doctors consider a second person in the room a time-consuming complication. The person might ask questions that have to be answered, and that takes time. They might have opinions to offer, and that takes time. Doctors seldom, if ever, actually want information from anyone but the patient. There is little recognition of the fact that illness is a family event. That it affects the lives, the emotions, the happiness of everyone living under the same roof. Or that family members develop instincts about the patient's condition and can offer the physician valuable insights. On the other side of the coin, the physician could offer the family confidence, good will, understanding, and relief in the sense of "you're not in there alone anymore; I'm taking care of him with you." But all of that takes time. And doctors see so many patients, they don't have time.

Anyway, I waited, but Ed told me everything when he came out. "He's attentive—he listened to everything I had to say. But I had to sell him. I liked him. But I had to sell him."

One thing Dr. Moore was for sure was quick. Ed was to check into the hospital the next day and begin his first round of chemotherapy with 5FU and Leucovoran.

June 25 to July 2

Ed fashioned himself a desk by lowering the bed table and pulling up the tiny hospital room's only chair. He had his briefcase open and his car-wash papers spread all over the "desk" and spilling onto the bed. He was doing income and expense projections based on the observations he'd conducted earlier in the month. Marty would be arriving around noon to go over the leases and other details of the deal. The way it looked now, we'd own the car wash and be operating it on the first of August. We'd definitely decided to go ahead.

I still didn't know what I'd do about running it if Ed wasn't able. We'd talked with Bob about a partnership and Bob had said "yes," but Ed wasn't at ease with this. Both men were used to being in charge, and when Bob disagreed with a couple of Ed's decisions, Ed backed away.

"I love your partner, Jean, but this is my thing."

"I know, Ed. It's okay." And then I'd feel the mud slide start to happen again.

"Look at this, Jean," Ed said from his hospital desk. "Expenses should average 45,000 dollars a month."

"Including debt service?"

"Including debt service. And, I figure there should be eight months with gross revenues of 70,000 dollars and four months with gross revenues of 60,000. That's a 29-percent return. It should be very good for us, Jean. Or, for you. I want you to be in good shape."

There was an IV tree beside Ed's chair, with a bag hanging from it. A tube went from the bag to a Heparin lock in Ed's left arm. The IV was dripping Leucovoran, in solution, into his vein. It took each bag about twelve hours to drip in. But the comment Ed made about leaving me in good shape was not necessarily weighted with awareness of that situation. Ed made it in the way any husband would make that comment to his wife when he was planning for the future.

Ed got up from his "desk" to get some papers off the bed, and I got up with him to move the IV tree. I was more worried than he seemed to be about the needle in his arm and about keeping the Heparin lock in place. As I pushed the rickety tree behind him, I looked up at the bag of Leucovoran—juice, the nurses called it. About half of it had dripped in. The liquid in the bag was absolutely clear. Colorless. But it had a sort of luminescence to it that separated it from water.

"This stuff looks like vodka," I said to Ed.

"I wish," he said.

I noticed a label from the hospital pharmacy stuck to the outside of the bag and picked up my glasses to read it. I tended to look everywhere for little clues that would give us the information that had always been so hard to get from the doctors.

"Oh, my God," I said, as I read the label. "Ed, there's a price on this bag. It says 35 hundred dollars."

"What?"

"It says 35 hundred dollars. Do you suppose that could be true?"

"Good grief, Jean." Ed picked up his pocket calculator and banged on it for a second. "If it is, it means this'll cost 42 thousand dollars a treatment."

"Just for the drug," I said. "God knows what the hospital is costing."

"It must be a mistake," Ed said. "No, wait. I know what it is. This is the first bag and they put the total cost of all twelve bags onto the first one."

"That must be it." I was relieved by that explanation, and yet a new fear began creeping up the back of my spine. What if insurance doesn't cover it? Does insurance cover experimental programs? Does the insurance have a cap on it? I remember looking at the policy early on and I seemed to recall a million-dollar cap. At 42 thousand dollars a treatment just for the drug, what had seemed to be a comfortably high cap could be eaten up in a few months.

We hadn't worried about money or insurance up to then. Ed was covered, as my spouse, under the policy through my office. It was a good policy, underwritten by Aetna through the American Association of Advertising Agencies. The insurance had paid for virtually everything—all the doctors, Kraft, Richmond, Bornstein, Ewen, and all of the care at the City of Hope, including two surgeries. Furthermore, the City of Hope had a policy that their care is free if insurance doesn't cover it. But this wasn't the City of Hope. I made a mental note to talk to Judith, our administrator, as soon as I got back to the office and get a clear understanding of the insurance coverage.

A nurse came in with Ed's lunch, and Ed was joking with her about the food. At many hospitals, it's a nutritional joke. Little, if anything, is fresh. Soggy carrots and faded peas come from industrial-sized cans. Canned fruit, loaded with sugar, is a staple, as are canned vegetables, which are loaded with salt. But the worst part is how everything is loaded with fat. I don't know how hospitals can serve bacon-and-egg breakfasts, tacos, pizza, meat loaf, fried chicken, macaroni and cheese, and spaghetti with meat sauce—and look themselves in the eye. I don't know how they can fill the trays with breads and rolls made from saturated fats like palm oil, or with whole milk, rather than nonfat milk, or with salad dressings—again loaded with oil, as well as salt. You'd think a hospital, of all places, would offer a diet high in fiber and low in saturated fat, salt, and sugar. I don't know their side of the story. I'm sure they have one. A complex set of issues bound up in the economics of running a hospital kitchen.

"Do you suppose that means 35 hundred dollars a bag, or is that for the whole treatment?"

"Hmmmm," she said. "That's a lot, isn't it? Well, I don't know. Ordinarily if it says 35 hundred dollars on one bag, that would mean one bag. I know the pharmacy had to special-order this stuff. That's why we started late. It hadn't gotten here yet." She shook her head and clucked her tongue. "It's experimental, this drug, and the drug companies try to recover some of their costs."

Leucovoran continued to drip into Ed's veins at about ten bucks a drip, I figured. Ed phoned the pharmacy about the price. They said they weren't sure yet down to the penny, but yes, it was going to be about 35 hundred dollars a bag.

Despite the shock of that tidbit, the time at the hospital took on the out-of-place but comforting aura of a summer picnic. I came over every day with bottles of Chardonnay and nice (nutritionally sound) lunches I'd bought at the take-out counter of a Gelson's near my office. Dr. Richmond came by to see Ed. He'd never heard of Leucovoran. "Sounds like a truck driver," he said. "Lou Covoran."

Dr. Kraft came by too. This was the first we'd seen of Dr. Kraft since he'd bolted from the hospital room at Cedars. "There are some spots on your lungs. We don't know what they are and you shouldn't speculate. All we know is there are spots."

Like hell that's all they knew. I had a feeling both doctors felt guilty about Ed. It wasn't as if he'd never seen a doctor. He'd had a physical every year from one or the other of them. Yet cancer of the colon that had matasticized to the lungs had gotten past them both.

But it was good of both doctors to come by. Ed, who was still coughing, joked with Kraft, "I have a cold complicated by cancer."

Marty was in and out, sewing up details on the car-wash deal. Bob dropped in. The nurses, unused to the cheeriness, the Chardonnay, and the camaraderie, kept saying to Ed, "What are you doing here?"

Dr. Moore dropped in every day, but there wasn't much to check on. The IV just dripped away. The side effects of the drug, if there were going to be any, as well as the efficacy of the drug wouldn't be known until later. Ed and I scratched our heads when Dr. Moore told him to expect severe side effects, because Dr. Ewen had told us the side effects were mild.

"Ewen wants to put things into a more positive frame of mind," was Ed's explanation.

"Ten different doctors will see things ten different ways," was mine.

The last bag of Leucovoran finished dripping in around midnight on the second of July. Ed had convinced the head nurse he could be checked out in advance, and we sat and watched the last of the liquid disappear down the IV tube, all packed, dressed, and ready to go. The minute the last drip of juice disappeared, I called the nurse and Ed began removing the Heparin lock himself. We bugged out of there in a flash and got home to Malibu about one in the morning, with yet another episode behind us.

July 4

THE AFTERMATH OF LEUCOVORAN. The Fourth of July had always been a big event at the Craig/McNeilly household in Malibu. Young people attached to one or another of the children would straggle in from various points up and down California. Friends of mine and Ed's would come from places like Culver City and Glendale, pleased to be invited to tan on the Malibu sand and sit on the deck and watch the parade of wildlife, human and otherwise, go by on the beach. To sit in the hot tub, drink Grand Marnier, and listen to me ask, as I always did in the hot tub, "What is the meaning of life?"

Ed would stand over the barbecue as the sun began to set, and burn chicken. He'd pass out pitchers of his killer margaritas. Frequently, he'd wander around with his 8mm Sony Cam Corder catching the usual silly mugging faces, which he'd then play back instantly on the TV screen. I always made a dessert called "red, white, and blueberries"—fresh strawberries, vanilla ice cream, and fresh blueberries—layered into brandy snifters. I dusted off dog-eared LPs to find John Phillips Sousa and usually had some contraband fireworks to sparkle up the deck. Around nine P.M., people would station themselves in little bouquets all over both decks to watch the fireworks shooting off on the beach. Ooooooohhhhhh. Aaaaaaaahhhh. The fireworks were never too spectacular. But the ambience was. Ohhhhh. Ahhhhh. What does Ed put in those margaritas? Ohhhhh. Ahhhhh. Did you notice Jean's red, white, and blue petunias?

But this year, there would be no party. We'd just gotten home from the hospital. Besides, we had no idea what kind of blows Leucovoran might deliver. There were bound to be side effects. You can't pump twelve liters of chemical into a human body and expect nothing to happen. Even mild side effects like diarrhea and vomiting are better handled in private. So no one was invited to Malibu for the Fourth.

None of the children were even around. Sug was still in San Francisco studying for the Bar; Chris was away on a camping trip; Erin and Rich had plans with some friends in Ventura; and Maureen, who'd decided to stay on the East Coast, had gotten a job, with Madeline's help, at Jordan, Case, Taylor & McGrath, an advertising agency in New York.

So, the Fourth of July was just the two of us. And it was too quiet. I suddenly understood the loneliness of holidays and why Christmas can be the worst time of the year for millions of people. Then, too, we were waiting for something to happen—we didn't know what. There was some fear. There was some dread. There was some feeling of being on a powder keg. It was a terrible weekend. I kept thinking of a recurring dream I'd had toward the end of Kevin's illness.

🐾 *The dream was always very vivid and real, rather than surrealistic like most of my dreams, gauzy and eerily mingled with mixed metaphors and mixed people. This dream wasn't anything like that.*

I was in the kitchen of our house on Benecia. I was wearing the butcher's apron I always wore; the door of the pale-yellow refrigerator was stuck full of notes, as it always was; the wrought-iron baker's rack for cookbooks was untidy and laced with an occasional schoolbook or library book shoved hastily into place by a child told to clean up the kitchen; the terrarium I'd made in a fishbowl had gotten damp and sort of gross on the inside. Terrariums looked good, I learned when they were in vogue, for a maximum of two days, and then they got gross.

All of these details were vivid and real. I was standing at the stove, sautéeing ground beef to go into lasagna, when the doorbell rang. I went to answer it with the spatula in my left hand. With my right hand, I pulled up the hem of the apron and dabbed the dew off my face, then made a futile effort to adjust my hair, which never seemed to look combed or tidy on the weekends. I opened the door and there was a large black dog there, a mean-looking sort of dog, like a Doberman. The dog had a wide collar, and somehow I knew that there was a tiny pocket concealed in the collar and inside the pocket was a message for me. The dog was growling and baring his teeth, but I knew he wouldn't harm me if I looked in the pocket for the message. I found a folded-up piece of paper, which I slowly opened. On it were the words "I've come for Kevin."

I slammed the door and the dog began to bark; then the barking would wake me up. One night, however, I didn't awaken, and the dog began to hurtle himself against the front door; I put my shoulder against it to keep it from opening. The force of the dog, or the force of something, hurled me back and the door opened, and that's when I woke up. I found myself, however, on the floor, and I could still feel myself being thrown there. I didn't fall there; I was thrown.

I never told Kevin about the dream. I never told anyone about it. ❧

To get my mind off things like that and to get Ed's mind off the Leucovoran sloshing around in his system, I went down to the video store and rented some movies. We watched nine of them over the course of a four-day weekend. Eventually, Erin and Rich came by. I'd never been so glad to see people in my life. Talk with them and some human contact chased away the demons.

July 6

THE EFFECTS OF LEUCOVORAN FINALLY HIT. Nausea. Disorientation. Fatigue. Blisters broke out all over Ed's nose and around his ear lobes, as if he'd been burned. He had no interest in food, yet an empty stomach brought on nausea.

I racked my brain for foods that would entice him to eat and turned to his childhood, because sick people often yearn for tastes they had as children from the kitchens of their mothers. It was especially true of Ed, because he adored his mother.

Ed was born in Okmulgee, Oklahoma, about 200 miles from where I grew up in Oklahoma City. Before he was a year old, however, the family moved to a farm near Pearl, Texas, about fifty miles west of Waco, dead in the middle of the endless Texas plains. His grandfather had a farm there and his own father was out of work. It was the Depression.

The extended family that migrated to the farm struggled through the Depression, growing their own food, raising a little cotton, and running a few cattle. Ed told me stories of the women picking cotton in the blistering heat of a Texas summer, of meals made up only of corn on the cob, of his Aunt Willie churning butter, and of milk "cooling" on the porch behind wet burlap catching the breeze.

They stayed on the farm until Ed was six or seven; then, like thousands and thousands of other dust-bowl families, George, Emily, and Ed McNeilly came to California. They settled in Burbank, and Ed's father got a job with Sears & Roebuck in the store at 7th and Western in Los Angeles, which is still there. He was a salesclerk in the major appliances department—washing machines and refrigerators. Ed was an only child, because, he'd told me, his parents felt they couldn't afford another one.

Ed had problems with his father. He told me stories of his dad beating up on him when he was a little boy. When he was sixteen and already six-foot-two, his father punched him in the face one night and Ed told his mother that if it happened again, the punching would start going in both directions. Shortly after that, he left home. The war was still on, but he was only seventeen, so he enlisted in the SeaBees and went to the Philippines. There was a rowdy crew aboard his ship in Manila Bay. He learned to use a six-inch stiletto knife and slept with it every night under his pillow.

When he came home in 1946, Ed spent half a year at Glendale City College, but the war had already grown him up, as it had so many young men of his generation, and he was too impatient to sit in school. He'd been a radio operator in the service, so he got a job in radio, and by the time he was twenty-one he was producing programs at a station in Bakersfield and trying to get into television. He finally begged his way into a job at a brand-new TV station in Los Angeles—KTLA—by offering to work for nothing to learn the business. Within a year he was producing and directing live television, especially commercials.

And that's what took him into the advertising business. He worked for a year for a Los Angeles agency called the Lansdale Company. (Ten years later, I came to Los Angeles as Mrs. Kevin Craig and got my first job at that same agency.)

In 1955, when I was graduating from high school in Oklahoma City, Ed joined Doyle Dane Bernbach in Los Angeles and became an account executive on the Gallo Wine account. (His first boss, Monty McKinney, is now Vice-Chairman of Kresser/Craig.) After two or three years at DDB/LA, Ed concluded that the mainstream of the advertising business was in New York and that if he wanted to make a mark he needed to be there. So he got himself transferred to DDB/New York, and after a short time, the Volkswagen account came to that agency.

Ned Doyle said to Ed, "Kid, you need some print experience," and put him on the VW account without even knowing of Ed's lifelong love affair with the car. As head of the VW domestic business, Ed rose to the top with the speed of a scuba diver running out of air. Within ten years, he was a Senior Vice President, a member of the Board of Directors, a major stockholder, and a wealthy man.

But his character was etched by the hot winds of the Depression blowing across a Texas farm, an unbending and angry father, and going to war at seventeen.

Ed adored his mother and spoke of her with the tenderness of a small child. He and Emily had formed an early alliance to shield each other from the harshness of George, a man scarred perhaps because of failed dreams and living on his father-in-law's farm. Even though Emily had been dead for ten years by the time I met Ed, he spoke of her often. "Jean," he would say, "I'm sorry you never met Mother. She would have loved you, Jean."

So when Ed couldn't eat or wouldn't, I abandoned the cooking he and I dreamed up while poring over issues of *Gourmet* magazine—steamed mussels in saffron and white wine, angel-hair pasta with fresh basil and tomatoes—and reverted to the repertoire of his childhood and mine. Of his mother and mine. Grilled-cheese sandwiches and Campbell's tomato soup. Macaroni and cheese. Meatloaf. Stewed tomatoes. Chicken-fried steak. I had never seen a time when Ed couldn't or wouldn't eat a BLT on toast, with a shake whirred in the blender. But this time, even that didn't work.

I was scared and worried. The snapshot of a life without Ed implanted on the back of my eyelids was coming into focus more and more. He'd do something like clean the filter on the hot tub, and I'd tell myself I should ask him to show me how, so I could do it if I was alone, but I'd choke on the words. He'd do something else, like write a caption under a photo in an album, and I'd know that every time I saw that caption for years, I was going to cry inside, because every time I saw Kevin's handwriting for years, I cried inside. Handwriting is one of the very few things a person leaves behind.

I was scared to death about buying the car wash. I was scared for Ed. For the first time, he had a sense of the fact that he could become very, very ill. That the future could hold things for him like pain, being in need, and the humility, in his eyes, of being brought down.

"I don't feel on top of this, Jean," he kept saying to me.

I phoned Sug to talk. And in a day or so, this letter came to Ed from her.

San Francisco
Monday, July 6, 1987

Dear Ed,
Here is a list of little annoyances of life:

1. *Parking tickets*
2. *Lines*
3. *Going to a party, when you don't especially like the host*
4. *Paying bills*
5. *Having nothing to eat in the icebox when you're craving a goodie*
6. *Having to go to work when it's a beautiful day outside*
7. *Feeling sick and blue when there are a bunch of things you want to do*

AND: here is a list of little pleasures—
1. *Waking up and seeing the ocean every morning*
2. *Watching nine movies on the VCR in one weekend!*
3. *Having a beautiful grandson*
4. *Frozen chocolate chips in the freezer*
5. *Having a big birthday bash where the guests are delighted to attend*
6. *A Bora-Bora room*
7. *A fine, fast car that many beautiful women would love to drive*
8. *Snorkeling in Bora Bora*
9. *Snorkeling in Fiji*
10. *Snorkeling in the Grand Caymans*
11. *Burning chicken when you barbecue it and everyone eating it and telling you it's superb*
12. *Cooking flank steak, and everyone telling you it's wonderful and meaning it*
13. *Thanksgiving stuffing contests*
14. *A wife who loves you to pieces*
15. *People who love taking care of you, like Momma and me*

So—live it up Ed. The goods far outweigh the bads. And you are loved so fiercely by so many people. We're all in there; not just you. Think of how strong that makes you.
I love you.

Sug.

The effect of one human being reaching out to another is enormous. When Ed got the letter, he called me at the office and read it over the phone. We both cried. And after that, the fatigue was less, the nausea eased, he could hold down tomato soup, and the eruptions on his nose started to clear up.

July 8

ED PICKED UP WHERE HE LEFT OFF on the purchase of Robertson Car Wash. There were meetings with the broker, meetings with Marty. The leases were very complicated and the details were endless. The broker and Marty both knew Ed had cancer, but they dealt with him as if he didn't, which was his wish, and the deal moved forward.

July 13

ED HAD A NOON APPOINTMENT WITH DR. MOORE. I walked into the lobby of the medical building to meet him and found myself standing in front of the bank of elevators with a crowd of people, one of whom was James Garner. You see a lot of famous people if you live in Los Angeles long enough. Their lives have been so public, you feel you know them. I wanted to walk up to James Garner and say, "Did you know you've always reminded me of my brother, Carl? And did you know that I'm an Oklahoman, like you are? And hey, what are you doing here? I hope it isn't serious."

But he got onto his elevator and I got onto mine.

There was that icy feeling again the minute I walked into Dr. Moore's office, as if it seeped under the door jambs and through the seams in the wallpaper, emanating from the pores of the people behind the glass partition. You're in alien country. You're an intruder.

Ed wasn't there, so I tapped on the window. I don't know what to do in doctor's offices other than tap on the window. The alternative is to shout through the window. Yet every time you tap on the window, you wait for it to open knowing the frozen face will tell you you're an interruption. The nurse looked up. She told me Ed was with the doctor and closed the glass. So I sat and waited.

When Ed came out he was smiling. The side effects had eased by then, the crushing fatigue had dissipated, and he was eating. But there was no report on the effectiveness of Leucovoran.

"It's too early," Ed explained. "It takes two or three months."

We'd gotten used to monthly X-rays, weekly blood tests, and the lab workup that were all routine at the City of Hope. They were a tangible monitor of what was going on. It was disconcerting to be without them.

"Well, they took some blood," Ed said. "But it's different here. They don't share the information with you. Dr. Moore did say we could continue the program."

"I didn't think there was any question."

"There isn't. He just doesn't understand me yet. The good news is he's going to look into some ways to handle the next infusion at home."

"Really?"

"Yes. There are some portable pumps they can use or some such thing. Anyway, I told him I wanted to be mobile and he said he'd look into it."

I recalled the IV trees, the bags of juice, the IV pump beeping when it got clogged and nurses coming in to do mysterious things to right it. I recalled the Heparin lock in his arm and the need to have the 5FU shots, as well as the Leucovoran infusion.

"What does he mean," I said, "a portable pump? How does it work? Who gives you the shot of 5FU?"

"I don't know, Jean. I don't know how it all works. He didn't explain. He just said he'd look into it. But it would mean the world to me to not have to go to the hospital every month."

We left and went to lunch at Islands and continued to speculate about portable pumps. Ed was feeling good. He was himself. He ordered the surfer burger, red wine, and french fries with the skins on them. It was his favorite lunch.

July 16

THE BILL CAME FROM CENTURY CITY HOSPITAL. The total was 35,105 dollars, for six days. Of that, 2,922 was for room and board. And 32,180 dollars was for drugs and hospital incidentals. Of that, 30,579 was for Leucovoran. The bags of juice cost exactly 3,057 dollars and ninety cents each.

The invoice indicated the insurance company had been billed. Judith had checked and found out it should be covered, but I was anxious to get the notice from Aetna that it had been paid.

Judith also told me the insurance had no cap, which was a relief. Who would have dreamed a million-dollar cap might be insufficient? The Aetna policy paid 100 percent of covered expenses. If we had a policy that paid 80 percent, which was more typical, we'd be short 7,000 dollars a month.

I wondered about all the people with poor insurance, limited insurance, or no insurance. I wondered if the care Ed was getting was available to everyone, or available only to people with good insurance policies and some financial substance.

You don't have to wonder too much. An insurance policy that will pay for a doctor of choice, like Dr. Moore, that includes 100-percent catastrophic coverage and that has no cap is simply not in the cards for someone like Alicia Lopez. Ed and I got the best that medicine had to offer and while I was glad for that, I was troubled by it. I don't like elitism, even when I'm the beneficiary.

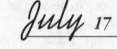 *July* 17

"WHAT ARE YOU DOING, JEAN?" It was a quiet question spoken softly in the quietude of dawn. First light was just beginning to dim the row of distant street lights that outlined Santa Monica Bay.

"I'm watching the sunrise," I said.

Ed got out of bed and joined me on the deck. Since he'd turned me into a morning person, we'd shared many beautiful sunrises, most of them on islands in the South Pacific or the Caribbean. A Los Angeles sunrise over Santa Monica Bay can be just as stunning as a sunrise seen from the island of Moorea, where it comes up over Tahiti. But somehow the encroachments of civilization change the mood. Instead of roosters crowing and mynah birds chattering, you hear, even at five A.M., the traffic on Pacific Coast Highway.

"Why are you up?" Ed asked, as he put his arm around me.

"I have some ARCO commercials due tomorrow and they're not done. How are you feeling today?"

"I'm feeling fine."

"Do you want to help me?"

A smile started at the corners of Ed's white moustache and worked its way into his clear blue eyes.

"I'd be delighted to help you."

We went downstairs and while I put on the coffee, Ed found a story-board pad and his magic markers, and the two of us worked from five A.M. until noon, with me as the copywriter and him as the art director.

We did three commercials for ARCO gasoline. That afternoon I took them to the office and showed Bob.

"These are wonderful," he said. He thought one of them was among the best commercials the agency had ever done. "How did you get these done? Who worked with you?" Ron, my art-director partner, was away on vacation.

"I worked with Ed," I said. "He wants to be an art director."

Bob looked at me and smiled with the warmth and understanding he always had for me. "We should hire him," he said.

That evening I told Ed that Bob was pleased and the commercials were going to the client the next day.

"We should start a new business," I said. "McNeilly & Craig, television commercials and car washes."

"No," he quipped back. "It's McNeilly & McNeilly."

July 18

ALAN & STACIE AND ERIC & MARY.
Kevin and I never hung out much with other couples. Never had much of a social life. There were lots of reasons. The children were with baby-sitters all week, for one thing, and it really bothered me to bring in a new bunch of sitters on the weekend or in the evening so we could go out. So we didn't.

But we did other things instead. We loaded everybody into the VW van or the Ford Ranch Wagon weekend after weekend and tootled around all over Southern California, up to Idyllwild or the top of the Grapevine to find snow, to see the wild flowers near Lancaster, to buy pumpkins in the Ojai Valley, to gather driftwood at Leo Carillo Beach, to the festival at St. Andrew's Priory near Valyermo, to see the railroad tracks from the top of the Cajon Pass, to picnic at Point Mugu, to find ghost towns off the Pearblossom Highway, to look at orange groves around Filmore and Santa Paula, and to the beach—always to the beach. Laguna. San Clemente. Santa Monica. Santa Barbara. Summers on Balboa Island. It was great. I loved it.

There were several families we spent time with when we lived on Bentley—the Ganezers, Bargeros, Ravens, and Herricks. But when we moved to Benecia, we didn't see them much anymore.

There was also the problem of Kevin. Being a postal clerk, there was some discomfort around my advertising friends. For him and for me. He was also embarrassing at times. He name-dropped. Made up stories. Tried to be the center of attention. The classic actions of a person trying to compensate.

When Ed came along, he and I, to my utter delight, started to hang out with other couples. Like Eric and Mary and Alan and Stacie. Both friendships came through Ed. Indeed, the genesis of both was the same. Eric Davison and Alan Pando both worked, as did Ed, at DDB/New York and then again at Della Femina in Los Angeles. We felt equally fond of both couples. But Eric and Mary knew about cancer. And Alan and Stacie did not.

Eric and Mary had a contemporary split-level house in Manhattan Beach, with a corner of an ocean view and two-story walls that held the art they had collected when Eric was working at McCann/Erickson in Paris and the art they had collected when he was working at McCann/Erickson in Mexico City. Their children were grown and gone, like ours. But unlike us, they'd been married almost thirty-five years and their rhythms were very in tune. Mary would make an almost imperceptible nod to Eric, who would disappear into the kitchen to put the fish onto the broiler.

"Why don't you do that?" I'd say to Ed afterward in the inevitable comparison people indulge in so they can make themselves miserable.

"Do what?" Ed would say.

"Broil the fish when I nod."

"For Chrissakes, Jean."

Me and Ed in the kitchen was no symphony. Spilling things. In each other's way. Criticizing. Ed had this particularly endearing habit of using nine pans when one would do.

Eric and Ed shared a lot of things. Cars. Being married to women they were crazy about. Antipathy toward Della Femina. Good champagne. The advertising business. The car wash. Restoring Eric's MG. They had lunch every other week or so and Ed told Eric about cancer from the start. So having dinner with them was a relief, because we could talk about it.

We'd talk about Ed's progress, about Leucovoran, Heparin locks, colostomies, the City of Hope. Eric and Mary were tentative at first, but as the months wore on, cancer became another subject, like restoring Eric's MG was another subject.

At least, it did on the surface. We'd talk about cancer with seeming ease, but underneath there was an ache. Like on this particular evening.

Ed must have gotten up fifteen times to use their bathroom, because Leucovoran was causing galloping diarrhea. As the trips out of the room continued, I saw concern begin to flash through Eric's eyes. Ed saw it too. When he came back into the room for the sixteenth time, he cracked a joke.

"I guess I'm just a party pooper," he said.

We all laughed like hell. And relaxed again to mingle talk of Dr. Porsche with talk of Dr. Ewen.

And that's the way it was at Eric and Mary's. We talked about cancer. And it was a relief.

Alan and Stacie didn't know about cancer.

We went to their condo near Sunset and Doheny two days later. If a journalist were to do a profile on contemporary life, Alan and Stacie would be described as a power couple. He was head of DDB/Needham in the Western United States. She had her own company, On the Scene Productions, a kind of video PR firm. But if you knew them well, you knew they were a mess, just like the rest of us. Alan was born in someplace like Iowa, but he grew up in Argentina and had the heart and soul of a Latin. He talked too much. Drank too much. Loved too much. Overdid practically everything in the most endearing of ways.

Stacie still hadn't gotten over her own success and liked to talk about how she could always be a hairdresser again, if On the Scene went off the scene. Theirs was a second marriage. A second for Alan, actually, who had grown children when he met Stacie, and a first for her. Socially, Stacie was Alan's Greek chorus.

"Alan is cooking tonight, if he ever gets it together."

"Stacie, don't say I'm not getting it together. Your job is the salad. One lousy salad, Stacie."

"You haven't even started the coals yet. The salad would wilt."

"Ed, would you remind Stacie that the refrigerator has been invented and that she could put the salad in there."

"He's just covering for himself. He can't even find his recipe."

"Why aren't we like that?" I'd say to Ed on the way home.

"Like what?"

"So much fun."

"For Chrissakes, Jean."

On this particular evening, Ed still had diarrhea and was using Alan and Stacie's john every fifteen minutes. But instead of concern, there was bantering, bordering as it usually did between Alan and Ed on ridicule.

"What's the matter with you, Ed? Are you going in there to use drugs or what?"

"I'm going in there because I'm fascinated by the condoms in your medicine chest. They're so small."

And that's the way it was at Alan and Stacie's. We didn't talk about cancer. And it was a relief.

July 20

A WOMAN PHONED ED AT HOME and identified herself as Maggie from Lifeline Homecare.

"Who?" asked Ed.

"Lifeline Homecare. Didn't Dr. Moore tell you I'd be phoning?"

"No."

"Oh, ... that's funny, ... well, ... I'd like to come by to familiarize you with the equipment for your home infusion."

"My what?"

"Your home infusion."

And that's how Ed learned Dr. Moore had put into place the method for getting chemotherapy at home. I don't know why the doctor let us wonder for weeks about home infusion instead of just explaining it. It's done all the time and needn't have been a mystery until Maggie phoned, or a surprise when she did. But we weren't in the mood to complain about Dr. Moore's methods. We were too delighted Ed didn't have to go back to the hospital.

Maggie came out to Malibu at five-thirty in the afternoon so I could be there and learn the system too. She was an off-beat sort of person. Her nurse's uniforms looked like tennis outfits one day and dance-class garb the next. But she was very accommodating and a consummate professional. She could get a vein on the first try without missing a blow in the recounting of her latest Saturday-night fiasco with some typically self-centered LA male.

Nursing organizations like Lifeline Homecare and nurses like Maggie make it possible for people who need all different kinds of medical attention to have it at home. Maggie told us about a patient of hers—a woman in her thirties—who had bone cancer, which is very painful. The woman had four children under the age of ten, the youngest three-year-old twins. Maggie brought her 70 milligrams of morphine a day, and they planned it so that part of the time she'd be weaned off the drug, in order to have quality time with her children.

Another patient was a pregnant woman who couldn't hold down food. She was fed intravenously every day under the supervision of Lifeline. But most of Maggie's patients had cancer and were getting morphine, chemotherapy, or both.

Maggie showed us the equipment and demonstrated how it worked. The centerpiece was a computer-run pump in a canvas case, about the size of a paperback book. The bags of chemical—like Leucovoran—were also housed in the case, with the pump on one side and a bag on the other. When the case zipped shut, it looked like a Sony Walkman. It was meant to be worn on the body, on a belt around the waist. Or, if you preferred, in a sort of shoulder holster, like a private eye might wear. A spaghetti-thin line with an intravenous needle at the end went from the case, around the neck, and down the arm, where the needle went into the Heparin lock, which shunted into the vein. The pump ran on batteries and sent the Leucovoran from the bag, down the line, to the lock, and into the vein—twenty-four hours a day.

Maggie showed Ed how to charge and change the batteries, how to set the computer on the pump to infuse at the proper rate, how to sterilize the needle and insert it into the Heparin lock, and how to start fresh bags of juice. If the lines got clogged or twisted, if the batteries got low, if the juice was running out—if any problem occurred—the computer would beep a warning. The system left a patient completely mobile. You could drive. Walk around. Go out.

"It all depends on how confident you are," Maggie said, and then she winked at Ed. "You look pretty sure of yourself to me." I thought she wiggled her miniskirted behind a little too much as she sashayed across the room. "Of course, if you're throwing up from chemo, it's a different thing all together."

Maggie went to work finding a vein, so she could put in the Heparin lock. I noticed her fingernails had flowers painted on them. She caught me staring.

"People look at my hands so much I thought I'd do something different. Whadaya think, Ed? You like the daisies?" She got her vein in about two seconds, then told us she'd be coming once a day for the next five days to give the shot of 5FU and bring fresh bags of Leocovoran.

"It doesn't keep very long," she said as if she was talking about a dozen eggs. "Put it in the fridge."

She left us with a toss of her mini and a boxful of supplies—alcohol-treated pads, surgical tape, intravenous needles, cotton balls, the pump, batteries, and a self-sealing container for disposal. I felt like I'd just been handed plastic explosives and an alarm clock by a terrorist organization, then told to build a bomb and go take out a bridge.

"This is complicated, Ed. It makes me nervous."

"I know. We'll get used to it. It's just a matter of familiarity." There was absolute determination in his voice. He didn't want to go back to the hospital for his infusion.

"We can make this work, Jean. I know we can."

July 21

HOME INFUSION STARTED, BUT THERE were problems. The Heparin lock infiltrated the vein without Ed realizing it and Leucovoran got pumped directly into tissue. He finally discovered it when his arm started to swell. He phoned Lifeline; they told him to stop the pump and were there in an hour to redo the Heparin lock. Later on during the day, the pump malfunctioned. He phoned Lifeline again, and after running down a checklist of possible problems over the phone, they decided to bring out a new pump and were there again within an hour.

Lifeline was like that. You called them and they were there. They were ready to come all the way out to Malibu at the drop of an intravenous needle, which gave Ed some feeling of security. Nevertheless, he was very stressed and phoned me at the office. It was hard to be home alone, with a potent chemical dripping into your veins.

"I feel like a time bomb," he said, "sitting here waiting for something else to go wrong."

"Would you like me to come home?"

"That would be great, Jean. I'd love you for that."

"Going to the beach, Jean?" someone called after me on my way out.

It was often that way. People would make a teasing remark at a time when teasing didn't feel good. But, how could they know?

Ed and I spent the afternoon and evening together, watching TV, staring at the pump, eating dinner, staring at the pump, looking at each other, checking the lines, checking the lock, figuring out how to sleep with it. It was a little like having a new baby in the house. Except you love a baby.

July 22

HOME INFUSION CONTINUED.
And it continued to be nerve-racking. Ed accidentally removed the batteries from the pump and caused its computers to lose the program. He called Lifeline and, working with them over the phone, he reprogrammed it.

"We all want to meet you, Mr. McNeilly," one of the nurses said. "Nobody's ever been able to do that over the phone before."

Ed beamed. He was determined to get comfortable with the equipment. But equipment wasn't the only thing he had to deal with. The side effects were starting. Horrendous diarrhea once again. And he wouldn't leave the house.

July 23

THE PUMP'S COMPUTER STARTED BEEPING
in the middle of the night. I woke up first.

"Ed, there's something wrong."

We worked together, the two of us, for about fifteen minutes, but we couldn't find the problem and the computer just kept beeping. The only thing we knew for sure was something was wrong. It was very scary. Finally, we phoned Lifeline even though it was three A.M. In thirty minutes or so, a nurse named Karen was at the front door and she found the problem. There were air bubbles in the line, which automatically shuts the system down, lest air bubbles get into a vein. Karen bled the lines, amidst sighs of relief. But between the loss of sleep and the emotional stress, I was exhausted by home infusion. Ed, however, was not.

"I'm going to get on top of this, Jean."

July 24

BEFORE I LEFT FOR WORK,
Ed asked me to help him rig a windbreaker so he could more easily carry the pump around without it showing. I enlarged a pocket in the

jacket, making a deep cocoon so the pump wouldn't fall out. Then, when Maggie came in the afternoon, Ed asked her to teach him how to bleed air from the lines himself.

July 25

IT WAS SATURDAY. ED HAD HIS JACKET. He didn't have diarrhea. He had a week's experience with the pump. And he had me. So he thought he could leave the house. We went, of course, to the Hughes Market and ran into Nancy Beck, the real-estate agent who had sold us our home. We started talking with the easy camaraderie shared by people who live in Malibu. Something is always going wrong, and we all stand around at the Hughes Market and talk about it. Rocks slide onto the Coast Highway and they close it down. The wind blows and the electricity goes out. Septic tanks overflow. The cable-TV company loses power about once a month. A high surf rolls in and batters a house or two. We chatted with Nancy, leaning against our shopping carts, about the current hot topic: sewers.

"If sewers come, a Sheraton won't be far behind," said Ed.

"It's the County Board of Supervisors that's the problem," said Nancy. "Too many of them are pro-development."

"They've got the construction industry in their pocket," Ed agreed knowingly. As we left the market, Ed skipped a little and took my hand.

"She didn't notice a thing," he said.

"Except your tan," I said.

Close to midnight, the last bag of juice emptied. Ed turned off the pump, disconnected the lines, took the needle out of the Heparin lock, and removed the lock from his arm.

"It's going to be okay, Jean. I can handle it."

There isn't anything this man can't handle, I thought to myself.

July 30

THINGS WERE MOVING FORWARD on the purchase of the car wash. Ed ran a daylong meeting with attorneys, accountants, the car-wash owners, and the broker. The escrow was supposed to close, but they still weren't able to sort through the leases. The closing was moved to August 10.

The car wash was going to happen. That was abundantly clear. And there wasn't going to be a partner. Bob or anyone else. It didn't make any sense to commit in the name of Ed's self-assertiveness and then create a situation that undermined Ed's self-assertiveness. So, we were going it alone. It was sort of like the decision I'd made more than once in my life to have sex under less-than-ideal conditions, and without benefit of birth-control measures. You know you shouldn't. You know it's a stupid risk. But sometimes you do it anyway.

And that is surely the first and last time in the history of humankind a car wash has been or ever will be compared to sex.

July 31

ED WOKE UP WITH A TERRIBLE PAIN in his mouth. His teeth and gums were aching. He could feel eruptions starting all over the inside of his cheeks.

"It's Leucovoran hitting," he said.

The drugs used in chemo go after the bad cells in the body. In the process, they can also attack good cells. The mouth is a prime target, because it's full of bacteria and the drug doesn't know the difference between good bacteria and bad.

Ed phoned Dr. Moore's office and spoke with Louise, the head nurse. She told him to rinse with hydrogen peroxide. It didn't help. He phoned again, but this time it was several hours before Louise called back. She talked to the doctor and he ordered a prescription. But by the time the pharmacy got the prescription and we picked it up, it was five in the afternoon and Ed had spent the entire day in unbelievable pain. His mouth was so sensitive, it hurt when he talked. Drinking water hurt. He walked around all day with his mouth open lest his teeth nick against each other to cause excruciating pain. The prescription didn't take the pain away completely, but it helped.

"Why didn't Louise send the prescription in the first place?" I asked Ed.

"I don't know."

"Did you tell her how much pain you were in?"

"Yes."

"Maybe the doctor wasn't there and she couldn't order it."

"He was there. She put me on hold while she talked with him."

"I don't get it. If they had something that helps, why did they wait?"

"I don't know, Jean."

"Well, I know," I said, venting my opinion. "She didn't really listen to you. They have a routine with this problem. And they follow the routine regardless."

"Maybe that's it, Jean, I don't know."

"They start with peroxide and if that doesn't work, then the prescription. It's the same thing every time. They treat the problem, not the person."

"Don't be angry, Jean. I need you to watch a movie with me and hold my hand and smile at me."

"Okay, Ed. I won't be angry."

But I got a knot in my stomach and struggled to push down the growing antagonism I was feeling toward Dr. Moore and the people in his office. The same disturbing situations were beginning to repeat, as with Kevin years earlier. I'd hoped things would be different. They weren't.

August 1

SUG CAME HOME. One of the most important things that ever happened to me in the half-century I'd been alive was that Sug came home. Shortly after I told her Ed had cancer, she phoned me one evening and said she'd quit law school and move back to Malibu to help.

"Law school isn't nearly as important to me, Mama, as you and Ed. I'll come home if you need me."

I didn't need her right then. Ed was fine. And I didn't want her to quit. It was her final year. But all these months, I'd harbored the hope in the back of my mind that she could come if things started to turn.

And now she was coming. We never discussed it. I never had to ask. But she knew and she was coming. She was that kind of person.

The favored memories I have filed in the cabinet of my mind labeled "Sug" have to do with nurturing. At two, she was putting dollies to bed in the tea-towel drawer. At three, she was holding Maureen and giving her a bottle. At five, she informed her kindergarten teacher on the first day of school that Chris was shy and should be handled gently. "Don't yell at my brother," she told Miss Feldman. When she was about ten, she baked, all by herself, a heart-shaped cake for my birthday, which began a habit of baking for people. Perhaps one million cookies have been baked since by Sug, for friends, schoolmates, boyfriends, and relatives, largely to note the kind of events that otherwise tend to go unnoted. And, Lord be praised, by the time she was twelve, she was packing everyone's lunch in my stead and more or less cooking the evening meal. When we moved to Benecia, she sat me down for a talk.

"Do we have to have babysitters anymore, Mama?"

"Don't you like Deva?" Every fall, we got a UCLA student to help at home. Deva, who wore a ring in her nose and chanted even though she was from Nebraska, not India, was this year's helper.

"I like her. She's nice. But Mama, I need to tell you something. I'm smarter than she is. I mean, she asks us to do dumb things. And I can cook better, too."

So we never had babysitters after we moved. The children and I divided up the chores. Everybody took his or her turn on the wash, vacuuming, cooking, and doing the dishes. We had a housekeeper—Rosa, who preceded Alicia—who came once a week. But with four kids, housekeeping is a daily event. And Sug, being the oldest, took the lead.

But behind the domesticity and the caring nature, a bright and very focused young woman was also developing. Sug won a city-wide speech contest when she was in the seventh grade beating out three other contestants, all of whom were high-school seniors, because of her greater poise. She started college at UC San Diego but applied for the Study Abroad program and spent her junior year, off on her own, in Birmingham, England. By the time she came home, Ed was spending a lot of time with us in the house on Benecia, and they fell for each other like a ton of bricks.

"I want a man just like Ed, Mama," she told me once.

"I've never met a person as easy to love as Sug," he told me once.

She finished up her last year of college at UCLA and became part of life for me and Ed. She got an apartment of her own, but she came over every weekend. Did her laundry. Suntanned. Stayed for dinner. Then she was off again to law school. Even then, she came down to see us every few weeks and lived with us the summer between her first and second years.

When she called to tell me she was moving home again, I asked about Jim. He was her boyfriend. We all called him "The Fireman," because he worked for the San Francisco Fire Department while he put himself through law school. He and Sug had been seeing each other, off and on, since their first year at Hastings.

"There's no commitment between him and me," she said. "He didn't give me a reason to stay in San Francisco, and there's plenty of reason to come home."

"I don't want to change your life, Sug, or have you take it in a direction you never intended."

"My family's in Los Angeles, Mama, and I think that's where I belong right now."

Her plan was to take a couple of months off. "Just hang around." And then get a job as an associate attorney. Or maybe she'd wait to see if she passed the Bar. She wouldn't know about that until after Thanksgiving.

But she was really coming home to share with me and Ed whatever the future held. One of the first things I asked her to do was take Aunt Maureen to dinner and tell her about Ed.

🐦 *Aunt Maureen was Kevin's younger sister, the ninth of the ten children in the Kennedyesque Craig clan. Like her four older sisters, Maureen went to college at St. Mary's in Leavenworth, Kansas. But unlike her four older sisters, she entered the convent there in her sophomore year to become a nun—a Sister of Charity of Leavenworth. They were a large community when she joined them, about 1,000 strong, running hospitals, schools, and senior citizen's homes all over the Midwest and doing missionary work in South America.*

I didn't meet Maureen until 1969, a dozen years after I got involved with her brother and nine years after I married him. Convent life was very restrictive in the '50s and early '60s, almost cloistered. Nuns wore long black habits with starched linen headpieces that dated back to medieval times. They were kept away from the world, except for their work. Maureen wasn't allowed to visit her family, so I never met her.

Then, in the late '60s, the winds of change swept through all our traditional institutions, including Catholic convents. The Sisters of Charity of Leavenworth stopped wearing their black serge habits and began wearing whatever they liked and could afford. They dropped their convent names—Sister Assumpta, Sister Immaculata, Sister Stephen—and went back to the names their parents gave them at birth. They were suddenly free to travel, see their families, take vacations, exist in the modern world.

One of the first things Sister Maureen Craig did was come to California to see Kevin and to meet me and the children. I'll never forget her arrival in our living room, as she shattered all of the children's preconceived notions about nuns.

"I bet you've always wondered if nuns wear underwear," she said to her wide-eyed nephew and nieces. "Well, we do."

Aunt Maureen was a nun, with all the traditional values that implies. She was also irreverent, witty, and very bright. When we first met her, she was teaching developmentally disabled teenagers at an inner-city high school in Kansas City.

She came to California in 1969 to be with me when Kevin had surgery. His "good" carotid artery—the one they thought would last only six months after his first operation in 1964—had now indeed gone south and was about to close off completely. He checked into the UCLA Medical Center, where they took a vein from his leg and used it to replace the clogged artery. This operation, unlike the one in 1964 that is still clouded with doubt in my mind, was a success. Indeed, it gave Kevin a new lease on life.

But a few months later, his brother Frank died. Frank was the youngest of the ten, two years behind Maureen and seven years younger than Kevin. He dropped dead on the golf course at age thirty-two of a heart attack.

Suddenly, Kevin's brothers and sisters gasped and took a look at themselves. Kevin had atherosclerosis. Frank died of a heart attack at thirty-two. John had died of a congenital heart defect at seventeen. Ricky had developed a blood clot on his brain after an accident and died from it six months later. Kevin's mother had died at age fifty-one, of a heart attack.

The brothers and sisters and their children began a parade to their family doctors, and it became clear that the family was riddled with coronary artery disease and related heart problems. Kevin's sisters—Therese, Rosaleen, Pan, Brenda, and Maureen—all had elevated cholesterol counts and evidence of the disease. Among them, they had twenty-four children and about half of them also had cholesterol counts in the 400s through 600s. Of the five brothers, only Kevin and Bill were still alive. Bill was okay, but two of his four children had the problem.

And that's the way it was in our family. Chris and Maureen had no evidence of familial hypocholesteremia. Erin and Sug did. At ages three and five we found cholesterol counts for Erin in the low 400s and for Sug in the high 400s. They became patients at the Pediatric Coronary Care Unit at UCLA. The entire family went on a low-fat diet. We learned to drink nonfat milk and simply eliminated things like red meat, fried foods, eggs, and butter from our menu. We still eat that way and have all become amateur dieticians. We know which cooking oils are really the lowest in polyunsaturates, how to bake a low-fat cake, and what to order off a coffee-shop menu.

Erin and Sug were taught the value of exercise in lowering cholesterol. Sug became a runner and Erin a swimmer. Dr. Fogelman told them it would add ten years to their lives if they never smoked, and of course they haven't.

They were teenagers, past puberty, when they started taking a cholesterol-reducing drug called Questran. It's a substance that looks sort of like cornstarch. It comes in coffee-sized cans, and you put a scoop in water and drink it down before every meal. It lines the walls of the stomach and stops the absorption of fat into the blood. Questran worked real well for Erin and less well for Sug, although it helped her too.

She also had more problems with it than Erin. "It's like drinking a cup full of sand," she told me. "It makes me gag." It can also cause severe constipation. But we developed a sense of humor about all those things. "I'm the only person at Uni High," said Sug, "with a box of dried prunes in her locker."

With diet, exercise, and Questran, Erin and Sug's counts were brought down considerably—to the low 200s for Erin and the mid-200s for Sug.

Some years ago, on The Today Show, I watched a family with the same problem being interviewed. They talked about the stress within a family when children are afflicted with disease. They talked about fear and depression. They talked about diets, deprived childhoods, and having to go to the doctor all the time. I was dismayed by their attitude.

Children rise to the level of your expectations. If you tell them they're deprived, that's the way they feel. In our family, we downplayed it. We tried to put familial hypocholesteremia in a league with, for example, wearing glasses. We didn't want anybody to feel deprived. We didn't want anybody to find his or her identity in illness. Drinking Questran in our home was as matter-of-fact as taking aspirin. When we had guests in for dinner, we never bothered to mention they were eating a low-fat menu.

Aunt Maureen was the closest link we had to Kevin's family. She knew, of course, all about him, his illness, and his quirks. She became an outlet for me and a good friend.

When Kevin died in 1977, Aunt Maureen made an effort to stay close to us. She had summers free from teaching and spent most of the summer with us in 1978 and again in 1979. Then Ed came into my life and that changed. "Who is she?" he'd ask. "She's your aunt?"

"No. She's the children's aunt. She's a nun."

"Jean, your kids in the house are one thing. But a nun . . . ."

So, she didn't come to California for the summer. Then, she got transferred to St. John's Hospital in Santa Monica. Her Order owned and *operated the hospital and Maureen was going to be stationed there for three years. Maybe more. So she started coming out to Malibu for Sunday dinner from time to time and for holidays. Ed didn't know what to make of her at first. But when she asked for gin in her tonic, talked about her experiences with drug-addicted teenagers, and pontificated with savoir faire equal to his own on the inadequacies of the Reagan administration, she won him over.*

"I never thought I'd know a nun," he told me once. "Much less like one."

"It's because she's second to nun," I said. But he didn't get it. I guess it's a Catholic joke.

Sug told Aunt Maureen about Ed and she began to share his illness with me, as she had her brother's. ❧

August 6

ED WENT TO SEE DR. MOORE, who finally had X-rays—the first taken since the Leucovoran protocol started. The X-rays made it clear. Leucovoran was working.

Ed was thundering in approbation, as exalted as if he'd just won an Olympic marathon. Which he had, in a sense. The doctor, on the other hand, made clinical comments tinged with mild surprise.

"There's no new growth," he said. "There's even some evidence of shrinkage and a bad spot in the kidneys is now looking good."

"How long do you think I can tolerate the chemo?" Ed asked.

"Leucovoran side effects are not necessarily cumulative. You may be able to tolerate it for quite some time."

"Jean," Ed was roaring over the phone. "Jean, the next treatment, I'm going to go to work wearing the pump. This is great, Jean. Let's drive up to Santa Barbara tomorrow and pick up the engine. I want to do things."

Ed had run across a garage in Santa Barbara that took the cranky engines out of the sexy bodies of Jaguar V-12s and replaced them with good old American engines out of Chevys. The garage had no use for the Jag engines it removed and just . . . well . . . threw them away. Ed had arranged to get one to make into a desk for the car wash.

It seemed to me that the transition from engine to desk required a certain leap in logic, if not design and engineering skill. But Ed had it all planned out on the drafting table in his mind.

So, here we were in August, just a year after we'd been told it was all over, about to drive up to Santa Barbara in a rented truck to pick up an engine to make into a desk to put in a car wash we were about to own.

Stick it in your ear, Dr. Bornstein.

August 10

THE ESCROW CLOSED on the car wash. We owned it. Holy shit, we owned it.

Robertson Car Wash. 2410 Robertson Boulevard, just east of Beverly Hills, on Robertson Boulevard, of course, not too far from the on-ramp to the Santa Monica Freeway. When Ed filed with the state to classify it as a Sub Chapter S Corporation, he made the official name Robertson Soap Opera Co.

About thirty people worked there. A general manager, a manager, two cashiers, a bookkeeper, a detail guy, and twenty-five more who washed the cars. Almost all the staff was Hispanic. The business was open seven days a week, with a weekly payroll nudging up against 7,000 dollars. My mouth flew open when Ed told me that, as my mouth flew open with practically everything I learned about the car wash.

The first thing that happened was that the manager, Domingo Chavez, took off for Mexico to attend a funeral. The second thing that happened was that the head cashier, Aurora Blanco, took off for Argentina on vacation. The third thing that happened was that the conveyer belt broke down.

"Ed," I panicked, "what're we going to do?"

"This is great, Jean," he bellowed, oblivious to my terror, "I've never had so much fun."

He began leaving the house every morning at seven-thirty. He was hiring cashiers, bringing in sign people, drawing up plans for a face-lift, redesigning his office, figuring out where to put his engine-desk, and reorganizing the way cars piled up on the apron.

"If I can put together a string of days like this one," he told me after the first full day of operation, "I can do anything."

The moment he said that, I never again regretted going ahead with it. But to my utter surprise, indeed, shock, I found the business to be a kick. I liked the people. I liked the immediacy of it. And talk about hands-on. The day's receipts came home every night in a brown paper bag on which Ed scrawled the day's date with a magic marker.

"Yeah. I thought about putting the money in like...a briefcase. But then I thought...why? This isn't the advertising business. I don't have to impress anyone."

It's hard to imagine two businesses as different from each other, yet as reflective of life in southern California as the two we found ourselves in: advertising and washing cars.

Advertising sits on the fringe of the entertainment business. Copywriters and art directors, educated at places like the Art Center College of Design in Pasadena, dream up commercials that become mini-films. There are producers, art directors, cinematographers. You rub elbows with people who wear Giorgio Armani suits and eat lunch at trendy places like Citrus.

What you're selling is the American dream. Better automobiles, the latest in fast food, the hot new components in home stereo systems. What you're trying to capture with your work is contemporary life, as the people with disposable incomes attempt to dispose of it.

At the other end of the spectrum sits the car-wash business, with its immigrant work force, washing the cars that symbolize the best of contemporary life. Most of the people who wash cars don't own one. They're part of the population flooding into southern California from Mexico, El Salvador, Nicaragua, and Costa Rica. Most of them don't speak English. Most of them are raising families on four dollars and twenty-five cents an hour, plus tips.

The first amazing discovery Ed and I made during our first weeks at Robertson Car Wash was our manager, Domingo Chavez. Actually, his name wasn't Domingo, it was Simon (pronounced See-moan), which I discovered one day when he asked me to write a letter for him to immigration.

"Domingo," I asked, "why does it say here that your name is Simon?"

"Because that is my name," he said.

"Then why did you tell us your name was Domingo?"

"Because that's what everyone calls me."

"Well, why do they call you that?"

"Sometimes they call me Paez."

"Now wait a minute, what's really your name?" I was getting frustrated. The Mexican route to logic is circuitous.

"Simon."

"Is that what you'd prefer to be called?"

"Of course, Señora, it is my name."

"Then why did you tell us your name was Domingo?" I said, realizing full well I was starting over.

"It is my uncle's name and I used it when I first came here."

Simon was around thirty years old. He'd lived in the United States since he was seventeen, working all the time at car washes. He supported an extended family—parents, wife, and children—who lived in a village near Guadalajara. He spoke English well, but he couldn't read or write it very well, although he tried to make it appear he could. He was a very proud young man.

There is a stereotype of Mexicans we all pick up somewhere, somehow. The word that comes to mind is *indolent*. I soon discovered Simon was a Mexican Sammy Glick.

"Simon," I said to him one day, "why are you here all the time? You're here on your day off. You're here at seven in the morning. You're here at six at night. You're here all the time."

He looked at me with that look people get when they've just discovered they're wiser than you are.

"But this is what I do," he said. "This is my work."

I watched Simon a lot those first days. He was a skillful manager of people.

"Some guys don't like to work in front, because they're afraid to try English, so they work on the line, but then they don't get tips. So I pay them more and give them more overtime, but I don't make friends with them because then the guys in front get pissed. The guys in front got to feel they're special, you know?"

"I know," I said, thinking of some art directors I'd worked with. They don't really like to go to the client, but they get pissed if you don't ask them.

Simon was a mechanical wizard. One day the air conditioning broke down (everything seemed to break down the first week), and Ed was going crazy because chemo was making him sweat. It was going to be hours before the electrician could come over and fix it, so Simon crawled up on the roof and fixed it himself. It was a five-ton system, installed in the 1960s, that chugged all day like an old Bendix washing machine.

"Have you ever fixed the air conditioning before?" I asked him.

"No," he said.

"How did you know how?"

"You must think like a Mexican," he smiled. "In Mexico nothing is new and nothing ever works, but you figure it out and make it work anyway."

Ed and I also watched him take abuse because he was Mexican.

One day, a customer got angry claiming we had knocked a piece of chrome off her Cadillac. She wanted us to pay to have her car repaired. But Simon was confident we hadn't done the damage.

"I have been in car washes since I was seventeen years old," he told Ed. "I know what damage we do and what we don't. What happens is people look at the cars for the first time in a week, and they see something wrong and they think we did it when we didn't. Besides," he shrugged his shoulders, "the chrome isn't here. If we had knocked it off, it would be here."

But the lady wouldn't accept his explanation and only got angrier. She got really stupidly angry. And left. But she came back in about fifteen minutes with a policeman. Or I should say, in this instance, a cop. The cop walked straight up to Simon and started yelling at him.

"Listen here, you Domingus or Domingi or whatever the hell your name is, you pay this lady what you owe her. And you better do it right now, Señor, or you're going to be up to your ass in green-card problems."

Ed and I, sitting in the tiny inside office, couldn't believe what we were hearing. But when Ed went out and identified himself to the cop, everything changed. Ed was white. American. No accent.

The cop suddenly became polite, calm, and reasonable. And so did the woman. They accepted Ed's explanation, which was no different from Simon's. And left.

"I don't worry about it, Señora," Simon said to me later. "It's no problem. It's life, that's all."

"Simon and I are going to be good partners," Ed told me. "I trust him. And if I can have just six months, Jean, I can make this a great business. It will be your legacy, Jean."

I kept recalling an old movie, starring somebody like Barbara Stanwyck as a toughened woman in the Old West who took over the ranch when her husband got sick and found herself boss over all the cowboys and Mexican vaqueros.

I thought of that movie every time Simon called me "Señora."

August 21

WE NERVOUSLY LEFT THE CAR WASH over the weekend with Simon, who was quite calm, got into the Porsche, and headed up the coast on Highway 101, toward Monterey.

We were going to the world-famous Vintage Car Races at the Laguna Seca Raceway, which happen every year on a Saturday in late August and are followed on Sunday by the internationally renowned Concours d'Elegance on the grounds of the Del Monte Lodge at Pebble Beach in Carmel.

The event in Carmel is the premiere classic-car event in the United States and brings together collectors from all over the world. One year, we saw Wolfgang Porsche, son of Ferdinand. Another year, the Ferrari family. Otis Chandler, the publisher of the *Los Angeles Times* and a well-known collector, never misses the event. Incredibly beautiful automobiles from the '20s, '30s, and '40s are parked in neat million-dollar rows on the grounds of the hotel, and the setting itself is stunning.

In the background, the Pacific Ocean roars into Monterey Bay, with its barking seals, it otters, and its shoreline fringed with gnarly cypress. The casual chic of the hotel, with its lawn sweeping down to the sea, is in the foreground. They put up green-and-white striped tents where you can buy champagne, cappucino, croissants, and fresh-squeezed orange juice. The rich and the cogniscenti spread quilts on the lawn and unpack their picnic lunches of paté, cold lobster, and fresh raspberries. And the men in their white linen suits with ladies on their arms in something oh-so-casual from Rive Gauche stroll among the cars.

There are Mercedes Touring Cars, American Roadsters, and Pierce-Arrows that predate 1915. There are Cadillac Dual Cowl Phaetons and Bugatti and Aston Martin racing cars from the '20s. There are the Dusenbergs, Bugatti Royales, Cords, Packards, Buick Brewster Town Cars, Delahayes, Talbot-Lagos, Auburn Speedsters, and Rolls Royce Phantoms from the elegant 1930s. There are post-World War II European sports and racing cars—the Ferrari GTO, the Lagonda, Alfa Romeos, Porsches, the Triumphs, Scarabs, Aston-Martins, and Hispano-Suizas. There are cars that make you gasp because they're so elegant. There are cars that make you tingle because they're so sexy.

Before we got into the Porsche, Ed put the top down. I noticed he had on his driving cap with the Cobra insignia as well as his belt with the Allard buckle.

"How are you feeling?" I asked.

"Fine," he said.

Another round of chemo was to start as soon as we got back. I wished he hadn't put the top down. I was worried about him catching cold and complicating things in his lungs. I was also worried about the dust at the racetrack, the chilly ocean air, and Ed being on his feet all day Saturday. I wished he would think once in a while about conserving his strength.

"Would you like me to drive?" I asked cheerily, thinking I was being subtle.

"Jean," he said my name with a great deal of tenderness, "I'm not an invalid yet. And you know how much I love to drive this car."

What he meant was, why didn't I knock off the worry-wart stuff so we could have a good time.

I obliged by turning up the car radio, and off we went with the top down and my hair blowing in the wind. A Beatles song from the '60s was playing on the Blaupunkt. "Let it be, let it be, let it be, let it be, whispering words of wisdom. Let it be."

At the races the next day, Ed ran into an old business associate from the days on Volkswagen in New York. The man was now the publisher of an automotive magazine. He was cool to Ed and didn't acknowledge me, turning to avoid my presence and shaking my hand. I knew it was because he was friends with Donna.

"I'm sorry, Jean," Ed said as we walked the other way.

"It's okay," I said, and then remembered how wise Simon had been when faced with a similar situation. "It's life, that's all."

Eric and Mary were at the races too. We sat with them, watched the antique cars roar around the track, and forgot about cancer, as well as social snubs.

August 24

ED MET WITH DR. MOORE, who gave him another good report. He didn't order an X-ray, which made Ed anxious. They were the surest way to tell what was going on and had been routine at the City of Hope. But Dr. Moore did run blood tests, which indicated less cancer activity. Arrangements were made to start another round of chemo. Another round of home infusion. Ed—feeling good, bullish and confident—asked Maggie to come out to Malibu in the evening to give him his shots and supply of fresh juice, so he could work all day at the car wash.

August 25

THE FIRST DAY OF CHEMO. Ed went to work with an intravenous needle in a vein on his left arm, a Heparin lock in the arm, and a line leading from the lock up his arm, around his neck, and into the case in the windbreaker pocket, which housed the juice and the pump. It was only his second round of home infusion, and he hooked himself up in the morning as casually as a person would put on a pair of glasses. I was so proud of him, I thought my Ed-owned heart would burst.

Midway through the day, however, there was penetration—the intravenous needle pushed through the vein. Lifeline came to the car wash to put in a new Heparin lock. Ed told Simon that Maggie was an interviewee for the cashier's job.

"I don't want Simon or the others to know I'm sick, Jean," he told me later. "It would undermine their confidence in me."

I also knew it would scare them. Ed and I had been to a clothing store together to buy him some pants. In the process, the clerk noticed the rig and I saw fright cloud his face. "Is he contagious?" I'm sure the clerk was wondering, "Is it AIDS?"

The pump, the lock, and the problem were too hard to explain. So Ed didn't. Even to Simon.

August 26

THE SECOND DAY OF CHEMO. Bob dropped by the car wash to say hello. Ed showed him the tunnel, the conveyer, the plans he had for the boutique, the office, the signage, the landscaping. He also showed him the windbreaker, the pump, the Heparin lock, the intravenous needle, and the bags of Leucovoran.

"It's the most guts-ball thing I've ever seen," Bob said to me when he got to the office.

That evening, when Maggie came to the house I looked at her records and found out that Lifeline Homecare charged 1,151 dollars for a bag of Leucovoran, about a third of what it cost at the hospital.

"Well,...beats me,...I guess hospitals mark it up," Maggie shrugged.

"I guess they do," I replied.

A five-day infusion through Lifeline cost 12,700 dollars, including nurses, home visits, and supplies. The same thing at the hospital cost 35,105 dollars.

I thought it curious that Dr. Moore never mentioned that in addition to being better for Ed, home infusion would cost 22,000 dollars less each month.

August 27

THE THIRD DAY OF CHEMO.
"Jean," Ed was phoning me from the car wash, "I feel like I've walked into a wall. Can I come over and lie down on your couch?"

"Maybe you should go home, Ed."

"I don't think I could make it. I don't think I could drive that far."

"Stay there, Ed. I'll come get you."

"No. It's okay. I can make it to your office."

He came over and slept for an hour on my couch. I closed the door, locked it, and sat there with him while he slept. Dr. Moore said that the effects of Leucovoran weren't cumulative. Then why was it hitting him so hard this time? I was worried, as I constantly was, that it wasn't just chemo, but cancer spreading again. When Ed woke up, however, he felt refreshed.

"The least you could do is take me to lunch," he said. So we went to my favorite—Harry's Bar.

Then he went back to the car wash.

August 28

THE FOURTH DAY OF CHEMO.
Kresser/Craig held its annual summer picnic on the Malibu beach near our home. Ed dropped in for an hour or so, his pump hidden in his windbreaker, his Heparin lock under his shirt, his chemical dripping into his arm, and laughed and joked and ate barbecued chicken as if he hadn't a care in the world.

Once again, I couldn't believe his poise. His determination. His courage. Ernest Hemingway, in an article in *The New Yorker* in 1929, defined courage—actually, he called it "guts"—as "grace under pressure."

That, indeed, was Ed.

August 29

CHEMO ENDED AND THE FATIGUE
seemed to end with it. The car wash was running okay. Sug, pooped from law school and taking the Bar, was off on a camping trip with a

friend. The house was quiet and the Labor Day weekend was coming up.

"I'm feeling okay, Jean," Ed told me. "I want to do things. I want to go see the kids."

September 4

MATTHEW RAY MCCLURE WAS THREE YEARS OLD. Not yet to the age of reason. But probably to the age of memory. I can remember when I was three. I can remember my mother telling me that peas and carrots make you grow, and then wondering why when I cut myself, I never found any peas and carrots in there.

I can also remember telling my mother one morning I wished the lady down the street was my mother instead of her. When Mama asked me why, I said it was because the lady down the street always had Cokes and we never did. To my toddling mind, that was very important. But my mother didn't really hear what I said about Cokes; she just heard me say I liked someone else better than her, and I saw a look of terrible hurt flash across her face. I didn't know it was hurt at the time, but I knew it was something, and the look etched itself into my brain, and I wonder sometimes to this day if that one childish comment didn't contribute to a distance between my mother and me when I was a very little girl, because there was one.

Another thing I remember is my grandfather. My mother's father. He came to visit when I was barely three, a dark and shadowy figure, stern, upright, righteous. I met him only that one time, as he died a few months later. But my three-year-old brain was bright enough to peg him. When I got old enough to know what "righteous" meant, I saw it sometimes in my mother and knew where it came from.

Ed and I talked a lot about three-year-old Matthew Ray McClure.

"I want him to remember me," Ed would say. "I want to be an influence for the good in his life."

But I had my doubts about how well it was going between Matthew and Ed. Their encounters, up to then, had been on the tentative side. Ed was awkward with Matthew. The little boy bossed his parents a bit, as first children often do with a young couple. But it made Ed uncomfortable, coming from a children-should-be-seen-not-heard generation. That had a negative influence on how he related to the child, which the child was smart enough to pick up on. Something like that was going on.

But so was this incredible urge to imprint. It was the one tangible way I saw Ed deal with his mortality.

"My God, Jean, I'd love to show him things. I'd love to show him the water. Take him fishing. Show him how to snorkel. But he's too young. I can't do the things I do well with him. He's still a baby."

To an eight- or ten-year-old boy, Ed would be a hero-grandfather. If he shared with a boy even the tiniest bit of what he knew about cars, the kid would idolize him.

But that wasn't going to happen with Matthew Ray McClure. You can't show a three-year-old an ad you just saw in Hemmings, or take him with you to Riverside, or show him how the gearshift works on a Porsche. So Ed was troubled as we sat together on Delta Airlines on our way to Orlando to visit Matthew and his parents.

"Help me, Jean. I don't know what to do."

I wished that Robin and Michael had been sitting in the seat with us. I wished they could have heard his voice when he said that. They'd have known how much he cared and how hard he was trying. But it never seemed to work just right.

"Dad doesn't do too well with Matthew," Robin would say after each visit.

"Ed," I lied, trying to give him confidence, "you're better with kids than you think. But you know, you shouldn't try to bounce him on your knee or do things you think grown-ups are supposed to do with kids. You should treat him like a person. Do you know what I mean?"

"I'm not sure."

"Remember when we were in Fiji and you let the little island girl use your camera? You showed her how like she was an adult, not like she was a child. Am I making any sense?"

"Yes," he said amazingly.

That evening when we got to Orlando, Ed let Matthew show him some dinosaurs he played with. And the next day when we drove over to the beach at Daytona, Ed let Matthew teach him how to build a sand castle. The two of them didn't exactly walk hand-in-hand down the beach into the sunset, but there was a moment or two, as the paper cups filled with sand were being turned into turrets, that I noticed the casualness of genuine rapport.

"Grandpa Ed, Grandpa Ed," the three-year-old bossed, "you're not doing it right."

"Yes, I am. We're doing it this way because we need a moat."

"We do?"

"Of course, we do."

Before Ed and I got on the plane to return to Los Angeles, Robin took me aside.

"Dad's doing so much better with Matthew," she said.

I don't know if Matthew will remember Ed any more than I remember my own grandfather, a shadowy figure I can barely dredge up from the near-subconscious of three years old.

But if Matthew Ray McClure ever does anything in his life that's lusty in its feeling and bold in its scope, or if he shows a great deal of grace under pressure, I'll recognize the imprint and know where it came from.

September 8

THE AFTER-SHOCK OF LEUCOVORAN waited to rumble over Ed until we got home from Orlando. But rumble it did. And it was devastating.

There were drenching night sweats. We started waking up to a bed that was soaked and pillows that had to be hung up to dry. The sweats were often followed by chills and terrible diarrhea.

"I wonder if this is what it's like to have dysentery," Ed mused out loud. "I was watching a hostage on the news who was freed by the Iranians, and he said the worst part was dysentery." That's the closest Ed came to complaining.

There were no problems in his mouth this time and no blisters on the nose. Leucovoran seemed to pick different targets each month. But Ed was fatigued and occasionally spacey. He went to the car wash every day but couldn't make it past one or two in the afternoon. He'd come home, almost in a daze, and collapse into bed.

Way, way back in the deep, closed pockets of my mind, I sensed an overall decline. There was a weakening I hadn't seen before. But I didn't acknowledge it. It was safer to ignore it and pretend chemo was the culprit.

It made me understand why people often see trouble coming but fail to respond. Why Jews stayed in Germany in the 1930s. Why parents fail to recognize drug-addicted children. Why husbands and wives ignore the tell-tale signs of a troubled marriage.

To acknowledge trouble, you must admit to fear. And fear is one of the most difficult of human emotions. What's more, if you acknowledge trouble, then you have to act. But most of us don't know what to do. So we don't acknowledge.

At least that's the way it was with me.

September 12

so he and I could spend the day talking about the company.

"Craig," he said, "we need to talk about our people, our accounts, where we're going. We'll do it on your deck. And we'll unplug the phone."

So out he came, wearing his beach attire. Orange nylon running shorts; a T-shirt with a Coors emblem on it, a remnant I suppose, from his days at Berkeley in the '60s; a baseball cap that read "I'm the boss at am/pm mini markets," and 400-dollar running shoes. His legs looked nine feet long in his running shorts, and he propped them on the table on the deck and unzipped his ratty nylon briefcase. He looked a little like Jimmy Stewart might look if he were playing the part of a bum.

But Bob was smiling his wonderful smile and waxing his boyish enthusiasm.

"Look at this, Craig," he said, putting in front of me the year-end projections. We'd been worried all summer. ARCO, our largest client, had cut their billing. Select-TV, another client, went bankrupt and owed us over 100,000 dollars. But we'd made some cuts and dug in on overhead, and it looked like things were going to be okay.

"Let's give some raises," he said with a grin. So we sat there for a couple of hours discussing each and every person on the staff, from Canary the receptionist to Paul the executive vice-president, more like we were parents than the owners of a company.

"John is bright, but he's lazy," Bob would say. "He gets a raise, but I also want to send a message that he needs to get off his ass."

"Mike is an unsung hero," I would say. "He's got a big hit coming." It had become a thing with me to not let squeaky wheels fare better than the quiet people.

As we sat there running the company, Bob's enthusiasm for our work, our partnership, our people, and each other oozed all over the conversation like the soft Malibu sunlight seeping through the leaves of the eucalyptus shading the deck.

"We're going to make it and we're going to make it big," he said. And then, to prompt me into letting him continue his thought, he asked, "Do you know why?"

"Why, Bob?"

"Because we're good people."

It was an ingenuous, endearing comment. He believed that he and I ran a better company than a lot of people in the advertising business.

But he honestly thought our real edge was that we had integrity, we didn't bullshit and we cared.

"The good people prevail over time," he said. "I really believe that." And he proceeded to paint a glowing picture for the future of Kresser/ Craig. But as I listened to the sweet, warm words of this unlikely advertising executive who I loved, I felt an overwhelming sense of irony. All the while the future of Kresser/Craig looked bright as hell, the future of Jean Craig looked as dark as the Malibu sky on a moonless, starless night.

"How can my life be going forward and backward at the same time?" I was asking myself as Bob waxed on. I thought about that for a moment and reached the inevitable conclusion. It wasn't going forward and backward; it was only going backward, despite my wonderful partner and his happy thoughts. There was no real comparison between the importance of my personal life and the importance of my business life. There wasn't then and there never had been. All the business success in the world would never fill a hole left by Ed.

It's easy to despair when you look at the future and see nothing but sadness. I knew I shouldn't look. How did I know what tomorrow would be? It hadn't happened yet. But the English language does have a common, everyday word for fear of the future. *Dread.* Everyone on earth has experienced it. People dread everything from IRS audits, to asking for a raise, to biopsy reports. But dreading doesn't prepare a person for a better outcome. It only prolongs the agony. Sometimes it leads to panic and makes the outcome worse.

What I needed to do was concentrate on now. To keep my thoughts in the present. To keep my mind from drifting to a future I couldn't foretell. "Try not to speculate," the doctors had said so many months before. I tried. But then I'd see Ed putting on the pants he'd bought to work in at the car wash and I wondered if I'd see him wear them out. I did my share of dreading. But something deep inside—an image of my mother, who never faltered, an optimism rooted in my own beliefs and values, the knowledge that Ed needed me, a distaste for self-pity—kept it from turning to panic.

Ed came home from the car wash around noon, as Bob and I were still working on raises. Ordinarily, he would have joined us on the deck to give his opinions, asked for or not. But he barely shouted hello to Bob and went upstairs to go to bed. Bob looked at me warily.

"He's not doing too well, right now," I said.

Bob looked away. There wasn't really anything to say or do.

September 14

ED WASN'T MAKING IT.
He wasn't bouncing back from chemo at all. He couldn't focus at the car wash and began to do worrisome things, like arrive home with credit-card slips, coupons, the daily cash-out sheet, and the cash—hundreds of dollars—shoved in a tangled mess into one of his brown bags.

"I couldn't count it, Jean. I couldn't make the bank deposit. I was just too tired."

I decided I'd better get involved at the car wash. So when Saturday came, Ed stayed in bed while I went over and talked with Simon.

"Ed has some problems with his health, Simon. He won't be able to be here all the time and you're going to be seeing more of me. I'd appreciate it if you'd keep in touch with me, let me know what's happening, and call me if there are any problems."

I don't know what it is about people that allows them to connect. What it is that causes them to see past each other's eyes and into the workings of the mind. There was no reason for there to be sympatico between Simon Chavez and myself. But there was. So many people advised me to be careful with Simon. My brothers. My business friends. Other car-wash owners I'd met. "Don't give him the run of the place. It's too easy for a manager to steal." Or, "You've only known him a month. Put some monitors in the place. Some checks and balances. I'm warning you." Or, "You're crazy to give him access to the cash. He has the combination to the safe?"

But I discounted all of the advice. I'd known Simon long enough to get a sense of his character. I knew he was a good person. I also thought that trust was a two-way commodity. You give it. You get it.

"I knew Ed was sick, Señora. It shows around his eyes. But you don't have to worry. I'll run this business like it's my own."

I believed he would.

When I got home, Ed was distraught.

"I feel so guilty, Jean. I'm not on top of this."

"Don't worry, Ed. It's going to be okay. I have a plan." I'd wondered what I'd do if Ed couldn't run the car wash and it fell on me. Well,... I was going to find out.

The plan was simple enough. Aurora, the grandmotherly cashier, was promoted to office manager. Her job was to bring order out of the chaos in the office. Joh Koppel, the controller at Kresser/Craig and a dear and good friend, spent two Saturdays with Aurora, teaching her how. Aurora, a Cuban refugee who'd come to the States twenty-five years earlier, was a fast study. The rest of the plan involved Chris and Sug. The car wash wasn't their business and Ed wasn't their father, but they were ready to help.

Chris would come by every day after work to do the cash-outs and make the bank deposits. In general, handle the money. In his heart, Chris didn't like the car wash and was reluctant to agree. Yet he did agree, because he loved his mother. Sug would put off looking for a job as an attorney and be the cashier until Aurora found someone; then she'd help out in the office until things got onto an even keel. Simon, of course, would continue to operate the business and get the cars washed. Ed would show up when he could. I'd be there regularly a couple of times a week to keep on top of things.

And that's the unlikely band that started running Robertson Soap Opera Co., dba Robertson Car Wash, with its 7,000-dollar-a-week payroll and its 70,000-dollar-a-month gross. Jean Craig, advertising executive; Chris Craig, hydrology technician with the U.S. Army Corp of Engineers; Deirdre Craig, attorney at law but not yet practicing; Simon Chavez, Mexican immigrant; and Aurora Blanco, grandmotherly cashier, now office manager.

Simon and Aurora were the only ones who knew what they were doing.

September 15

ED WOKE UP YELLING FROM A SHARP, stabbing pain in his lower back. It came and went, but he talked about the "taste" of cancer in his mouth.

Leucovoran was due to start again on the twenty-first. But he obviously hadn't recovered from the last treatment yet.

"Are you sure you want to start chemo again?" I asked.

"I don't want to back off, Jean."

September 19

SUG WALKED INTO THE LIVING ROOM carrying a cake she'd baked. As she put it on the coffee table to the oohs and ahhs of the group we'd gathered, she glanced at Erin.

"You can get married at the car wash," she said. "You can walk down the tunnel like it's the aisle."

Erin and Rich were leaving for the East Coast to go back to school and get their Master's degrees. Hers from MIT. His from Dartmouth. We were having a little party to see them off, and we took the occasion to start planning their wedding.

"Erin, I'm fifty-four years old and I've never been a bridesmaid." It was Aunt Maureen. "I think you ought to give me that chance. I'm your dear Aunt, Erin. I'd look so cute...."

"The car wash is perfect," said Chris. "We wouldn't need a band. We have Musak."

"I don't know," I said. "When Erin gets back from MIT, she'll be a nerd. She won't want a nice wedding."

"Erin," went on Aunt Maureen, "if you let me be a bridesmaid, I'll bring all the other nuns and line them up and when the wedding's over, we'll give you a twenty-one-nun salute."

"Nobody's asked Rich what kind of wedding he wants," said Sug.

"Who's Rich?" said Ed.

"Sug, have you told everybody about the guy in the Mercedes?" I asked, deciding to give Erin mercy.

"What guy?" It was a chorus.

"Well, there's this really attractive guy who comes into the car wash all the time...."

"He drives a white Mercedes," chimed in Ed.

"And he started stopping at the cash register to chat with Sug. Then the other day, he asked her out."

"Are you going?" asked Erin.

"Well, I don't know," said Sug. "He has this funny business card with Roman columns on it. In gold."

"Wouldn't it be funny, Jean," said Ed, "if after UC San Diego, England, UCLA, and law school, Sug finds Mr. Right at the car wash."

"I could wear blue, Erin," said Aunt Maureen. "It's my best color...."

And so in the midst of chemotherapy and a worsening condition, life continued.

September 21

I WENT WITH ED TO KEEP his ten-o'clock appointment with Dr. Moore, determined to find out what was going on. Actually, I had yet to meet the doctor. I was never invited into the examining room when I went with Ed for office visits. And when Ed was in the hospital, the doctor never happened to be making his rounds when I was there. So even though he'd been caring for my husband in a life-and-death situation for four months, I had yet to look upon his face. Or he upon mine.

But this time, I felt I needed to be with Ed, whether the doctor preferred it or not. Ed had a downhill curve going on and I needed to hear what the doctor said. I needed to know what the doctor thought.

The nurse behind the glass partition opened it but didn't really look up as she motioned us to a seat. After twenty or thirty minutes, Louise called Ed to an examining room. When I said I wanted to come too, she simply said, "okay."

Louise was, I thought, the only RN on Dr. Moore's staff. I called the lady behind the glass partition a nurse because she was dressed like one, but she was more likely a receptionist/typist in a white uniform. The other "nurses" were more likely "medical office technicians." It takes about six months' training to become an office technician. You learn to take blood, give shots, take blood pressure, run an EKG—do the routine things.

But Louise was senior to the others. A fortyish woman, her features were attractive and she went to some trouble to find nurse's uniforms that helped lengthen a fulsome look. Her manner was polite but distant, as if she was afraid of real human contact or didn't have the time for it. And while she'd occasionally offer a slight smile or a pleasant word, she had the demeanor of a perpetually beleaguered person.

I asked her once if she had had a nice weekend. She answered, "Yes, my family came to visit, but I never stopped cooking."

She was a "yes . . . but" person. "Yes, something good happened, but believe me, there was bad news too."

I wanted to like Louise and I wanted her to like me. I wanted to make her my friend so in days to come I could turn to her comfortably when I needed her. But it never worked. Louise was careful to keep me at my distance. To keep me from penetrating her professional reserve. I could understand that. People in medicine can't let every single patient into their emotions. But Ed was making such an extraordinary effort, I thought he and I might be one of her exceptions. We all hope to be the exceptions.

Louise was also careful to let me know she was terribly over-worked. Maybe she was. She probably was. The problem was, like many people in medicine, she thought she was the only one in the world who was.

I was surprised when Dr. Moore walked into the examining room. Ed had told me he was young, but I wasn't ready for the unlined features, the youthful eyes, the flush on his cheeks that made him appear callow. I was also surprised by how little he looked like a doctor's supposed to look. His was a face without prominent features—no craggy eyebrows, jutting chin, or broad forehead. No piercing eyes, unruly shock of hair, or bookish beard. None of the features that brings character to the faces of doctors in literature and story. This was not Dr. Schweitzer. This was not Dr. Casey. This was not even Dr. Kildare. He looked more like an MBA, or an accountant.

He got a phone call right after we got settled, and he took it. The examining rooms were so small, phone conversations were shared whether you wanted them to be or not. I felt that made him uncomfortable and his end of the conversation was stiff. Across the small room, I could hear the sound of noisy children coming through the mouthpiece.

"How old are your kids?" I asked cheerily when he hung up.

"They're in elementary school," he said as he picked up Ed's file.

"Where do they go to school?" I pressed on, trying to make a bond.

"How are you feeling, Ed?" he said.

"Where do your kids go to school?" Ed picked up on my question.

He finally answered by naming a school in a very expensive part of Los Angeles County. I couldn't decide if he'd ducked my question because he wanted to keep things impersonal, because he wanted the focus in the room to be between him and Ed, or because he was embarrassed to admit he lived, at his tender age, in such luxurious sweetness.

The meeting with him was disconcerting to me. Throughout the half-hour we spent in the examining room, he never turned toward me as a person might do to let it be known I was included in the conversation. He never even glanced at me. I knew he wanted to make it clear the relationship in the room was between him and Ed. I also thought he was trying to avoid giving me openings—for questions, comments, opinions—because he didn't really want them and because if I started talking, as well as Ed, it would take a lot more of his time. It was a way of working I'd seen in doctors over and over again.

I wondered whom he thought he'd be working with to care for Ed in the months and weeks ahead, if not me. Florence Nightingale? But of course, doctors don't consider themselves working *with* anyone, neither the patients nor the families. They're in charge. They run the show.

But more importantly, the meeting was also disconcerting to Ed. He went down a litany of symptoms and problems that had plagued him since his last visit to the doctor. The chills, the sweats, the diarrhea, the heaviness in the chest, the stabbing pains, the taste of cancer in his mouth, the coughing, the fatigue, the spaciness, the nausea.

Dr. Moore took notes and said nothing. He never said what any of it meant or put it into perspective or made any comment at all. Ed and I were both anxious for an overview of his condition, but the doctor was a master of noncommittal answers. He said things like "That's interesting," or "We'll see how that goes," or "Those symptoms are common in your condition."

Ed tried to press, with specific questions like "Do you think it's chemo that's been making me so sick, or do you think the cancer is spreading?"

But the doctor would give only vague answers. "There's so much going on, I can't tell for sure."

Ed needed to hear how he was doing. If he was doing well, he needed to be told that. If he was doing badly, he needed to be told he was putting up one hell of a fight. That he was a goddamn hero for going to work wearing his pump, that he'd beat the shit out of cancer for a year, and no matter what happened next, he and the doctor were going to link arms and continue to beat the shit out of it.

"I don't need to be told I'm fighting a good fight, Jean," Ed said to me later, "although it would be good to hear a doctor say that. I know I'm fighting a good fight. What I need to hear is that he's fighting with me. I want somebody who's involved with me. I don't want a goddamn observer. I don't want a note taker."

We left Dr. Moore's office feeling frustrated and in the dark. Chemo was to start again that afternoon. Was it chemo that was making him so sick, or was it the onrush of cancer? I wondered why Dr. Moore didn't order an X-ray and take a look at the growth in the lungs. It had been a month since he'd done that. I wondered if Dr. Moore thought it didn't really make any difference what was going on or what was causing what. The only option left was to continue to treat with chemotherapy, no matter what an X-ray showed.

I'm not sure what Dr. Moore thought or what his medical opinion was, because he never shared it with us. Did he share it with his colleagues? When we left the office, did he share it with Louise? As he took off his lab coat, did he turn to her and say, "Ed seems to be slipping. The blood test shows increased activity and I didn't like what I heard in the lower left lung"?

Did he turn to a colleague later in the day and say, "I saw Ed McNeilly again today. You wouldn't believe the amount of growth he has in the lungs. But he's still strong as a bull. The bastard's still going to work."?

The stubbornness with which doctors withhold information from their patients is arrogant on the one hand and patronizing on the other. It's an attitude that may once have been widespread but has all but disappeared in other professions.

Banks and lending institutions used to hide things like true interest rates in the voluminous fine print of their thick, creamy documents. "Lay people can't understand APR," they'd say. Or, "You can't let a customer know he's really paying 18 percent. Monthly payment is all that counts. If he sees the percent, he'll panic."

Then, full-disclosure laws were passed. The lending institutions had to reveal the true facts up front. Wondrously, the American public coped.

The same thing happened in the food industry with truth in labeling, in the automotive industry with Monroney stickers on the windows, and in TV advertising with substantiation requirements. The right of the consumer to know is one of the good things that happened in our country in the 1960s and '70s.

Full disclosure opened up the musty insides of every business in America, from General Motors to General Mills. Today, you know exactly how much interest you pay over the life of a car loan and just exactly what the nutritional content is of a bowl of Wheaties.

But the one profession that's gone absolutely untouched is medicine. Doctors and hospitals are not required to tell you what tests they're running, what they're for, what they cost, or what the results are. They're not required to tell you how many operations the doctor who's going to cut you open has performed or what his success rate is. Even your own private physician, the one who's your buddy, your golfing partner, perhaps, would be reluctant to show you his notes or share with you his write-ups.

A breath of fresh air needs to blow through the medical community. It needs to join the rest of us here in the Information Age. It needs to lose its fear of the people it serves.

To be as human as the people it treats.

September 22

CHEMOTHERAPY STARTED. I WAS AT HOME when Sharon, a new nurse from Lifeline, came to the house with the now-familiar bag of juice, the pump, the case, and the sealed container for disposal. I watched with a terrible foreboding as she put in the Heparin lock and started the treatment. But Ed was certain and sure.

"I'm fine, Jean. It's for the best."

September 24

ED WOKE UP SICK. The minute he got out of bed, he went to the bathroom and threw up. Then there was a terrible coughing spell. He wanted to go to work, but I eased him back into bed.

"I have to go, Jean," he said. "It's payroll day and Aurora isn't authorized at the bank."

"It's okay, Ed. I'll take care of it."

I went to the car wash and learned Aurora needed a special key, matched by a key at the bank, in order to get the payroll released. The key was in Malibu in Ed's pants pocket. Shit. I drove back out to Malibu and got it, then went with Aurora to the bank, introduced her to the manager, and got her authorized to handle payroll. Then I went to the office, where Bob had gotten an angry phone call from one of our clients over a mistake we'd made in television production. He was pacing up and down waiting for me. Shit. Then there was an important meeting at ARCO at two in the afternoon. We were presenting new creative. It didn't go well. They didn't approve anything. Shit. Then that evening, there were focus groups. One at seven P.M. and another at nine P.M. I didn't get home until after eleven. Shit.

Sug was with Ed in the evening, and I talked to him a number of times on the phone. But he hadn't eaten all day. He said he couldn't. Diarrhea was continuing. Coughing was continuing. Sharon came for his shot of 5FU in the late afternoon and Leucovoran was continuing to infuse. He was weak. He was exhausted. I was exhausted.

The stress I was under was high. It usually is when patients and their families are dealing with serious illness. Lives don't stop when illness starts. People still have jobs, children, responsibilities. They often begin to have work or financial problems because of the illness. They often have problems in the home. Illness can ruin a marriage. It can require more of people than they're equipped to give. It can create enormous problems that go beyond being sick.

But no one in Dr. Moore's office ever said to Ed or to me, "How're things at home? How're you guys managing?"

They did, however, frequently make it clear to us that they were under stress themselves.

The next morning I phoned Dr. Moore's office to report on Ed's worsening condition and heard Louise struggling for patience, as if I shouldn't have phoned, as if she was busy and tired and I should have known by then that there were limits to what she and Dr. Moore could contribute. The pointed politeness in her tone of voice punctuated her message.

"Mrs. McNeilly, you have to expect chemotherapy to take its toll."

"But this is different. It's never been this bad."

"Well, of course, there is progression, Mrs. McNeilly."

"I have a feeling there are complications beyond chemo."

"Dr. Moore is doing everything he can." There was great weariness in her voice.

"Will you tell the doctor I'm concerned?"

"Yes, Mrs. McNeilly."

"Will you ask him to phone me?"

"I'll do that, Mrs. McNeilly."

He never phoned.

September 25

IT WAS FRIDAY AFTERNOON, and I left work early to be home when Sharon got there at five. She gave Ed his shot, then took me aside.

"The decline is really noticeable," she said. "I'm going to phone the doctor."

"Oh, Sharon, I wish you would." I thought he would respond to her as he had not to me.

"The change since Monday is shocking. I've never seen such a decline."

"I think there's something going on besides chemo," I said. "He's been running a fever. Chemo doesn't make a fever, or at least it never has. I think he has an infection of some sort."

"Let me phone the doctor. Maybe we can start an antibiotic."

"You won't get him any more this afternoon."

"Then I'll phone him Saturday morning," she said, "and he'll phone you back."

That night, Ed coughed so much, he didn't sleep more than a couple of hours. Neither did I.

September 26

IT WAS SATURDAY MORNING, and Chris, whose apartment was near the car wash, had been opening on Saturdays. Aurora didn't work weekends and Simon couldn't work the register, so someone had to be there to open it and make sure there was plenty of change. But Chris was away on a field trip for the Corps of Engineers, so Sug ran into town to take care of things. Ed was miserable, worried. And difficult.

"Why are you letting Sug do that, Jean? She doesn't have enough experience to set up the register. You should do it yourself."

I got angry, because he didn't seem to understand the strain I was under. He didn't realize I was exhausted and afraid. We talked about it. But he ended up being surly and abusive and I ran upstairs crying.

When Sug got back, Ed asked her to get him some coffee and then chided her when she didn't do it fast enough. He had her on the verge of tears as well.

Then Alicia came. In addition to taking care of our house plus two others, Alicia worked in a nursing home. She was there six nights a week from eleven until seven in the morning, sleeping on a cot in the office in between calls from the residents.

"Alicia," I said to her one day, "how in the world do you manage to work at night and then clean houses all day?"

"It's not so bad, Yean," she said. "Some nights I only have to get up two or three times."

At six every morning she started the day at the nursing home, taking juice to everyone and administering their medications.

People like Alicia, whose lives are hard, seem to know more than the rest of us about human nature. Alicia was only twenty-nine years old, but she was wise far beyond her years and had a capacity to see very quickly into people's souls.

"You son is quiet," she'd tell me, "but he's afraid right now. I can see it in his eyes."

"Why is he afraid?"

"He's afraid for you."

On this particular morning, Alicia immediately sensed the dynamics in the household and went to work to change them. She looked for things to do for Ed. She ironed his bathrobe, clipped flowers from the Plumeria in the greenhouse, and put them where Ed could see them. She told me to get out of the house for a while.

"Go down to the beach," she said. "I'll take care of Ed."

She also had a talk with Sug.

"Shu-gar," she said, bringing her own pronunciation to my daughter's name in the way she'd changed mine to Yean. "Shugar, you have to understand that sick people have all of this anger inside. They're angry because they're sick. And because of the pain. Ed isn't being unkind to you. He loves you. But he is so angry."

"At the nursing home where I work," she went on, "people throw things at me sometimes when I bring the medicine. But it's not because of me or because of the medicine, it's because they're so angry. You just have to ignore the anger, Shugar. They can't help it."

"God," I said to myself, when Sug repeated the conversation to me, "she's so right. He's angry and there's no one to be angry at."

I told myself I had to remember Ed wasn't always himself anymore. If he became abusive, as he did that morning, it wasn't really Ed, it was the anger. Or the pain. And I shouldn't react as I might have before. I had to learn to not be hurt. To just walk away. It was one of my more important lessons from Alicia Lopez.

Saturday went by and Dr. Moore never phoned. The Lifeline nurse who came at five was a new one, because it was Sharon's day off. She said she didn't know if Sharon had phoned the doctor, but Sharon would be working Sunday and we could ask her then.

I was feeling my own share of anger. My own brand of anger. Toward the doctor. Toward cancer. Toward life. That evening when I couldn't get the VCR to work, it was everything I could do to keep from pulling it from the wall, like Ed had pulled the phone from the wall at LAX.

September 27

CHEMO ENDED. WHEN SHARON CAME to give the last shot, she asked if Dr. Moore had phoned.

"No. I thought you must have talked to him and the two of you decided not to do anything over the weekend."

"I don't understand," she told me. "I never talked to him, but I left a message with his service to phone you or me immediately."

"It's Sunday," I said. "Maybe he's out of town for the weekend."

"But there should have been someone on call. I'm sorry, Jean. I'll phone him first thing tomorrow morning and make sure he understands."

"It doesn't make any difference now," I said. "Our regular appointment with him is on Tuesday."

September 28

THE COUGHING GOT SO BAD DURING THE NIGHT Ed couldn't lie down. Every time he lay flat, he'd get mucus in his throat and start to gag and cough. What little sleep he got was fitful dozing for ten or twenty minutes at a time in between coughing spells. All weekend, he was at his wit's end. Coughing. Coughing. Coughing. Fever. Nausea. No food. Weak. Stir crazy. I'd never seen anyone so miserable. Sug and I were both showing the strain of worrying for him and caring for him. Not knowing what to do.

There was a distinctive odor to the mucus Ed was coughing up and it had a brown color. I knew it had to mean something, but I didn't know what. I was sick that Dr. Moore hadn't responded to Sharon. My instincts told me Ed had an infection and needed an antibiotic.

I should have phoned the doctor myself and been persistent until he responded. I felt guilty because I hadn't. The coughing had gotten so much worse over the weekend and the mucus had turned brown over the weekend, whatever that meant.

I went to work for a little while to brief a new copywriter for some work on ARCO and then to the car wash to go over applications with Aurora for a weekend cashier, then came back home to help Ed get ready for the trip to Dr. Moore's office. It took all the strength he had to get himself up, dressed, and shaved.

At the doctor's office I was told by the nurse they'd received no message from Lifeline about Ed over the weekend.

Did the message get lost between Friday night and the weekend? Did Dr. Moore see the message and not connect Sharon with Ed? Was the message garbled by the answering service? Did Dr. Moore self-screen his calls by responding only to those who called him back several times? Did he get the message and make the judgment there wasn't much he could do for Ed, he was going to see him Tuesday anyway, so why bother over the weekend? Did Louise, on the other hand, get the message and decide not to bother the doctor? Was the message simply ignored?

I don't know what really happened. But no matter what the excuse, it wasn't good enough.

The meeting with Dr. Moore wasn't very good either. He took blood tests and X-rays, but he didn't prescribe anything or suggest anything.

"I'm very concerned," he said, "but I can't determine exactly what's going on until I get the tests back."

"When will that be?" I asked.

"Thursday."

"Well, could you start him on an antibiotic now?"

"There's so much going on, Jean," he said.

By now, there were chills, fever, sweats, strange shooting pains in the back and pains in the rectum, nausea, and inability to eat. And something new: badly swollen feet.

"I'd rather not prescribe anything until I know. There may be an infection. I tend to think it's increased cancer activity. It may be both."

"But what's the downside risk of starting an antibiotic?"

"What do you mean?"

"If he needs one and you start it, he gets help. If he doesn't need one, it won't hurt him, will it? I mean, there's no downside risk in giving him one."

I had clearly irritated him. I was trying to be the doctor.

"Let's get the test results back, and you bring him in again on Thursday."

So we went home. But the agony of the situation was enormous. Every few minutes there were painful, hacking coughs, with the brown mucus coming up and the odor like sour milk. The whacks created by the coughs would cause Ed to double up. Sometime during the past few days, he'd herniated the wall of his stomach, weakened by the two surgeries at the City of Hope. So now when he coughed, a ball would poof out from his abdomen, about the size of a grapefruit.

He desperately needed sleep, and I knew there would be two more sleepless, hacking nights before we saw the doctor again.

"I think I could sleep, Jean, if I was sitting up. If we had a recliner, I think I could sleep in that."

So we went to the RB Furniture store on Pico in West LA to find a recliner. When I told the salesman we wanted to take it right then, right off the floor, he said we couldn't. It was against company policy. I asked him to speak to his manager. I motioned toward Ed. "He's very sick. He can't sleep lying down. If we can't take it home with us right now, he'll have to sit up all night." The man looked at us, trying to decide if he wanted to get involved.

"You know, they don't like us to ask for exceptions. We aren't supposed to do it."

"Please." It's all I could think of to say. I'm a shy person. I don't speak well when my own emotions are involved. The word came out strangled and tense. The salesman bit his lip and left to talk to his manager. When he came back, he said it was okay. I felt like hugging him.

Annie met us at the store with her truck, as did Chris, who'd finally come home, and we loaded the chair and took it home. Ed slept in the chair that night in the living room and I slept beside him on the couch. It wasn't a good night, but it was better than sitting up in a chair.

September 29

WHEN I GOT UP IN THE MORNING, Ed was worse. His feet were terribly swollen now, the coughing was continuing, his fever was up, and he was beginning to hallucinate.

I called the doctor's office. They told me they had some of the tests back, but not all of them.

"I can't wait for any more tests!" I shouted at Louise into the phone. "I can't wait until tomorrow. He needs to be in the hospital."

Louise talked to the doctor while I waited on hold, and when she came back on the line she said to bring him in. The doctor said he'd seen some of the tests, and there was fluid in the lungs.

It was all Ed could do to walk the fifteen steps from the car to the elevator in the parking garage under Dr. Moore's office. As soon as the doctor saw him, he ordered hospitalization.

"Don't go home first, Jean," he said. "Take him over right now. We need to drain off the fluid in the lungs and find out what's causing it."

The hospital was in the same complex where Dr. Moore had his office. I took Ed down the elevator and headed for the patio that separated the buildings. But Ed couldn't make it. He was teetering on the verge of falling over, passing out, or both. I sat him down on a couch near the elevator and ran into the hospital lobby for a wheelchair.

An orderly saw me struggling and came with a wheelchair to help. We got him through Admitting and into a room, where they immediately started an IV.

I left him for a few minutes, went to the ladies' room, and locked myself in a stall. A single thought was pounding inside my head: "This is the beginning of the end. The beginning of the end. The beginning of the end."

September 30

THE FIRST TWO DAYS ED SPENT in the hospital blurred together like double-printed images on film. Chris and Sug bringing dinner. Holding my hand. Phoning Maureen, Erin, and Robin. Phoning Carl. I ran out to Malibu to get Ed his things. I ran over to the agency and talked to Bob.

"I don't know how long I'll be gone."

"Of course you don't," he said. "Don't worry about anything here."

Ed was taken in and out of his room constantly for tests. I'd get there and he'd be gone, so I'd run to the car wash to handle something and come back to find I'd missed the doctor.

Dr. Moore had called in a lung specialist, but I had yet to meet him and had heard nothing conclusive from Dr. Moore. I found out from one of the nurses that the IV was an antibiotic, and they were giving him Demoral for pain. The coughing had let up a little, and he was sleeping.

Early in the afternoon on the second day, I went to a nearby coffee shop for some lunch and when I came back, Ed was in his room, awake and lucid.

"Dr. Kanon was just here," he said.

Dr. Kanon was the lung specialist.

"He told me," Ed continued, "that he didn't know what was going on in the rest of my lungs, but in the lower right-hand corner, it was pneumonia."

Pneumonia.

Late that night, I got home to my beloved house and in the hollow unreality created by Ed's absence, I walked straight to the guest room with the built-in bookcase. On the middle shelf was the four-volume *Illustrated Medical and Health Encyclopedia.* I'd ordered it years before from the Book-of-the-Month Club because I'd been so frustrated by Kevin's doctors. I found I could learn more by looking something up in my encyclopedia than I was likely to learn by asking them. The encyclopedia also helped me know what to ask. I picked up Volume 4, "Pleuresy to Zyme," and turned to *pneumonia.* This was what I read:

In the symptoms of a typical case,... a shaking chill may be followed by a sharp stabbing pain on the side of the chest, with coughing and expectoration of brown sputum.

When I read "brown sputum," all my senses froze and my body turned to ice. Ed had coughed up brown sputum for five days before Dr. Moore sent him to the hospital or prescribed an antibiotic.

October 1

I STILL HADN'T SEEN DR. MOORE or spoken with him since Ed had been hospitalized, and I was determined to talk to him face-to-face. I got to Century City Hospital by eight A.M., hoping I'd arrive before he made his morning rounds, and I did. Ed told me he hadn't been there yet. I sat with Ed and waited. He was asleep most of the time.

By eleven, the doctor still hadn't come. I had to run over to the agency. There was something urgent Bob needed to see me about. I'd also gotten a call from Aurora and needed to go by the car wash to sign checks. She reminded me that if I got Chris authorized to sign checks, it would help. I also needed to get some lunch.

But I didn't want to miss the doctor. So I phoned his office and spoke to the receptionist.

"When do you expect Dr. Moore to be making his rounds today at the hospital?"

"I don't know, Mrs. McNeilly."

"Could you check?"

"The doctor's tied up with a patient."

"I didn't mean for you to bother him. I thought you'd know his routine."

"It's not always the same."

"Look, I'm not trying to be a problem. It's just that I have a business. I work. I'm also running my husband's business right now. I can't always stay at the hospital the entire day and I keep missing the doctor."

"But Mrs. McNeilly, I really don't know."

People often say that they don't know when they do know, or at least know more than they're acknowledging, because they feel they shouldn't be asked. But I was persistent.

"Well, . . . could you tell me if he'll be here closer to noon or closer to six o'clock this evening?"

"Could you hold a moment?" she said with a sense of defeat in her voice.

When she came back on the line, she told me the doctor would be there between twelve-thirty and twelve-forty-five.

"Thank you," I said, relieved. I phoned Bob and told him I'd be at the office around two, after I'd seen the doctor. Then I phoned Aurora and told her I'd be at the car wash around three. Sometime in between the doctor, the agency, and the car wash, I'd get lunch.

But the doctor didn't arrive at twelve-thirty. Or twelve-forty-five. He arrived at three o'clock. I sat there and waited. Nervous, agitated, depressed, weary. I wished I could burn the car wash down. Walk out of the agency and not come back. Take Ed away with me, take care of him myself, and at least be in peace.

I believe doctors begin to think, as medical students—indeed, I believe they're taught as medical students—that their calling separates them from the rest of us. They believe that the nature of what they're doing with their lives is, in itself, an entitlement. That the word *doctor* calls for preferential treatment and accommodation by everyone else.

I discovered at Robertson Car Wash, when handling the cash register, that doctors include "M.D." in the imprint of their names on American Express and Visa cards. "John French, M.D.," the card will read. I know of no other professional people who identify themselves on a credit card. Lawyers don't do it. Clergymen don't do it. Congressmen don't do it. Professors don't do it.

But doctors do it.

Why?

So you'll know who they are and honor their entitlement. You should wash my car faster, the "M.D." is supposed to communicate, because I'm a doctor and you shouldn't keep me waiting.

Dr. Moore, I'm sure, was late for a good reason. I didn't think he was schmoozing over lunch at the Bistro. He probably had an emergency. But his receptionist didn't have an emergency. Nevertheless, her telephone would have turned to salt before it occurred to her to phone me back and let me know.

The onus is all on the patient. It's an attitude inbred in the profession, and it's been that way so long and is so universal they don't even know they're doing it anymore. When Dr. Moore finally arrived at three o'clock, he walked into the room, glanced at me, but spoke to Ed.

"You have an infection," he said. "We're treating it." He then exchanged a few pleasantries and turned on his heel to leave. My mouth flew open and I raised my voice to stop him.

"Wait a minute. Is that all you're going to say? Is that your conclusion? I haven't seen you since this started. Where are you going?"

I couldn't believe he was going to leave. That all I was going to get from him after all that had happened was a one-liner. Not only was he late, it didn't even register with him that he hadn't spoken to me since Ed was admitted. Or else he didn't want to speak to me. But he saw the look on my face and motioned me into the hall. Since I'd pressed, he'd respond.

"There's an infection and fluid in the lungs, which we drained," he said. "But there wasn't as much fluid as we expected. There may be a mass, a tumor behind it, which is the cause of the infection. I'm very worried about Ed. His breathing is very labored."

I believed he was worried. I believed he was a good man. But somehow, his profession had screwed him up. I found it curious that he kept referring to an "infection" rather than pneumonia.

"The X-rays seem to indicate," he continued, "that there's growth in the other nodules, which means Leucovoran has lost its effectiveness. First we need to clear up the infection; then we can tell better."

It crossed my mind to confront him about the brown sputum. But the freight train was roaring in the back of my mind. The noise was deafening. I thought my head might explode.

I told him instead that as soon as he could give me one, I needed a short- and long-term prognosis.

"I have Ed to care for. My business to run and his business to run. I have family and resources to call upon, but I need to know what to expect, so we can cope."

"I'll have a better picture by Monday," he said. "All I know for sure, right now, is the antibiotics are taking hold."

"Ed isn't coughing anymore," I said. "Doesn't that mean the infection, rather than the spread of cancer, was causing the coughing?"

"Not necessarily," he said. Then he repeated himself. "First we need to get the infection cleared up. Then we can decide what to do next."

He left, and I spent the rest of the afternoon fighting off sleep. My brain was fried. Ed, cancer, the doctors, the uncertainty, the office, the car wash, home. I'd let the insurance lapse on Ed's Porsche. Things were intense at Kresser/Craig. The moody copywriter had quit. I needed to replace him but couldn't even begin to address the matter.

We still hadn't gotten new work approved at ARCO. The problems were creating tensions among our own staff. I was yelling at people. They were yelling at me. I felt absolutely beleaguered and was near desperate to slip into the escape of sleep. But I couldn't even do that. Ed's room was so tiny it held only his bed and a couple of straight-back chairs. To keep my wits about me, I spent the afternoon writing in a notebook, and what came out was anger. At Dr. Moore, but most of all, at his profession.

Twenty-five years earlier, the doctors at UCLA guarded information just as he did. Shut me out, just as he did. They performed a summerful of tests on Kevin, not one of which was ever shown to us when it was completed or discussed with us beforehand. They'd whisked Kevin out of NPI to Cardiology without even telling me. They'd performed twelve hours of surgery and not even met with me afterwards.

Doctors just do what they do.

My brain flooded with less important incidents over the years. The skin specialist treating Chris' acne. It wasn't improving. Chris told me he never saw the doctor, only the nurses. I went to see the doctor to ask about it and he got incensed. And the Beverly Hills gynecologist. He literally told me to "sit down and stop asking the questions, I'll do the explaining" and tried to tell me I wasn't going into menopause, when I knew I was. (You only have to have one hot flash to know what it is.) And the internist caring for my mother. Her bowels weren't working. My brothers thought there was something the matter. The doctor said, "Yes, she's old." It turned out to be an obstruction.

I remembered, with both Kevin and Ed, doctor after doctor after doctor coming into the hospital room to do something and asking me to leave.

"But I'm his wife."

"I know."

I remembered being told countless times by irritated doctors and nurses, as I tried to do it: "You aren't allowed to look at his charts."

Why does a spouse have to leave the room? Why can't people see their charts?

The anger that tumbled out wasn't really at Dr. Moore. It was at Everydoctor. Here we were in the Information Age and there was still the "know-it-at-my-largesse" attitude. The power in medicine is in the hands of the doctors. Shouldn't it be shared with the people occupying the bodies they're treating?

In my opinion, patients and their families should see a printout of every test run on an individual every day and should have the specific results of those tests, not a verbal summary. They should see a listing of the drugs being administered, the procedures being performed, the X-rays being taken, the IVs being infused. They should have access to the doctor's notes if they want to see them.

I can hear the medical profession now screaming bloody murder.

"But people wouldn't know how to interpret," they're crying. "A little learning is a dangerous thing," they're warning. "They wouldn't know what any of it meant," they're defending. "It would only scare them," they're condescending. "I don't have time to answer their questions," they're whining.

People will surprise you. They'll handle it well. You're underestimating them. They'll return the confidence in greater measure. You'll come to prefer it.

That's what I'd shout back at them.

October 2

SUG, SENSING MY DISTRESS DURING THE WEEK, dropped what she was doing and joined me at the hospital on Friday. She brought lunch, along with a brown bear for Ed to hug. She also had a bagful of Halloween goodies.

"This is for you, Mama," she said.

It was a red wax moustache, the kind you hold in place by clamping it between your teeth.

"It makes you look like Ed."

I put it on and he tried to laugh through the cobwebby consciousness that surrounded him.

Sug's boyfriend, Jim the Fireman, was flying down from San Francisco later that day. Their relationship had heated up since she'd moved to Los Angeles. (I wasn't surprised. Women often have to go to great lengths to get a man to realize he's involved.) They were on the phone all the time and seemed to be crazy about each other. I'd met him, but I didn't really know him.

"He wants to come by and see Ed," she said. "Is it okay?"

"Sure, it's okay. I'm sorry the circumstances aren't better."

"Well," she glanced at Ed, who'd drifted off to sleep, "this is who I am right now, and he needs to know that."

She'd been at my side a lot the past few days and had slipped into the role of caretaker with poise and grace. Ed had accepted her and she was beginning to share the more intimate and less pleasant aspects, physically and mentally, of a worsening condition. She'd said to me earlier in the day in a soft, sweet voice, "Ed doesn't mind anymore if I help him." In addition to being a caring person, she had a lot of guts.

I'd phoned Eric that morning and asked him to phone a list I'd made of Ed's friends to finally tell them Ed's whole story. Then I phoned Robin and asked her to talk to her mother and her sister. Ed had written to them, but I thought they should know he was in the hospital and that the situation wasn't promising.

Robin called me back an hour or so later and said both Kim and Donna already knew how serious it was. Kim, who was a media planner at my old alma mater, FCB, had overheard rumors about Ed being terminal at a media luncheon, from someone in my office who didn't know who she was.

I didn't mention any of that to Ed. He was still sleeping most of the time and was light-headed when he was awake.

October 3

IT WAS SATURDAY MORNING AND THE PACE at the hospital slowed. There weren't many patients on weekends, so the nurses had time and were generous in giving it. Nadia was especially dear. She was from Belize, a country on the eastern coast of Central America, and had the soft, easy manner of a Caribbean person as well as the Caribbean lilt in her voice.

"I like your husband a lot," she told me as she took special care with Ed's bath. "He reminds me of my husband. My husband is seventy-four years old, so I know how to take good care of an older man."

I grinned at her and tried to guess how old she was. Thirty, I decided. Maybe a little more.

"Nadia," I asked, "why did you marry a man so much older than you?"

"Because he loves me," she shrugged.

I thought that to be a fine answer.

Dr. Kanon, the lung specialist, came in. He seemed easier and more accessible than Dr. Moore, so I asked him about Ed's condition, but he was evasive. "I'm not the primary care doctor," he said. "But," he went on, "I can tell you about the pneumonia. I think we'll get it cleared up in three or four days and as far as I'm concerned, Ed can go home."

It was the first positive news I'd heard. I allowed myself some quiet optimism.

"Your husband worries a lot about bowel movements," Nadia was chattering on. "When you're married to a seventy-four-year-old man, you learn a lot about bowel movements."

Sug came by with The Fireman. Jim Bustamante. We chatted for a while and I found him to be a macho but sensitive young man. He had the olive-skinned good looks of his Latin heritage—his parents were born in El Salvador—and he was taller than I expected, brushing six feet. He had a moustache. "All firemen have moustaches," Sug told me. "All firemen all over the world." We talked about how he was combining law with being a fireman.

"I'm a lawyer," he explained, "and that's what I want to do with my life, but I love being a fireman. It's exciting. There's a sense of contribution, and as long as I can do both, I'm going to."

I thought that, like Ed, he combined manliness and gentleness in one person, and the two men would like each other a lot. It was sad they were meeting under these circumstances. Ed hardly knew Jim was in the room. Jim was seeing this great bull of a man down on his knees.

Sug and Jim left, and the day dragged on. I picked up a Raymond Chandler novel, one of his famous Phillip Marlowe murder mysteries set in Los Angeles in the '40s. The Santa Ana winds were blowing, and LA always felt more present and in focus to me when the winds came in off the desert. It was a perfect day to read Raymond Chandler, but my mind kept drifting to better times.

I recalled a day not long after Ed and I had started seeing each other when he decided to storm his way into my emotions without an invitation and assume the consequences. He'd been away on a business trip and when I picked him up at the airport, he got into my car waiting at the curb, and as I pulled into the jumbled traffic at LAX, he turned to me and said, "I love you."

"What!" I said, more as an exclamation than a question.

"I love you."

"You can't say that."

"I know I'm not supposed to say it."

"I can't say it back, Ed."

Since I'd been "dating" after Kevin's death, I'd learned to put a limit on my involvement and my feelings, because there is a fear of people who are needy and a fear of people who are givers, lest there be an expectation of giving back. I'd learned not to care, but to be interested more in companionship and not look for anything beyond that. Now here was a man turning the tables.

"I thought about it the whole time I was on the plane, Jean, and I decided to go into a free fall, to just jump with no parachute. That's the way I feel and I decided to tell you. I don't know what it means and I don't know what the consequences will be and you don't have to do anything about it, but I had to tell you. I love you."

I was so unprepared and shocked, I almost wrecked the car. I think all women dream quiet dreams of being overtaken by a man. I was so lucky to have had that happen with Ed.

Around four in the afternoon Ed came out of one of his hazy sleeps and sat up in bed, as if an engine inside his body had suddenly turned on.

"Come here, Jean," he called softly to me. I came over and sat beside him on the bed.

"I love you," he said. He wasn't coughing. He wasn't running a fever. "I'm hungry," he said. "Do you suppose you could call Chris and ask him to bring me a hamburger from Islands, and Jean, could you turn on the TV? We're missing 'Magnum.'"

There's an irrepressible spirit born into every human being. Most of us lose it or get it beat out of us by the time we're adults, but some of us have it forever.

Ed did.

October 4

ED AND I SPENT AN OPTIMISTIC SUNDAY at the hospital. The nurses took him off the IV and reduced the oxygen. He was feeling good enough to walk to the rec room, where we watched the premiere episode of "Star Trek, the Next Generation." I was a Trekkie and it was hard getting used to the Captain—he was so different from Kirk. But I did like Lieutenant Commander Data.

Drs. Moore and Kanon both came by early in the day, and they seemed to be sharing an encouraging prognosis. One thing I must give doctors credit for is the long hours and the weekend work. Dr. Moore said they might give Ed "localized X-ray treatment." There was a big tumor near the pneumonia that could be contributing to the blockage of air passages. He'd know more after X-rays were taken on Monday morning.

Somebody taught Dr. Moore to use euphemisms, I thought to myself. First he calls pneumonia an infection. Now he's calling radiation a localized X-ray treatment.

Sug and Chris came for dinner, which we ate as a picnic in the rec room. They brought chicken from Jimmy's Ribs at the Beach, Ed's favorite take-out place in Malibu. Chris had spent the day at the car wash. He'd begun opening it on Sunday mornings, as well as Saturdays, and was staying to give the cashier her lunch break and do the cash-out. I'd never really asked him to work weekends. He'd just seen the need and done it.

"How many cars?" Ed asked him.

"Three hundred and fifty."

"That's great for a Sunday in October."

A funny smile flashed across my son's face. I had the feeling he hated the car wash. He hated the responsibility, he hated interrupting his weekends, he hated the constant problems with customers. But he also liked it, because he liked the involvement and liked being needed.

Nothing is simple. There are opposing forces at work in life all the time. Love/hate relationships. Trends and countertrends. You hate your job one day, you love it the next. As Charles Dickens said, "It was the best of times. It was the worst of times." Right on, Charlie.

October 5

THE OPTIMISM OF THE QUIET SUNDAY at the hospital turned on Monday into a new sense of dread. I'd thought Ed and I might have a window of time. He might get over his pneumonia and be well again for a while. But the window seemed to be slipping shut, and once again there was a climate of uncertainty. I was stunned by the change and felt like someone had pulled an unseen plug in my body and drained its energy, like oil from a car.

X-rays were supposed to be taken in the morning. When they weren't, Ed spoke to the nurses and the doctor on the floor, then called Dr. Moore's office to discover he'd forgotten to put in the order. When the doctor came by at two-thirty in the afternoon, Ed chided him.

"I don't feel you're being aggressive. You have to understand I don't want to let up. I want to get over my pneumonia and resume chemotherapy."

"5FU and Leucovoran may have run their course, Ed."

"How do you know if you don't run the X-rays?"

"We'll run the X-rays this afternoon."

Ed had a long, low, wheezing cough. It sounded different from any cough he'd had before. His color was also different. Ed had a deep natural-hued tan with a reddish cast, unlike the neon tans you often see in Los Angeles that come from tanning salons or skin creams. He was one-sixteenth Cherokee Indian, which perhaps accounted for the hue. But suddenly, his color was tending toward yellow. It was a little thing, but you become sensitive to little things. And you get feelings. I got the feeling there was something going on we weren't privy to. Drs. Moore and Kanon knew something or suspected something they weren't sharing with us. The feeling simply added to the stress. In the midst of it all, Maureen phoned from New York.

"What's going on, Mom?" she asked. "How's Ed doing? I feel so far away."

Her voice sounded small and hollow. I pictured her alone in New York, afraid to call, afraid not to call. When I thought of the possibility of this child losing her father again, my heart flew into my mouth. Then I caught myself. When I had to face the fear of losing Ed, I put it in terms of the children, because I couldn't stand to put it in terms of myself. I talked about my fear for Maureen but what I was really expressing was my fear for myself.

Ed fell into a wheezy sleep. I kept hearing myself think. I don't understand. I don't understand. I don't understand. I didn't understand why this was happening. Why I had to lose two husbands to debilitating disease. The Catholicism in which I was raised teaches there's a reason, an intelligence behind everything. That it's all part of a larger picture. But sometimes mortal man is not supposed to understand.

It's God's will, first-graders are taught. When you don't understand, you must accept God's will.

It's easy, then, to lump everything that can't be explained into one convenient catch-all—the God's will in-basket. I didn't buy it anymore. What's more, if it was God's will that Ed be sick, I didn't like God. What kind of God would cause the beings He created to suffer? No. God's will had nothing to do with it. It was just random. Random bad luck. And trying to understand it or find a reason was, as Cynthia Root and I had agreed, a waste of time. And a cause of pain and frustration.

Late in the evening, around seven o'clock, Dr. Kanon came by. The X-rays had finally been taken, he'd looked at them, and he had for us, at last, some hard information. He wanted to do a bronchoscopy, a procedure where they put a fiber-optic tube down the throat and look into the lung.

"The X-rays show the pneumonia isn't clearing up," he told me. "We need to find out why."

"What do you expect to see in the lung?" I asked. I liked Dr. Kanon. He didn't try to candy-coat his information.

"We might find pus, water, hardened mucus, but options one through ten," he continued, "are we find a tumor blocking an air passage."

"Okay," I said calmly. But I was scared to death.

All my life, I've been afraid of showing my own emotions. Not reluctant. Really afraid. I can cry at movies or at someone else's problems, but not my own. I can get angry with others, but not on my own behalf. I find it easy to say "I apologize" but very difficult to say "You hurt my feelings." If I'm to be honest with myself, I must admit it's a fear of being vulnerable. I hide my wounds like a shy child crouching in the dark.

I don't know where that comes from. I just know I have the problem, and one of the reasons I loved Ed so much was he saw through it from the start. "You're part little girl," he said, and in so doing gave me permission to act like one. But most people, even some who know me well, don't know I need permission. They see my calm face and think I'm tough. But all the people who put on calm faces when they're scared to death inside know how much more lonely it is when what you're really doing is hiding.

October 6

IT WAS A TERRIBLE DAY. Ed was very agitated. Very much in pain. I sat beside his bed all afternoon crying. They'd taken him off Demoral because they didn't want to slow his respiration, and he was groaning from pain. I was so scared I couldn't focus. I couldn't read. I couldn't make phone calls. My hands and legs were unsteady. My brain was rattled.

We waited all day and they finally ran the bronchoscopy in the early evening and found what they expected: a tumor had spread and was blocking a vital air passage.

"There are two options," Dr. Kanon told us. "We can attack the tumor with radiation or with a laser beam." He was leaning toward the laser beam.

"It's a little more dangerous, but there are fewer side effects. Not many tumors are treatable this way," he went on.

He explained that the doctor to do it was a surgeon who'd made techniques with the laser beam his specialty. The doctor and the equipment were at Cedars, where the whole saga began. Ed would have to be transferred there.

"But I want to talk to Dr. Moore," the doctor said. "We can all decide in the morning."

"Let's do the surgery," said Ed. "Let's do it right away."

A lot of people phoned that evening. Madeline, Annie, Carl. Eric. Bob dropped by the hospital. I had a long talk with him about whether I needed time off, how to handle things at the office, how he could help.

"I think you should stay involved at the office," he said. "It keeps your mind occupied. It's better for you."

He'd talked to many of Ed's friends. And many of them were phoning. Alan and Stacie. Monty. Jack Reilly. Wonderful John Tripp. Dan and Ann Mahan.

Robin phoned and said she was keeping her mother and sister up to date.

It sounded like a soap opera.

October 7

IT WAS WEDNESDAY MORNING. The decision was made to do the laser surgery, but we were told it couldn't be done until the following Monday.

Ed was angry. "This is life and death, Jean. I'm in pain. I can't breathe. Why do I have to sit here and wait for five days?"

"I don't know, Ed. I guess the doctor's booked. They were vague about why."

"I don't wait well, Jean. I never have."

I sat beside Ed and tried to calm him and in the process calmed myself. I felt better. There was a plan in place. We had to wait, but at least we knew where we were going.

Eric came and spent a lot of the afternoon with Ed, to help with the waiting. Then Alan and Stacie came in the evening. Alan talked with Ed as he would have talked with him over lunch during better times.

"They're driving me crazy in New York, Ed. They think they know about the VW business out here, but they don't."

It brought Ed out of himself. It helped.

Then Eddie phoned from New York. I watched my husband's eyes mist over as he talked to his friend. If I'd watched that moment in a TV movie, I might have thought it was sappy, but somehow when you're living the moments, there's nothing sappy about them.

Eddie phoned again a couple of hours later and said he was coming out. He'd arrive in Los Angeles the next afternoon. No. I didn't need to pick him up. I didn't need to do anything but just let him come.

October 8

PUNDITS WHO COMMENT ON THE INTRICACIES of human relationships are wont to say that men are given to easy, casual good fellowship with other men. That men are generally good at camaraderie and just enjoying each other. "Male bonding" is the term they like to use. Women, on the other hand, have relationships with other women that are deeper and more enduring. It's women who really talk to each other, get to know each other, share each other's lives.

One of the most moving things I ever witnessed was the conventional wisdom of that attitude being shot to hell in a hospital room in Los Angeles by Eddie Russell and Ed McNeilly. I saw a friendship between these two men that seeped from the very marrow of their bones. I saw an intimacy that would make a woman ache and a tenderness that would make a woman weep.

Eddie arrived early in the afternoon. He was a tall, handsome man— elegant is a word that fits—in his early sixties. Witty, charming, and poised, he would flirt with my twenty-five-year-old daughter and I wasn't surprised when she flirted back.

He breezed into Ed's hospital room dressed in corduroy trousers and a hunter's padded vest from L.L. Bean, looking for all the world as if he lived like a country gentleman in a converted barn in Pound Ridge, New York, which indeed he did. He was carrying a huge pink box, which we soon discovered held a buffet luncheon from Scandia, a favored restaurant of Ed's.

"I brought you the Smoorgasbricke," Eddie grinned. We opened the box to find Gravlax, pickled herring, Danish sausage, paté, and the other Scandinavian delicacies Scandia was famous for.

We spread it out on Ed's bed table and the three of us nibbled while the two of them talked. They'd shared the better part of thirty years, these two. But it wasn't just their history together that made them close. There was a oneness of spirit. They were men who were some-what larger than life. Men cut from the cloth of the khaki uniforms of World War II. Men who'd learned to be daring. To take risks as human beings. Who found some of their manliness in going too far, then taking the consequences, good or bad.

As the afternoon wore on, I watched in wonder as a phenomenon began to happen. Eddie began to tend to Ed, as naturally as a new mother begins to tend to her child. He was helping him out of bed, helping him onto the portable commode, helping him handle the spit tray—helping him do the rather nasty things only the nurses, Sug, and I had done up to then.

It was touching to see these two men who'd shared the boardroom of an international advertising agency and the barrooms of Wolfsburg, Dusseldorf, Stuttgart, New York, and the world put their arms around each other and struggle to get Ed to the toilet.

Eddie Russell had cut a wide swath during his years with Ed McNeilly at Doyle Dane Bernbach. He was an irreverent man given to grand gestures. He liked to live well. He liked to drink champagne. As with Ed, some people didn't approve of the style in which he lived and some people didn't like him.

But as I sat there that afternoon and watched him wash my hus-band's face and shave his day-old beard, I thought I'd never loved any-one but Ed as much as I loved Eddie at that moment.

October 9

IT WAS A SLOW, SEAMLESS FRIDAY afternoon, with the day-to-night hospital atmosphere causing time to lose its boundaries. Eddie, Ed, and I were sitting and talking about something. About nothing. Just talking. Trying to pass the interminable five days until Monday. Suddenly, a woman came into the room. She just stood there for a moment. She looked distressed. Ed didn't say anything. Eddie didn't say anything. In a heartbeat, I realized who she was, and blurted out.

"Oh my God, it's Kim."

Ed hadn't seen his daughter in three-and-a-half years and his senses were dulled by pain and drugs. Eddie hadn't seen her in many more years than that. I was the first to recognize her.

Ed looked at her and simply said her name. She went to the side of his bed, took his hand, and started to talk. Eddie took me by the arm and we left the room.

Kim. Ed's younger daughter. Twenty-six years old, married to Mark, living in Los Angeles. Working in the advertising business like her father. Close to her mother most of her life, but in temperament more like her dad. Kim. The daughter Ed lost when he left Donna.

The estrangement between Ed and Kim didn't happen abruptly. It just slipped into place. Ed and Kim saw each other from time to time after Ed moved out, but Kim was understandably angry and there was tension. The times together were unsettling. She was there watching once when Ed and Donna had a terrible scene over the financial settlement. Then Kim had gotten married without letting her father know. She'd fail to return Ed's phone calls and had responded to his overtures half-heartedly or not at all.

"She's punishing me," Ed had said after he'd dropped a Valentine's present at her office and she'd never phoned to thank him. He'd kept trying and there'd be an occasional glimmer from her, but when she let his birthday go unnoted one spring and let Father's Day go unnoted as well, Ed told me he was giving up.

"I can't be punished forever, Jean. I'm not going to get on my knees to her. Something has to come from her."

So the weeks slipped by with no communication. Then weeks became months, which wore into years. Robin, who'd managed to handle the divorce and stay on good terms with both her parents, wouldn't get into it with Ed and Kim. "It's between Kim and Dad," she told me once. "I can't get in the middle; it wouldn't help anyway." Robin did keep her father informed about Kim. "Kim got a new job," she'd chat in a breezy way on the phone.

I tried to do something once or twice. I phoned Kim's husband, Mark, to see if he and I could have lunch and perhaps find a path that would work for his wife and my husband. It took me weeks to stick my finger in the dial and make the call, but he was away on vacation. I didn't phone again. It bothered me a lot to act behind Ed's back. But, thank God, Kim finally decided to just show up.

It was two hours, maybe more, before she emerged, tearful but smiling, from her father's room. She found me and Eddie at the coffee machine and brought us back. Ed was tearful and smiling as well.

"Kim and I had a wonderful talk, Jean. We talked about everything. About the divorce. About Donna. About the anger. About cancer. Kim is back, Jean."

The room would have been awash in the sentimentality of the moment if Chris hadn't walked in with a pizza and a sheepish grin.

"This is Kim, Chris," Ed almost shouted. "This is Kim and she's back."

"I knew who she was," said Chris. "Anybody would know. She looks exactly like you."

October 10

NOTHING HAPPENED IN THE HOSPITAL on Saturday that had to do with medicine, but a lot happened that had to do with life. Eddie was there every minute and Kim came again. This time with her husband, Mark. Though we didn't know each other very well, Mark and I had always had a good rapport and liked each other a lot. The rapport picked up where it had left off three years before. He took me into the hall and told me Kim had been in agony over what to do. "Why doesn't Dad phone *me*?" she'd been crying.

"I told her," said Mark, "it was time to stop playing those games, and get her ass to the hospital and I wouldn't go with her, either. She had to do this one on her own. It took a lot of guts for her to come, Jean."

"I know it did. Ed knows too."

Eddie told me Donna also wanted to see Ed. I told him he should talk to Ed about it. He said he would, but he didn't want to talk to Ed without talking to me first. I said it was fine with me if Donna saw Ed, as long as it was fine with Ed.

Robin was in constant touch over the phone. Her voice broke when I told her Kim had come. "She did, Jean? I'm so glad."

Sug came while Kim was there. They'd never met, but they greeted each other with warmth. Sug, who'd long since joined me in the role of nurse to Ed, helped him with a difficult and unpleasant coughing fit. He was spitting phlegm into a spit-tray Sug held under his chin. As I eased people into the hall until the moment passed, I saw recognition in Kim's eyes that my daughter was more intimate with her father than she was.

It was a difficult moment for Kim. Sug told me later it was a difficult moment for her as well. "I don't want to feel guilty because I love him so," she said.

October 11

WE MOVED ED TO CEDARS.
Cedars-Sinai was not that far away. But moving Ed was an ordeal that not only took all day but also made me realize once again how difficult it is to be sick.

Ed had to be bathed, shaved, and dressed—things we all do every day without thinking. But when you can't do them for yourself, the time and effort they require is surprising. Ed insisted on brushing his own teeth, but his stamina was low and his focus fuzzy, so it took him fifteen minutes. His feet were still swollen and none of the soft shoes or slippers I'd brought from home would go on. Eddie slipped out and came back from somewhere with big white socks. It was difficult for Ed to raise his arms over his head to pull on a T-shirt. He had to be moved onto portable oxygen equipment. He had to be put into diapers. He wasn't incontinent, but he was concerned about diarrhea and being unable to control it. Orders for his medication had to be written up. Release papers had to be signed.

The most difficult part was getting him out of bed and onto a gurney. Every move was painful, but, more important, he wanted control of himself and would't let the orderlies lift him. It's very difficult for institutional staff members to bend in such a situation. They have a way of doing things and they mean to do them that way.

But Ed was struggling for control and his own sense of self. "I'm still a man, for Chrissakes," he seemed to be saying. "I'm still using my brain. I'm still capable of thought. I will get out of bed and onto this gurney like a human being and not like a piece of meat."

Ed won. He got onto the gurney his way, while the orderlies sulked. Eddie buckled the straps for him and winked at me.

Then Ed spent forty-five minutes lashed into place while we waited for the ambulance, which somebody had said they'd ordered but hadn't. The ambulance finally came when we ordered another one. Two of the nurses, Patti and Nadia, saw us off.

"Good luck, Mr. McNeilly. Let us know what happens."

"Your husband is an unusual man," Patti said to me as she handed me the release papers. "We've all admired him. Most people as sick as he is are beaten down. I hope things go well for you and him."

It's funny, I thought to myself, that I get acknowledgment from the nurses. From Renee at the City of Hope. From Betty, the bag lady. From Sharon and Maggie with Lifeline. And now from Patti.

But I never got it from the doctors. None of them ever said to me the things Patti said: "Your husband is an unusual man. He's putting up quite a fight. We admire him." I thought the reason was that they didn't see him as a person. To them, he wasn't Ed McNeilly, keeping his dignity and being a man while he struggled for his life. To them, he was an aeodinocarcinoma of the seigmoid colon with metasteses to the lungs.

Eddie rode with Ed in the ambulance to Cedars and I followed in the car. When we got there, we had to go through the bedeviling process of admitting. With Eddie beside him, Ed sat lashed to his gurney, while they sent me to the fifth floor; but there wasn't anyone at the desk, because it was Sunday, so I went back to the first, then back to the fifth, and so on. We finally got Ed into his room around four in the afternoon. The move had taken eight hours.

We were all exhausted. Ed, me, Eddie. When Eddie took me to dinner at the Hamburger Hamlet across the street from Cedars, I thought we were both going to end up asleep at the table with our faces in the No. 11 Quarter-Pounder with bacon and cheese.

October 12

ALL OF THE PROFESSIONS IN THIS COUNTRY, for reasons I don't understand, have quit using the English language and adopted a technolanguage of their own that only they can understand.

On an airplane, for example, you don't "get off." You "deplane." I once heard one flight attendant ask another where she was "domiciled." That means "Where do you live?" Morticians would die these days before they'd use the word "die." Instead, they say "expire." Advertising media people never talk about getting a large audience. They talk about "maximizing the reach and frequency." Teachers don't talk about math and English. They talk about "numerical skills" and "language skills." One of these days, the gardener is going to come to do some trimming and ask if he can "degrowth" the trees.

And, of course, the medical profession has refined technolanguage to the point where even they don't know what they're talking about. The dehumanization of language has come about to shield us from things the technocrats don't wish to confront. When the flight attendant says over the microphone "In the unlikely event of a water landing...," we all know she means "crash," but for Chrissakes, the technocrats argue, you can't SAY that.

So when the medical profession means "it's an emergency," they instead say "Code 10." When they mean "there isn't much we can do," they say "you need to look at *your* options." And they refer to everything they do, from putting on a Band-aid to taking out your liver, as "the procedure."

The doctors at Cedars kept referring to Ed's laser surgery as "the procedure." We're going to do "the procedure" at noon. The anesthesiologist will be here soon to discuss "the procedure." We'll put you on medication prior to "the procedure." You can't eat until after "the procedure."

The "procedure" finally happened at noon, after an interminable morning. Ed, Eddie, and I sat there with the knife edge of worry taking each minute and ripping it into strands that stretched for hours. The laser surgeon came early in the morning. Dr. Tuchman. He looked to be about thirty. He was excited about the surgery and even referred to it as "the surgery." He thought it would work. He thought it would really help. He was pleased he could do it. His enthusiasm and openness were refreshing. I couldn't quite place his accent. Middle Eastern, I guessed. Probably Israeli.

"He's acting like a person," I said to Eddie, "because he wasn't trained in the U.S."

By the time they took Ed to surgery, Sug and Chris had joined us, and the four of us left the hospital and went to lunch. Eddie told stories about his youth and falling in love with Mary Jane that charmed my daughter, chagrined my son, and caused all of us to forget "the procedure" for a couple of hours.

Around five in the afternoon, we were back at the hospital and scrunched into Ed's tiny room when Dr. Tuchman burst in. If he were a dog, I thought to myself, he'd be barking and wagging his tail.

"Everything went beautifully," he said. "It was easier than I expected. There were no complications. We removed a blockage about the size of a quarter."

Sug and I crawled together into Ed's empty bed and hugged each other. When Ed was finally wheeled into the room on a gurney, his cheeks were pink and he was breathing so much easier.

"I feel better, Jean." He looked at me for confirmation through hazy half-conscious eyes.

"I know you do, Sweetheart."

But the relief of the moment was to be just that. A moment.

Around six o'clock, Dr. Moore came into the room. He checked Ed's charts and spoke to him for a minute or two. When he turned to leave, I followed him into the corridor. I knew he wasn't going to speak to me or tell me anything unless I asked. But I wasn't even mad about it anymore. I couldn't waste my energy on being mad. And while Dr. Moore never offered anything, he would answer my questions if I initiated a conversation. And so I did.

"Dr. Tuchman said the surgery was successful."

"Yes. It was successful. The obstruction is gone. However, the walls of the lungs are embedded with tumors. I'm afraid it's going to be one thing after another from now on."

I took a deep breath. "Could you give me a prognosis?"

"It'd just be a guess."

"It may be a guess, but it's an educated one."

"If we can get him past this and get him home, he might have ninety days."

I could feel the bullet inside my head again, banging against the backs of my eyes, making them smart. I blinked quickly to keep the projectile from bursting through, pulling me with it.

"But it won't be life for him as he's known it before. He might be able to get up to go to the bathroom. Or to sit in a chair for a while every day. He'll need to be on oxygen."

"Will there be pain?" It was a question strangled through the tightness in my throat and the dryness in my mouth.

"We'll try to manage it. You should think," he went on, "about how you want to handle this. Some families want people at home. Some don't. It's a big strain on a family. There are hospice situations you can look into."

"Ed still thinks we can resume 5FU and Leucovoran."

"Obviously, they're no longer doing anything. We're running out of things to do. There are one or two more things I can try. And Ed will feel better if I do because it's his nature to want to be doing something, but I feel they won't work."

We talked a bit more. About home nursing care, hospice care, and hospital care. But I finally ended the conversation and walked away by myself down the corridor. Cedars is a big hospital. I walked along corridors until I didn't know where I was, until I was lost and faceless and nameless among people I had never seen before and would never see again. I'd read an article the day before, while we were waiting around, by Stephen Hawking, the brilliant English physicist. In it, he described black holes in space as matter turning into itself until it becomes so dense, it disappears. I wanted to turn into myself like a black hole and disappear.

I was sitting in a small reception area somewhere on the fifth floor, under one of the zillion paintings that line the walls, when Sug came and found me.

When I told her about the ninety days, she took my hand and sat down beside me. She was quiet for a long time, struggling through the moment as I was. She loved him too. She finally said the best possible thing in the world for her to say. The thing I needed to hear from her because she was involved as deeply as I was. The thing she knew I needed to know, even though I'd never asked, as if our shared gene pool had mingled for a moment. "Mama, let's take him home as soon as we can," she said. "You and I and Chris can take care of him at home."

Me and Sug and Chris. The two of them had been a handful, twenty-five years earlier, when they were born. Now, it seemed, they were going to give it back.

❧ *Kevin and I were married in December 1960. In February of 1961, I had a miscarriage. We must have gotten pregnant on our wedding night, which we spent in a motel in Shamrock, Texas on our way to California. That was our honeymoon—driving to California, where Kevin had taken up residence and where I was going to join him as Mrs. C. Kevin Craig. We were married in Oklahoma City in my parish church, the Cathedral of Our Lady of Perpetual Help. Father Bob, my brother, performed the ceremony. Marta, my sister, was my bridesmaid. The reception was at home, in our big, rambling frame house at 3100 North Olie—a wonderful family home with five bedrooms and a big front porch—even though it was across from Fairlawn Cemetery. Carl, Marta, and I had used the cemetery like a park as children. We'd stolen pecans from its trees in the fall, played tag behind tombstones, and dared each other to go on walks on moonless Halloween nights.*

Kevin and I were driving to California after the wedding in my 1954 Chevy coupe. The day before, Bob had used the car to go to the corner grocery and get a quart of milk and came back saying, "You can't drive to California in that. The brakes are about to go out." So my three brothers got my car fixed in the nick of time; nevertheless, a tire blew in Albuquerque, and the twenty dollars we spent on a new one taxed the honeymoon budget.

When we had the early miscarriage, the doctor told me that it wasn't a big deal. "It's nature's way of correcting problems. Every woman has two coming to her." And by June, I was pregnant again. I was working at my first job in advertising as a copywriter for Phil Lansdale, and by October I was having trouble finding maternity clothes big enough to work in. I'd already put fifty pounds on top of a skinny 115-

pound, five-seven frame. The doctors decided something was up and X-rayed. Lo and behold—twins.

They were due in mid-March and I quit working for Phil on January 31, so I'd have six weeks to get ready. But lo and behold again—they were born the next day. February 1, 1962. Kevin and I hadn't done a thing to get ready for them, as I was looking forward to doing it at my leisure after I quit work. We didn't have one diaper, one T-shirt, one blanket, or one bottle, much less two of anything. We didn't even have cribs. He went out and charged it all at Sears in Santa Monica while I was in the hospital. He had no idea what to buy, but some woman at Sears took pity and he actually did just fine. We brought the twins home to a tiny one-bedroom apartment in West LA, and they slept in little baskets on wheels in the living room. I didn't have any help. Indeed, it was a different era and it never occurred to me to get help. It never occurred to me I needed it. I mean, that's what women did. You had babies. You took care of them. I was twenty-four years old. Kevin was thirty-one. We had no idea yet he had atherosclerosis.

They were small—Sug was five pounds, Chris was five pounds seven ounces—so they had to be fed every two hours. And being small and less than full-term, they got colic and cried a lot. I didn't get enough sleep. I didn't know what I was doing, actually. If the pediatrician hadn't given me a paperback copy of Dr. Spock, I think I might have drowned the children at bath time or overfed them into insensibility. After a few days, our landlady, Paula, noticed what was going on and circled me like Indians circling the wagons. She was a Swedish woman in her seventies, long widowed and on her own but a mother of six in her time. She got into the habit of dropping in every morning, and again around noon, sizing up the situation and pointing me in the right direction.

"They don't have to sleep right next to each other," she'd say. "They wake each other up."

Or, on the other hand, "If you gave them a bath at the same time, it would save you work."

Paula helped me a lot. Indeed, she saved my life and (maybe theirs) and became part of our family—a grandmother away from home—until she moved away to Laguna Beach some years later.

I tried to dress the twins alike at first. Little-boy pants in blue, without ruffles. Little-girl pants in blue, with ruffles. But I quit it when Kevin said to me one day, "How'd you like to go through life, if you were a boy, dressed like your sister?"

People didn't notice as much that they were twins when they weren't dressed alike. I missed the attention for a while. But I finally decided one of the reasons twins are dressed alike to begin with is so the parents will get the attention. What other earthly reason is there to dress two children the same? After the first few months, when we'd had time to think about it, we cut out as much as we could of the "twin" business, because we thought it far more important to stress their differences than their sameness. They each had a right to be an individual child and shouldn't be raised as part of a twosome. We hardly ever referred to them as twins, just as my little boy and my little girl. In about a year, Chris was a lot bigger than Sug was and they quit being noticed as twins. When they started school, we were careful to see they never shared the same classroom. By the time all four of our children were born, people who knew we had twins often thought the twins were Erin and Maureen, who were only sixteen months apart and looked a lot alike. People still ask me today, "Now, which are the twins?" I think that's good. I think it's healthier if twins are allowed to just be two children, like any other two children in a family.

But they knew, of course, what they were. And the bond between them, while not fanatic, did exist. To this day, Sug understands Chris better than anyone, perhaps, save me. And he has a loyalty to her more fierce than to anyone, perhaps, save me.

Twenty-five years earlier, as Kevin and I shared two A.M. feedings, he holding one child and I the other, in the tiny apartment in West LA, no one could have dreamed up or believed the events that would lead me, my little girl, and my little boy to Cedars-Sinai and Ed McNeilly. ❧

October 13

FLORENCE WAS A NURSE ON THE FIFTH FLOOR. She was a six-foot-four black woman and while she was changing the bed, looking for all the world as if she could pick up the mattress with the same ease she picked up the pillows, I asked her why Ed seemed weaker today than yesterday.

"Shouldn't he be stronger today? The doctor said the surgery went beautifully. There were no complications."

"The first day after any surgery is a bad day," she said. "He's fine. Don't you worry."

"But he just doesn't seem right to me. He's so hyper."

"It's mental," she said. "He's afraid."

Ed was exhausted, but he couldn't sleep. I thought Florence was probably right. He was afraid. Afraid to shut his eyes. Afraid to go to sleep lest he not wake up. Afraid to cough. Afraid he'd gag in his sleep.

Eddie was still in town, spending his nights at the Westwood Marquis and his days with me and Ed at Cedars. We worked the *New York Times* Sunday crossword puzzle and worried that Ed was so edgy.

By nine o'clock at night, Ed was crawling the walls. He was in pain. He was exhausted. He felt no one was responding. I went to look for Dr. Kramer, the resident on the floor, but she was handling an emergency. Ed insisted that the head nurse phone Dr. Moore at home. She didn't want to. He kept insisting. And finally, she did. Dr. Moore ordered morphine.

Eddie and I were still there with him. Eddie was beginning to look as exhausted as Ed, but he never left my side and he never stopped helping. "I'm scared for him to start morphine, Eddie," I said. "Once you start morphine, you can't stop."

"It's okay. He'll sleep. I think it will be good. You have to take things one day at a time."

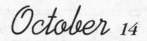

October 14

ED PHONED ME AT SIX-FIFTEEN in the morning. I could barely hear his voice.

"Could you come?"

I got scared and phoned the desk to talk to the nurse. She told me that even with the morphine, he hadn't slept through the night.

I skipped the niceties of getting dressed, threw on some jeans, and rushed to the hospital. Ed was very weak and mentally hazy, but the nurse said there were no new complications, nothing much had changed. Eddie came around nine o'clock. He was leaving at noon. We had one good, last talk. We talked about death, pain, and the days ahead. We talked about the ad agency, my children, Donna, Kim, Robin, the divorce, our marriage, all of it.

"Take care of yourself," Eddie told me before he left. "Don't take on the responsibility of Ed's children, or their mother, or their relationships with each other or your children. They're all adults. Take care of yourself."

I sat there by myself after he left and stared out the window. I could see the twin towers of Century City on the other side of Beverly Hills. I thought about what was going on at my office. I was missing a big-deal preproduction meeting, but I suddenly couldn't remember why it was a big deal or why anyone thought it was important that I be there. All I could think about was Alan Fogelman saying those same words to me ten years earlier.

✐ "Take care of yourself, Jeanie," Dr. Fogelman had said as I left his lab. "You have a lot going for you. Take care of yourself."

I'd come to see him a few weeks after Kevin died, at his invitation. He wanted to talk to me about Kevin and the children.

I followed the familiar color-coded lines up to the fifth floor at the UCLA Medical Center to the outpatient clinic in the Coronary Care unit.

"I'd like to see Dr. Fogelman," I said to the nurse behind the glass partition.

"He doesn't see patients on Tuesdays."

"I'm not a patient. I'm here to see him personally."

"May I have your name, please?"

"Mrs. Kevin Craig."

"Oh. I know your husband."

"My husband died a couple of weeks ago."

"Oh." Her voice sounded genuinely shocked and sorry. "I didn't know he had expired. He was a nice little man."

It startled me to hear Kevin referred to that way. A nice, little man. I must not have noticed how much his illness shrank his body during the last months. Or how much it shrank his inner person.

After a few minutes, Dr. Fogelman came to the waiting area and took me with him into the labrynthine recesses of the fifth floor till we found the dark and quiet of his lab.

Alan Fogelman at that time was head of Cardiac Research at UCLA. He was a slight man, thirty-seven years old. Shy. Quiet. He'd been Kevin's doctor for the past seven years. Being a researcher, and head of a department, he wasn't really anyone's doctor anymore. He had largely quit seeing patients, but a bond had developed between him and Kevin, and Alan had remained involved and kept Kevin's routine monthly appointments at the Med Center.

I found in Alan the differences I'd found all my life between doctors who are researchers and doctors who are in private practice. Like Dr. Ewen at the City of Hope, and Dr. Beckman at UCLA, Alan was a fighter. He wasn't in medicine to treat but to win, to beat the shit out of heart disease and get rid of it. He also took a personal approach to his patients and got to know them as people. At least he did with Kevin. Somehow, he got to know him well enough that he never saw him as a postal clerk, who wore clothes that never fit and who did odd things like carry this big black bag full of stuff.

He got to know him well enough to see the same things in Kevin that I did. A mind so strong he could lose Lord knows how much of it to atherosclerosis and still function. A passion for life that literally kept him alive. An understanding of the human heart, including mine. And the ability to see things in this world that others don't, like fear preventing a six-year-old from putting on new glasses at school, not orneriness like the teacher said.

During the time he was Kevin's doctor, I carried with me all of Alan's phone numbers: his office, his lab, his home, his private line in Cardiac Research. He made me feel I could call him anytime. And I did from time to time. When Kevin went on Questran and we discovered it was going to cost several hundred dollars a month, Alan phoned me and told me how to get it cheaper. He got our children into the Pediatric Coronary Care Unit and kept up with them, as well as with Kevin. He took a personal interest in Aunt Maureen, and also in Kevin's father when he ended up at UCLA.

We took Kevin to UCLA Emergency the morning he died and after a few minutes, it was Alan who walked into the waiting room and found us. It was Alan who told us that Kevin was dead. He was crying when he said it.

We sat down in his lab on that morning and he began telling me about the research he was doing.

"Atherosclerosis isn't really a blood disease," he said. "It's a cellular dysfunction. The cells don't do what they're supposed to do in processing fats. It's like diabetes, where the cells don't do what they're supposed to do in processing sugar."

He drew some diagrams of a cell and showed me how it all works.

"I don't want you to be worried about your children," he said. "We're working on it. And we're getting close. In time, we'll have a drug for atherosclerosis just like we have insulin for diabetes."

"See that they take care of themselves," he went on. "I can guarantee them ten years more life if they never smoke. Make them stick with their diets. Encourage them to exercise. By the time they're as old as you are now, we'll have an answer for them."

Then he told me some things about Kevin.

"We did an autopsy. His arteries were in such bad shape. More than you could imagine. All over his body."

"Alan," I said, "I feel so guilty. I feel like I didn't call the paramedics fast enough. I thought he was having another seizure. I didn't know he was dying."

He took my hand. "Oh Jeanie, his situation was so tenuous. Any little thing could have caused him to die. For years and years and years. He finally had a heart attack. There's no way he could have survived it, no matter what you did."

He paused for what seemed like a long time. And when he spoke *again it was as if he were telling me something that was a newfound truth for him. A fresh revelation. A belief he had not always held.*

"I want you to tell your children something. Tell them that there's only one reason their father lived the last five years of his life. It's because he decided to."

We talked a few more minutes; then he guided me through the rows of beakers and Bunson burners and test tubes, back out to the reception area.

"Remember to take care of yourself," he said. "I know how much you have going for you. Kevin talked about it all the time. Take care of yourself." ❧

I was shaken from my reverie when Dr. Kanon came into the room. I was so glad to see him, I wanted to shout. Eddie was gone. I was alone. There was some reason Ed wasn't improving and I was afraid we wouldn't have even the ninety days. I had no one to talk to. I didn't know what to do. Dr. Kanon took one look at Ed and then looked at me.

"We have a problem here. There's something the matter."

He moved quickly and did an examination.

"There's fluid in the lungs," he said. "We're going to drain it right now."

"Right now?"

"Right now."

"Right here in the room?"

"Right here in the room."

Suddenly the room was filling with people—nurses, technicians, and young Dr. Kramer, who was going to assist. They were moving like the players in an intricate Japanese drama. There was a scenario in place but I was the only one who didn't know what it was. I asked if I should leave.

"No. Stay here. He's more relaxed with you here."

God, I liked Dr. Kanon.

So I watched while they inserted a long needle into Ed's lungs, right through the skin in the middle of his back. In about an hour's time, beginning to end, they removed two liters of reddish-brown fluid from his lungs.

"No wonder he was weak," said Dr. Kanon.

"Is he going to be okay now?"

"I wish I could tell you, Mrs. McNeilly, that the fluid is the aftermath of the surgery, but I don't think it is. The tumor is just spreading to beat hell. I'm not sure, but it might be one thing after another now. You may not be able to take him home."

The wallops were coming so fast, one on top of the other. He's better. He's worse. He's got a window. He doesn't. He can go home. He can't. I didn't even feel them anymore.

Ed was sitting up on the edge of the bed while they drained the fluid. When they were finished, he needed to use the commode. Florence was helping him walk the one or two steps toward the commode when he collapsed first into her arms and then crumpled to the floor. He was gasping for breath. The room filled up again with people. Doctors and nurses descended from all over. An oxygen mask went onto his face. An oxygen-monitoring device went into his arm. The strain of sitting up and trying to take a step had been too much.

Dr. Moore came a few minutes later.

"Ed is very weak, Jean. There's a limit to how aggressive we can be. I need to know how you feel about life-support systems."

"What?"

"Life-support systems."

"What do you mean?"

"Machines to keep him alive."

"Oh." I was so startled. For the first time, I realized—really understood—that Ed was near death. "I, well,...of course, no. No. We don't want to put him on machines."

I walked in a daze to the pay phone in the hall and called Sug.

"Can you come?"

"I'm on my way, Mama."

I phoned Robin in Florida and told her to come. I could hardly talk when I told her. I phoned Marty and told him Ed might not make it through the night and if there was anything that needed to be done regarding his will, he'd better do it right now. I phoned Chris. Eric, Kim, and Mark. I phoned Maureen in New York and told her to come. We couldn't find Erin in Boston, but Chris began phoning and leaving messages all over the East Coast. I phoned Longview to find Carl, and Jacque went out to get him off an oil rig. When he called me back, he said they were already on their way. I asked him to phone our brothers and sister, Howard in Dallas, Bob in Oklahoma City, and Marta in Iowa City. I asked him to ask Bob if he would do the funeral service. I phoned Bob Kresser. Annie. Alan and Stacie. Monty. Brantz and Wendy.

I sat with Ed all afternoon. People and friends I'd phoned and people and friends they'd phoned began quietly showing up in the hall.

Jack and Nancy Foster. Marge Powell. John Tripp. At one point, Ed pulled me close and said, "I know what you're doing. You're gathering the family. I love you." Eric took me out of the hospital for an hour to have dinner and asked if I'd tended to financial things and whether there was anything he could do.

The things were happening, the questions were being asked that a woman dreads all her life—have you made a will? is there insurance? does your lawyer know? what about a funeral? a cemetery? is there anything I can do? Somehow, we all expect to outlive our men.

Around nine P.M., Chris, Sug, and I were alone in Ed's room and we decided to spend the night.

"I can't go home, Sug."

"I'll stay with you, Mama."

"So will I, Mom."

Chris piled up blankets and pillows and slept on the floor, beside Ed's bed, while Sug and I took turns napping on a couch down the hall and keeping a vigil in the room. Every now and then, Ed would wake up and look around to see if we were there. He seemed to feel he could sleep because someone was in the room. Then, around three A.M., the vomiting started.

Ed had on an oxygen mask and threw up into the mask. Sug and I were both there and ran to help. He was too weak to push his buzzer for a nurse. If we hadn't been in the room, that would have been the end of it, right then. He'd have suffocated in the mask.

The fluid he was throwing up was bile. I recognized it from the post-op period at the City of Hope. It's a bright-green fluid you don't forget. He began throwing up more and more of it, about every fifteen or twenty minutes.

Sug, Chris, and I became a team with Olga, the night nurse. She was a tiny woman, really tiny—four foot six. But she became a big hero. As I watched her I knew if she hadn't done what she did, Ed would never have made it through the night. She decided to take him on and simply made up her mind to stop the vomiting.

What's astounding and frightening is that it was more or less her choice. No one would have criticized her if she'd chosen to be less aggressive. No one would even have noticed. Cedars is terribly under-staffed when it comes to nurses. Not because they don't have the money, but because they don't have the nurses. Olga was stretched thin as a penny rubber band that night. Every time she took care of Ed, she was being called to go someplace else. She didn't know what was caus-ing the vomiting. It seemed impossible to stop. The residents on the floor were unavailable. She had other patients who were just as sick. But, like I said, she made up her mind to stop it. And she did.

First she tried a nausea depressant you take by mouth. When that didn't work, she found Dr. Kramer, who was handling an emergency, to see about a tube down the throat to drain the stomach.

"I don't know why he's throwing up," Dr. Kramer said. "But it seems to mean there's liver involvement. And considering the condition he's in right now, a tube down the throat would be too invasive. I'm afraid it would do more harm than good."

So Olga came back and tried suppositories. But that didn't work either. She gave him morphine to calm him, thinking that might work. She tried suppositories again.

She finally got Dr. Kramer to order an injection of a nausea-suppressing drug. And that did it. Ed fell into a deep sleep and didn't throw up for a couple of hours.

He made it through the night. But he was obviously getting weaker and weaker.

October 15

ALL DAY LONG, ED WAS DYING. Chris, Sug, and I took turns going home for a few minutes, as dawn began to break. Ed could barely lift his hand when I came back into the room after the trip out to Malibu and back.

Alicia phoned the hospital when she arrived at the house and found everyone gone.

"I think he's slipping, Alicia."

"Oh no, Jean. It can't be." I heard genuine agony in her voice. "Can I come, Jean? Can I stay with you at the hospital?"

"Of course you can."

The doctors came and went—Moore, Kanon, Kramer, Pinella. Then a woman came, walked toward me, and suddenly put her arms around me. I didn't know who she was, but something made me realize after a few seconds that it was Donna. "No one knows but you and me what a dear man he is," she said. Then she added, "If only I'd had some warning, if only I'd known. I'm so unprepared."

She asked if she could see Ed and the question put me in a quandary. I certainly thought she had a right to see him and could understand her wanting to. But I was afraid she'd be a jolt to him. I thought about going in with her, but the melodrama of the wife and the ex-wife who'd never met now standing at the foot of the bed was demeaning. Then I remembered Kim was on her way. I asked Donna to wait a few minutes for Kim to arrive so she could go in with her daughter. She went to the waiting room to do that, but when Kim came and went to look for her, she was gone.

I felt badly that she left. She must have felt rejected. On the other hand, she could have phoned or come with Kim instead of just showing up like that. The whole thing left me shaken. And I didn't know who I felt worse for. Her or me.

Sug and Chris were there all day. Maureen arrived from New York around noon, looking as haggard as a twenty-one-year-old could look. We sat in Ed's room and spilled over into the hallway. Stunned. In shock. Alicia, with dark Spanish eyes deepened by the harshness of her twenty-nine years, looked like a pain-ravaged waif as she sat on the edge of his bed and held his hand. I looked into the faces of my children and saw the raw edges of grief. I thought I'd never seen so much hurt or emotion in the eyes of my son.

"I think sometimes," Sug said to me, "it was planned that Ed should be with us when he died, because we love him so."

Mark and Kim stood with me in the hall and I asked them some questions about a funeral. I wanted them to know I'd respect their wishes as well as my own. I found myself to be amazingly calm. Like the eye of a tornado. Or perhaps I'd removed myself from the scene. I was physically there, but my heart and soul were in a netherworld where there were no feelings.

The day dragged on. People came and went. Ed would slip in and out of consciousness. Then, sometime during the late afternoon, something changed.

It's hard to know what happened. It's like the moment in time when the tide that's been coming in with the momentum created by a hundred thousand square miles of water pushing toward the shore stops coming in. And in a split second, starts going out.

During the eternity of some unknown split second that Thursday afternoon in October, the tide of Ed's life reversed.

He was no longer dying. He was rallying. He stayed conscious, started to talk, could lift his arm to take my hand, asked for water.

"It's like his body just kicked in," was the way Chris put it.

By the time Robin arrived at six in the evening, our grief had changed to hope. The whispered droplets of conversation that had sustained us during the day turned to tiny puddles of talk.

Annie gathered up my family and took them home to dinner. The friends and relatives who'd kept vigil quietly dispersed in relieved groups of twos and threes.

By nine o'clock, I was alone with Ed when Carl, who'd come straight to Cedars from LAX, came tentatively into the room. He was clutching Jacque's hand and my big brother and his wife looked at me like two small, frightened children.

"How is he, Jeanie?"

"Oh, Carl," I said. "I'm so glad to see you and Jacque. We thought he was going to die today, but then he didn't." They stayed with me until midnight. Jacque held my hand and stroked my hair; then I stayed the night again. But there was no throwing up. Ed slept. And so did I, on a chair that turns into a bed, brought to me by Olga from some secret resource known only to her.

October 16

ED WAS BETTER. His arms and legs, which had become grossly swollen because his liver wasn't working, began to return to normal. He hadn't thrown up for twenty-four hours. He was conscious. He recognized people. He could talk. His color was back.

"I'm not making any more guesses about Ed," Dr. Kanon said when he made his rounds. "He proves me wrong."

Kim and Robin spent the morning taking care of him as a team and Ed was beaming. It was the first time the three of them had been together in six years. The rest of us got out of the way and let them have him.

My children were all gathered around. Erin had finally arrived from Boston at midnight. People were phoning. There was a sense of elation, even more than a sense of relief. I began telling everyone who phoned to join us for "dinner at Cedars." And that evening, a wonderful, loving melee of family and friends crowded into Ed's room and the adjoining waiting area. We ate designer pizza from California Pizza Kitchens and drank the good red wine that Alan and Stacie brought by the caseful. Simon came from the car wash, wearing a suit and carrying the largest bouquet of flowers I had ever seen.

"How many cars today, Simon?" Ed rasped as Simon entered the room.

"Four hundred and twenty, Ed. It's a record for a Friday."

Ed sent a clenched fist into the air. The whole room cheered.

October 19

THE WEEKEND CAME AND WENT. Friends and family came and went. Ed was up and down. Carl and Jacque took me to lunch at Trumps before they went back to Longview. "Take it one day at a time," they advised. Eddie phoned from Pound Ridge. "Take it one day at a time," he advised.

Ed had rallied on Thursday, it was now Monday, and the days were getting seamless again. I'd spent every night in the hospital, sleeping on the chair/bed. Ed didn't seem to be getting any better, but he didn't seem to be getting any worse. I was the one who was getting worse. I was pooped. I hadn't seen Dr. Moore since Friday. Dr. Kanon, Dr. Kramer, and Dr. Pinella, the resident on the floor, were all involved, but I concluded they didn't know any more about what was going on than I did. That's why everyone kept saying "take it a day at a time."

By the time Monday morning came around, I knew what I wanted to do. "We're getting you out of here," I told Ed. "We're going home."

Whatever happened next—good, bad, or indifferent—I wanted it to happen at home. A hospital is no place to be sick and it's a rotten place to die.

Cedars was crowded and chaotic. It was noisy and unnerving. There weren't enough nurses. They didn't have time to sit at Ed's bedside and help him eat, and try as they might, they couldn't check often enough to keep his bed dry. His monitors would beep and not be noticed. I'd been spending the night because I was afraid to leave him alone. What's more, the sense of turmoil was so constant. The night seemed to be almost as frantic as the day.

I didn't know how we'd manage to care for Ed at home, but I knew that's where he needed to be. And that's where he was going.

October 21

IT TOOK ME TWO DAYS, with Chris and Sug's help, to make arrangements at home.

Ed couldn't walk or get to the bathroom. He was on oxygen, which required equipment—morphine, antibiotics, and an array of other drugs to control nausea, diarrhea, edema, and other problems of the moment. He had a huge bedsore at the tip of his spine. He was wearing diapers. We were going to have to turn the house into a mini-hospital and I barely knew where to start. So I phoned Robin and over the phone from Orlando she helped me figure out what equipment we'd need. She advised me to get full-time nursing care, at least to start.

A social worker at Cedars put me in touch with a nursing service as well as Bowers, a medical-supply company, and that is the sum total of the help they offered in transitioning Ed to home. Nobody told me what to expect, gave me any advice, or even handed me a brochure. I got no instructions, no tips, no nutritional information, no lessons in emptying bedpans, no education on the drugs he was taking, and very little encouragement, one way or the other. A nurse named Carol was to come into the picture and be of enormous help, but nobody told me about Carol to ease my mind and let me know help was on the way. Like Maggie and home infusion, we didn't know about her until she showed up at the front door. But despite the lack of help, we managed.

In retrospect, so much of nursing and caring for the sick is common sense. My Aunt Viola was a nursing nun for fifty years, and I kept recalling her making that comment to my mother. The memory helped and gave me courage. But what helped most of all were Chris and Sug. They took on their stepfather's problem with me, as if it were their own.

Bowers was terrific. A few hours after I talked to them on the phone, they delivered the equipment we needed to turn our house into a clinic: a hospital bed, a bed table, a commode, a walker, a wheelchair, and oxygen equipment. We also got boxes and boxes of plastic pads to keep the sheets dry, plastic buckets, bed pans, urinal bottles, spit trays, plastic cups, glasses and straws, a thermometer, a heating pad, and an ice bag. We got the long plastic tubes that go from the nose to the oxygen tanks. We got single-bed sheets, because I didn't have any, plus blankets and smaller pillows. Sug went out and bought the supplies and arranged to be at home when Bowers came with the big stuff.

The oxygen equipment scared us at first. Bowers dropped off a huge tank of compressed oxygen, plus two smaller, portable units that could be filled from the larger tank. The tank was full of gauges and dials that monitored the flow, the richness of the mixture, and let you know when the supply was low. The tanks were marked with warnings and they hissed and hummed. It was like dealing with a bomb. Touch it wrong and it'll explode.

The Bowers technician, who arrived with the tanks, trained Sug to use them, and she trained me. It wasn't that hard, really, but it was scary enough that nobody else in the family ever got near them. In time, Sug and I kicked the tanks around like you kick around your car when it won't start. But at first, we were scared and felt any wrong move would affect Ed's well-being, if not blow up the house. Sug had a lot of poise, and I kept remembering Aunt Viola.

Then, there were the nurses. I discovered later on through Aunt Maureen and St. John's that there are excellent, really excellent nursing services, but the one the social worker at Cedars put me in touch with was not one of them. She should have given me a list, as St. John's ultimately did, but she gave me one name. And that's who I called. What did I know?

A good nursing service will send a supervisor to meet the patient, discuss the case with the doctor, and look over the situation in the home. Then the supervisor will help you work out what you need. Instead, I had only a disconcerting talk over the phone and was pummeled with questions I wasn't sure how to answer.

"Do you want three eight-hour shifts? Two twelve-hour? Or a live-in?"

"Do you need an RN? An LVN? Or a nurse's aide?"

"What will your insurance company cover?"

"Is the patient on heavy or light medication?" It was all heavy to me.

"Do you need cleaning and cooking, as well as nursing?"

We finally worked it all out, but I felt like I didn't know what I was doing or what I was getting into. We agreed on a live-in, six days a week. Sug and I would handle the seventh day. I was told the nurse's name was Jessie.

"Do I get to meet her first?"

"Well, no, … she's working someplace else right now. But she's quite competent."

I had to assume she was. Assume we'd like her. Assume Ed would like her. Assume we could live with her six days a week.

Then, there was the question of where to put Ed and the hospital bed. All the bedrooms were upstairs. But even if there hadn't been the problem of the stairs, putting the bed and patient in a bedroom takes them away from the center of things. Out of the action, so to speak. I talked with Chris and Sug and we decided to set Ed up right in the middle of the living room.

"He should have life going on around him," I said. "He should be in the center of things."

They were sympatico and we rearranged the house. We moved living-room couches into the dining room and put side chairs in the garage. If there were people in the house not involved with Ed, they could conduct their business or their visiting in the dining room or the kitchen. When people came to see Ed, I didn't want to escort them to a darkened bedroom, off to the side. They'd find Ed McNeilly in his living room, holding court, with his TV clicker in one hand and his portable phone in the other.

So the hospital bed, the commode, the oxygen tanks, the urinal bottles—all of it went into the living room, smack in front of the fireplace. We started answering the phone "Cedars, Malibu."

Dr. Kanon came to Ed's room right before we left and drained fluid from the lungs one more time. I looked at him, the intern, the nurse, the oxygen monitor beeping beside Ed's bed, the inhaler, the IV trees, the jungle-gym of equipment that surrounded the bed. "Nobody at Cedars Malibu knows what the hell they're doing," I mumbled to myself. "Stick with me, Aunt Viola," I mumbled to myself.

From the time we decided to take Ed home on Monday until we left the hospital on Wednesday, I didn't see Dr. Moore. I had no idea how Ed was going to be handled by the doctor while at home. When the nurse at Cedars handed me the release papers, she said, "Dr. Moore said for you to call about bringing Ed in for an appointment in a week or so."

"Bring him in for an appointment? My God, he's going home in an ambulance. He's on oxygen. He can't walk. How am I going to bring him in for an appointment?"

The nurse shrugged her shoulders. "All I know is that's what he said to tell you."

And so we took him home. The ambulance followed me to La Cienega, to the Santa Monica Freeway, to Pacific Coast Highway, to Malibu. When we got to the house, a pink 1970 Cadillac was parked in the driveway and Jessie was standing in front of it.

Ed saw her, saw the car, and laughed out loud. Being a car nut, the classic pink Cadillac established a bond, even though he'd never met her before.

"Get that Cadillac out of my way, Jessie," he called to her. "I'm coming through." The ambulance drivers carried him on the gurney into the house.

And Cedars Malibu was in business.

October 22

IT WAS GOOD HAVING ED AT HOME.
I had my feet on my own turf, for one thing, and my head on my own
pillow at night. And so did he. He could look out the window and see
the things he loved. The ocean, the Plumeria, the trumpet vine. He
could eat off his own dishes, drink from his own glasses, wear his own
pajamas. He could feel the bustle of Sug running the dishwasher in the
kitchen, rather than the bustle of a nurse running an IV in the next
room. In the normalcy of being at home, he quickly became less sick.
He stopped being stressed and hyper on the one hand, or hazy and half-
conscious on the other. He started sleeping at night. He started trying
to eat three meals. Even though there was a hospital bed in the middle
of the living room and a nurse in the house, the normalcy was a million
times greater than that at Cedars, and Ed responded.

I never doubted the decision to bring him home. That doesn't
mean it was easy.

Item No. 1 to get past is the gross stuff. Bowel movements and the
attendant problems of bedpans, urinals, adult diapers, diarrhea, accidents, and messes, as well as dealing with vomiting, giving shots, and
putting salves on bedsores. It may seem a big barrier at first, but it's a lot
like having a baby in the house. You clean up messes of all sorts with
babies, but after a while you don't even think about them. In time, Sug
and I were more concerned about keeping messes off the bed, so we
wouldn't have to change it again, than we were about the mess itself—
whatever dire source it came from.

Item No. 2 is fear. You're afraid you're going to do something wrong.
Medicate too much or too little. Hook up the oxygen wrong. Cook the
wrong foods. Handle the equipment improperly. Nobody told me it's
okay to make a mistake, but it is. You can screw up once in a while, and
it's okay. If you give morphine twice in a row because you forgot, the
patient won't die. If you set the oxygen meter wrong overnight, which I
did, he won't die either. If his fever shoots up and you can't reach the
doctor, it's no mistake to medicate on your own, using your own common sense. Give him aspirin and sponge him with cold cloths, just like
you did when your kids were little. As a matter of fact, I dug out my dog-
eared copy of Dr. Spock and used it as a practical guide for dealing with
tons of little everyday problems, like constipation.

Item No. 3. It's all a lot of work. Physical work. You need to be ready
for it and it's a factor in whether to bring someone home. There's a lot of

laundry, meals have to be served on trays, and the patient has to be shaved and bathed in bed. We learned early that Ed didn't like to be left alone, even for five minutes. He was afraid because he was immobile and helpless. I remember my mother feeling the same when she was bedridden. So someone has to be close by all the time. And that person is doing a lot of lifting, running, jumping, and fetching.

And then there's the mental stress. Most sick people are demanding rather than grateful. They're very focused on themselves and their bodies. They become inward and sometimes unpleasant. They're also bored, and they want your time. But all of those things happen whether or not you bring someone home. You need to be prepared to be very patient. In fact, I don't know how "patient" became the term for the sick person, because he certainly isn't. It's the caretaker who needs to assume the demeanor of Job.

But I asked Sug once how she felt about having Ed at home, and she said, "Mama, that was a very happy time for me. I felt so fulfilled."

The first thing we did with Ed was try to get a routine going. That was very important. And again, it's just common sense. First, breakfast. Then, the bath. Then, time to get him sitting up in a chair. There's security in a routine for the patient and less stress for the caretaker. It's like running anything—a home, a school, a business—it works better if there's some order to it.

I slept beside Ed on the couch in the living room and Jessie slept in the guest room, because I wanted to tend to him myself as much as I could. In the mornings I fixed his breakfast, while she did the routine of bath, changing the bed, shaving, brushing teeth, and medication.

Jessie was a black woman who had grown up in rural Arkansas. She spoke with the colloquialisms and casualness of that part of the world. By the time I'd known her fifteen minutes, I knew all about her divorce, her married daughter in Missouri, and what she thought about nursing at Cedars.

"My Lord, it wore me out workin' there. I took it for six years, but you know they don't care about people. You work a twelve-hour shift, they ask you to stay another four. They don't care. Goodness knows, they don't."

I went back to work. Actually, I'd been in and out of the office all along, but I went back now to a regular day. Jessie, who was a LVN, took care of Ed and the laundry and the meals, which had been a question. A lot of LVNs won't do anything but nurse. And nurse's aides, who will do whatever you ask, aren't usually covered by insurance. Insurance companies argue that a patient must be sick enough to require an RN or LVN before they'll pay for home care. But in my opinion, most home care could be well-handled by a nurse's aide, at about a third of the cost.

Alicia was also there two days a week, and she reported to me on Jessie. Whether I asked her to or not.

"Jessie is okay, but she talks a lot and tries to tell Ed what to do. Nobody can tell Ed what to do, Jean."

"I know, Alicia."

"I can take care of Ed, Jean. Anytime you want, I can do it."

"Alicia, you'd have to quit your other daytime jobs."

"That's okay, Jean."

"And you'd have to stay until I got home from work. Alicia, I don't get home sometimes until after six."

"It's not for the rest of my life, Jean. And I know more than Jessie."

I suspected that she did. Although in the first few days, we all learned a lot from Jessie—the nitty-gritty, so to speak, of home hospital care. We learned the inestimable value of Lysol and Mr. Clean through-out Cedars Malibu. A little in the urinals and commode and frequent use in the bathroom got rid of odor problems. Jessie taught us how to give a bath in bed. That you'd better write down every pill you gave, and what time you gave it, or you'll get confused. She set a routine of check-ing certain things every four hours. Temperature. Oxygen. Blood pres-sure. She taught us it's always a good idea to have a plastic bucket near the bed for accidents. We learned about dusting talcum powder on bedpans. Ed dubbed his urinal bottle "the pissoire." We learned it's smart to keep two of them handy, one hooked to each side of the hospital bed.

Ed, who had enormous candor in intimate moments, was nonethe-less a modest man during our marriage. He used the bathroom by him-self. But now, he lost all sense of modesty with me, which might be expected. But also with Sug. It was surprising to me how he let her tend to him. It was equally surprising to me that she did it.

"I love you, Sug," I told her one morning, "for helping with Ed the way you do. But I'm surprised you can do it."

"So am I, Mama. I don't think I could for anyone else. Maybe you," she smiled.

Partly by instinct, partly by design, Ed quickly made an effort to take control of his situation, his home, and Jessie. Being Ed, he was successful.

"It's time for you to take your medication now, Ed," Jessie would say.

"What are you giving me?"

"This red pill is morphine, the little tiny one is Ativan, and the capsule is Dulcolax. If it was me, of course, I wouldn't give you Dulcolax. I'm a strong believer in Metamucil, but...."

"I don't want any more morphine."

"Now Ed, you know I've got to give you what the doctors at Cedars said to give you. I don't like to argue now, with the doctors, Ed. Lord knows, I could get in trouble, Ed, ... now, just let me...."

"I'll take the Ativan and the Dulcolax, and you write down that I didn't take the morphine and you ask me again in four hours if I want morphine and I'll let you know."

He sent Chris out for a fifty-foot telephone cord so the phone could sit on his bed.

"Now that's not a good idea, Ed," said Jessie. "That fool thing'll wake you up every time it rings."

"I want to answer the phone myself," he said. "I don't want you to answer it for me and take messages. If I want you to take it away so I can sleep, I'll tell you."

I thought Jessie was probably used to a more conventional environment, where the nurse was left alone in the bedroom with the patient and had control over everything that had to do with the patient.

That was not the case with us. We didn't carry on separately. Ed was in the middle of the family life and family life was in the middle of Ed's illness. And it was somewhat disconcerting to Jessie.

I got home from work early one Friday evening. "I'll cook dinner, Jessie."

"That's fine. I'll just fix something for Ed and me."

"No. I'll cook dinner for all of us, and I'll take care of Ed the rest of the evening."

"But that's my job. You shouldn't be doin' that."

"I want to, Jessie. I want to take care of Ed every chance I get."

"All right," she sulked. "I'll be in my room."

"No. Come on, have dinner with the rest of us. Then we're going to watch a movie."

So Ed and me, Sug Chris, and Jessie ate Mom's pot roast and watched *Hoosiers* together on the VCR. Jessie was a little uncomfortable at first. But by the end of the evening, I thought she was buying the program. Ed was going to be involved in the family. The family was going to be involved in Ed's care. The nursing staff needed to adapt to that way of doing things. Institutional people have trouble bending. But Jessie had to admit she did like the movie.

October 23

ED PHONED DR. MOORE'S OFFICE
("I'll do it myself, Jean. I can do it.") to get his appointment for Monday.

"I want to get back on a program. I don't want to lie here and do nothing. I want him to do whatever's left."

When Ed talked to Louise, he was told he couldn't come in on Monday. They were booked. It would have to be Tuesday. Ed was frustrated and really angry when he got off the phone. He beat his fist into a pillow and let flow tears of rage.

"How can they not make room for me on Monday? They're responsible for me and I'm not being treated. No one wants to take responsibility, Jean. It makes me so angry."

There was anguish in his voice along with the anger. He'd hoped that Dr. Moore would phone him. That he would say, "Ed, here's how I want you to handle things for the next few days until you can come see me. But I want to see you as soon as possible, and we're going to put you on a new program. In the meantime, hang in there, Ed. You pulled yourself through at the hospital. You're doing great."

I hadn't told Ed about the ninety days. He wouldn't have believed it anyway and I wasn't sure I believed it myself. But I thought Dr. Moore believed it, which, of course, he had every right to do. And that because of it, he'd made Ed a low-priority patient. Which he hadn't any right to do.

I think everybody who sees a doctor has a right to the best the doctor has to offer. Perhaps when you're dealing with advertising campaigns or selling insurance, or putting in plumbing systems, you can have A, B, and C jobs, or clients, or tasks. But you can't do that when you're dealing with people. It's not fair. Nobody has the right.

When is a practice too big? When is a doctor spread too thin? How many patients and cases are too many for one day? How many operations? There are no guidelines. There are guidelines for how long a pilot can fly a 747 without rest. No more than so many hours. No more than so many days a month. That's because people's lives are involved. Yet in the profession where people's lives are at risk more than any other, there are no guidelines. Medicine and the people in it do what they want. And much of the time, in order to spread themselves over a caseload that's just too big, they prioritize.

Isn't there some better way than that? Shouldn't a patient, even a dying one—especially a dying one, some might say—have the best that medicine has to offer?

Shouldn't he?
Shouldn't he?

October 25

IT WAS "OH, SHIT!" WEEK AT THE CAR WASH. Aurora would phone. "Jean, something came in the mail and it looks like Ed never took out a business license for the City. Do you think he did? My goodness, it looks here like we're nine weeks late."

"Oh, shit."

Chris would phone. "The cash register broke. We're trying to take money by hand, but it won't work for long. Do you have any idea who to phone?"

"Oh, shit."

Joh Koppel, our controller, would phone. "Do you realize that Aurora hasn't been paying Workman's Comp or State Equalization taxes? That's a felony, you know."

"Oh, shit."

Sug would phone. "Mama, this man is threatening to sue because he says we ran his car into the telephone pole across the street. And his insurance company wants to talk to our insurance company. Do we have an insurance company?"

"Oh, shit."

Prudence, the bookkeeper, would phone. "Uh...Jean, I just want to tell you...uh...there's only 1,800 dollars in the checking account. I'm sure you know. But, well...that's not enough for payroll...."

"Oh, shit!"

Finally Simon phoned. "Señora, I think you and Chrees (he always called my son Chrees) need to come on Saturday for a staff meeting."

"A staff meeting?" Just like the advertising agency.

"Yes. These guys are driving me crazy. We need to talk about company policies."

"Company policies?"

"We need to get some things straightened out. Can you and Chrees be here when we close on Saturday at six?"

A staff meeting at the car wash. "We'll be there, Simon," I said.

So at six on Saturday, Chris and I arrived. We did some business in the office. I looked over the books. Scary. Simon told us we needed to talk to the men about overtime, wearing uniforms, and rotation for tips; also, Joe Wright, the assistant manager, had some things he wanted to get off his chest.

The men assembled in the car-wash boutique. About twenty-five Latino guys. Simon. Joe. Me. Chris. Simon started the meeting. I was ready to be the wise Señora. Sorting out problems. Bringing judgment to bear. Benevolent, but firm. You remember—Barbara Stanwyck on the ranch.

But the meeting was all in Spanish and I didn't have the least idea what was going on. Simon was pounding his fists. Then one of the men got the floor and said something that made the others cheer.

"What're they saying, Simon? What're they saying?"

"Not now, Señora. I got to handle this." There was more shouting and waving of arms. One guy walked out. A couple of others started waving their red wiping towels. Then Simon gave the floor to Joe Wright. He was the only non-Latino on the crew, a handsome, hard-working, fiftyish black man. Joe was speaking English and I understood what he was saying, but nobody else did. Well, Chris did.

"Simon, you've got to translate."

"It's not necessary, Señora. Joe always says the same thing. And the men know."

"Oh."

"But it's important he gets to say it, you know?"

"Oh."

Then, suddenly, the meeting ended. Everybody seemed happy. A lot of the men came up to me and smiled, or said, "Buenos tardes, Señora."

"Simon, what happened at this meeting?"

"No problema, Señora. We worked everything out."

"Worked what out? Why was I here, Simon?"

"It's good you were here. It means you back me up. It means you care about them, you know."

And suddenly I did know. Robertson Car Wash may not have been IBM. But to the men who worked there, it was close. It was the company they worked for and its senior management was me and my son. Seeing us was important to them. Smart man, Simon.

But it was still an "Oh, shit!" week at the car wash.

October 27

THE TIME HAD COME TO TAKE ED TO THE DOCTOR. First of all, I borrowed Bob's Ford Bronco, because I didn't think Ed could get in and out of my small car, nor did I think that I could get his wheelchair into it. Then I asked two young men from my office to meet me at the house at eleven A.M. with the Bronco. It took Jessie and me from eight until eleven to get Ed ready. It was the first time he'd been dressed in street clothes since the twenty-ninth of September, when he was admitted at the hospital. It was very difficult for him to put on underwear, a T-shirt, and socks. Jessie and I struggled, because while he'd lost a lot of weight, he was still a big man. His pants wouldn't stay up and I didn't have smaller belts. I finally had to tie his pants on with an old necktie.

We filled both of the portable oxygen tanks. But it was the first time we'd used them and we weren't exactly sure what we were doing. Each tank was good for only two hours and Ed was panicky we'd run out, because it was a forty-five-minute drive each way.

When Darryl and Jerry got to the house, they got on either side of Ed as he sat on the edge of the bed, picked him up, carried him to the Bronco, and lifted him in. Then we loaded up the wheelchair and the oxygen, plus Ed's medication, boxes of Kleenex, extra diapers, just in case, and extra oxygen lines. When we got to Dr. Moore's medical building, they picked him up again and lifted him into the wheelchair. Then one of them pushed him while the other followed with the oxygen tanks. We got him to Dr. Moore's waiting room; then they waited in the coffee shop downstairs while Ed saw the doctor. Then we reversed the whole process when we took him home. We didn't get back to the house until around two, with the oxygen barely lasting.

I wondered what people do who didn't have the resources. I had a company and could ask two people who work for us to take off the better part of a day. I could ask Bob for his Bronco. I could take the day off myself. If someone less fortunate than I had to get Ed to the doctor that day, what would she have done? How would she have managed?

No one in Dr. Moore's office asked me how I got him there or seemed to give it any thought. Nor was there any comfort in the rest of the visit. The doctor and his staff handled Ed with detached politeness. Dr. Moore asked Ed how he was feeling, did a cursory examination, and turned to leave.

"I want to start whatever you have left," Ed said.

"We will, Ed. But you're still too sick. I'll see you again in a week and we'll talk about it then."

And that was that.

November 2

SOMETIME DURING THE FIRST WEEK
or ten days after Ed came home, a circle of light came into our lives. The
dark fears I had about caring for Ed on my own were chased away. A
door opened and the stormy clouds of anger toward the medical profession were scattered amidst patches of sunshine. There was a radi-
ance. A new feeling of hope. The splendid gleam of trust. It was all in
the form of a person. A nurse named Carol.

Carol was from Lifeline Homecare. She was to call on Ed twice a
week, more if needed, and make reports to Dr. Moore. She just showed
up one morning, I'm sure at the behest of the doctor, but unknown to
us. Very quickly, she became more Ed's doctor than his doctor, in the
old-fashioned sense of that word. She became the one human being in
the complex matrix of medical professionals caring for Ed who was
truly involved, not just with an aedinocarcinoma that had metasticized
to the lungs, but with a man.

I think Carol was Jewish, but she reminded me of women I've
known who are nuns. She was ageless, as most nuns are, somewhere in
the middle. Maybe thirty-five. Maybe forty. She was motherly, but there
was an underlying firmness in her that told you that while children of
hers would be loved, they would also mind their manners and make
their own beds. She was very professional as well, like the nuns who
run high schools, or Sister Marie Madeline at St. John's. She knew her
business. She had her standards. And you could never put one over
on her.

When she came to see Ed, she was always dressed a certain way. She
never wore pants; she never wore tennis shoes, like other nurses who
came to the house. She always wore skirts, stockings, and shoes with
heels. It was a reserved look, but I thought she wanted to be regarded as
a professional and had found a way of dressing that reflected her position yet allowed her to work.

From the beginning, she was completely involved with Ed, from
the inner fierceness of his mind to the most mundane functions of
his body.

"I think you need to trim Mr. McNeilly's toenails," she said to Jessie
the morning of her first visit.

Then she set to work clearing up the deepening bedsore that was
still open and raw at the base of his spine. Like Dr. Moore, she got involved in everything that was high-tech, such as pain management and

the use of morphine. But she also got involved in everything low-tech. Toenails, dry skin, bowel movements, coughing, how to get out of bed without falling. It may be high-tech that saves a patient's life, but it's low-tech that's on a patient's mind.

Carol's methodology was based with simple and unerring precision on the most infallible method ever used in medicine. She listened.

Every Tuesday and every Friday when she came, she began by listening. And anything Ed wanted to tell her was relevant. She let him tell her, in his own way and in his own time, about everything that was happening to his body. And in that way, she came to know his soul.

"This is an unusual situation," she told me one day. "This isn't like other homes I come into. I usually walk in...and, you know...kind of take over. But Mr. McNeilly is in control. I've never seen anyone fight so hard. He's very special."

Carol found Ed, as a person, from the beginning. And she's the one who gave him a most precious gift that November.

His dignity.

November 3

JESSIE LEFT, BECAUSE SHE HAD TO GO to Missouri to be with her daughter, and the nursing service replaced her with Georgetta. We'd gotten more comfortable with each passing day, and the fear of screwing up with the oxygen tanks or the morphine, of being unable to handle a crisis or reluctant to handle a mess had gone away. So Georgetta worked from eight-thirty to five-thirty Monday through Friday, and Sug and I did the rest.

Sug had gotten a position, somewhat to her shock, with a law firm in Westwood.

"Mama, they offered me the job," she'd screamed into the phone when she told me the news. "And if I pass the Bar, I'll get a 5,000-dollar raise. Maybe I'm a lawyer after all."

The lawyer and I planned our time so that one of us would always be home with Ed when Georgetta wasn't. If I had to leave for work early, Sug would wait for Georgetta. Or, If I had to be late, she'd get home to relieve her. I asked Ed after two or three days how it was going with Georgetta.

"Jean, she's stupid. She watches 'General Hospital' and can't keep up with the plot."

I laughed, but I'd noticed a couple of things myself. She was bringing a thermos from home, because the Krups coffeemaker in our kitchen was beyond her. I asked her where she got her LVN.

"In Britain, during the War," she told me. But she was very short on specifics. In her spare time during the day, she was crocheting a purple-and-yellow doily of the kind you see under vases with plastic flowers, and she read a lot—*People* magazine, the Bible, which she brought with her, and my cookbooks, which fascinated me, because she fixed Ed's lunch primarily by opening cans.

It finally dawned on me that I was the one who was stupid. This great man of mine, Ed McNeilly, was not going to spend these precious days in the company of a woman who crocheted purple-and-yellow doilies.

He was going to spend these precious days with me.

I began to make arrangements to replace myself at the agency for the month of December. Jocelyn Weisdorf, a senior freelance writer with creative-director experience, was available and could pick up the slack while I was gone.

"I'm aware of your problem, Jean," she said when I phoned her. "I'm flattered to be asked."

That evening, Ed was in his hospital bed in the living room and I was making up my bed beside him on the couch. I'd told him about Jocelyn and being home in December. Actually, I was very excited. The prospect of being a housewife for a while felt terrific.

"Maybe I'll take six weeks, Ed. Stretch it a little. Start the week of Thanksgiving and stay gone the first week of January."

"Jean," he called my name. "Jean."

"What is it, Sweetheart?"

"Nothing. I just want to say your name. It gives me strength."

All of the struggling, all of the fighting, all of the not giving up, all of the treks to the City of Hope, all of the nights sleeping in the chair at Cedars, and all of the problems with home nursing care were worth it for that moment.

November 4

WE MADE OUR SECOND VISIT TO Dr. Moore's office, but it was easier this time, because Ed could walk a little. He hadn't started walking far enough to make it to the bathroom, but he could make it to the portable commode near his bed, and that was a big deal for all of us. We'd gotten him a fifty-foot extender for the oxygen tubes so he could walk to the Lazy-Boy recliner and spend part of his day sitting up. We made an effort to get him dressed every day, in things like jogging pants and loose shirts, so he could stand up to greet visitors, looking and feeling more like a person.

We'd had a weigh-in and he was down to 205 pounds. For him, that was thin, and he suddenly looked much taller than six-two looked when he was 240. His face had become gaunt, bony, and drawn. His hair had thinned. The great blue eyes were far away in the depths of the sockets. One of the people from my office came to see him and was visibly shaken at the sight. But I don't think Ed ever perceived himself as different. He never apologized for the way he looked or was reluctant for people to see him. He paid attention to himself every morning—shaving, trimming his moustache—as he always had. He wanted me to go shopping for clothes that fit him better. Ed was wounded. But he was never beaten.

There was a long wait for the doctor and Ed got quite uncomfortable. Sitting up was hard, his rectum was sore, and he was edgy. Dr. Moore finally came in, did the examination, and told Ed we could start a new chemotherapy program. Ed looked at me and threw a clenched fist into the air. The drug was called Mycostatin and was considered a secondary line of defense, a backup to 5FU. We had to wait some more while Louise prepared the injection, and Ed was starting to lose it.

"Help me, Jean. I can't sit any longer."

I stepped out of the tiny examining room to find Louise. She saw me coming, read the look on my face, and in a biting ten seconds not only prevented any contact on a human level but also dashed my fragile demeanor to bits.

"I know you're going to ask me to hurry, Mrs. McNeilly, but don't. I am well aware of the tensions you're under, but I'm under tension too and I'm working as fast as I can."

I blinked my eyes and bit my lip to force back the tears, turned around, and ducked into an empty room. Ed wasn't defeated, but I often was. Every encounter, especially in Dr. Moore's office, was negative. I felt that to Louise, I was the enemy. I went out into the corridor and got Ed a drink of cool water from the fountain. At least I could do that, and it gave me a moment to compose myself.

Louise finally got the chemicals mixed, but then she couldn't get a vein. After two or three unsuccessful stabs, she left to talk to the doctor.

Ed was in anguish. He wanted the injection. He wanted to start a new program. But the physical and mental duress of vein stabbing always took their toll. Louise came back into the room.

"The doctor thinks we shouldn't try any more today. We'll see you in a week and try again then."

Tears welled up in Ed's eyes. Louise thought they were tears of relief. But I knew they were tears of disappointment.

That night after Ed had gone to sleep, I thought about Louise and Dr. Moore. "I should talk to Ed," I told myself, "change doctors. Find someone different." But I had an overwhelming sense of defeat. Dr. Moore was Everydoctor. There wasn't anything different.

I though about phoning Alan Fogelman for advice, but he'd been an exception at UCLA. Kevin and I had had the same problems with most every doctor we saw there, except him. And there was an emotional barrier. I knew I'd never get the words out on the phone. "Alan, yes, it's been ten years. I'm calling you because my second husband is dying of cancer." My throat strangled at the thought of it.

I thought about going back to the City of Hope, but it was physically too far for Ed by then. And Hope had put us in touch with Dr. Moore to begin with. I thought about calling Phillip Richmond, but he was the one who'd sent us to Dr. Bornstein, the finest, he'd said—and we'd fired him on Day One.

I didn't think Ed was getting bad care in a technical sense. The efficacy of the treatment, while not perfect, was as good as you're going to get. Dr. Moore was highly qualified, and highly recommended. He'd made some mistakes, but I think most doctors would have defended his reasoning. "He was doing the best he could under the circumstances."

That, indeed, was the problem. Ed was getting the best medicine had to offer. Yet it was failing him. That's why I was defeated. Not because one doctor was remote. But because I'd come to believe the entire profession was.

I had no hope. No hope of finding a doctor willing to get involved in the emotional needs—in the link between body and spirit of a cancer patient given ninety days to live. I wasn't even sure I could find a doctor willing to get involved in his physical needs. When you already have too many patients, do you want an Ed McNeilly, diagnosed as terminal fourteen months before? After two operations? After months of debilitating chemotherapy? I had no hope.

Dr. Moore didn't return phone calls; wasn't always up to speed; didn't form a partnership; didn't engage the spirit; ignored the family;

was too busy; was protected by his staff; hoarded information; communicated poorly; treated disease, not the person; had nurses on power trips; all of it. But so does Everydoctor.

I was disheartened and defeated. It would be physically hard on Ed to change at this point. To withstand the tests and exams that form a new information base. To disrupt chemotherapy. To enter new surroundings. To go through the emotional drain of starting a relationship. What's more, it was medically problematic. And if I had no real hope of unearthing a doctor significantly different from Dr. Moore, what was the point?

We had medicine at its finest. That was the problem.

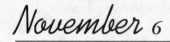

November 6

IT WAS FRIDAY EVENING, the weekend was trying to start, but I was delayed at the client and didn't get home until after eight. When I got there, Sug and Ed were waiting for me with the looks on their faces children get when they do something for the first time. "Look at me, Mom. Look at me. I can swim." Sug blurted out their news.

"We went to Pep Boys."

"What?"

"Ed and I went to Pep Boys. The rear-view mirror fell off my car and Ed said they had a special glue at Pep Boys, so we went and got it."

"You took him with you to Pep Boys?"

"Yep."

"How did you do that?"

"Well, his wheelchair fit in my car and he said he could hold the oxygen on his lap. And he said he could walk to the car. So, we went."

Ed and I had shared a lot of adventures together. Tahiti. Fiji. Bermuda. We went to London once for the weekend. We flew to San Francisco once for dinner. But I couldn't remember an adventure that had ever put more delight in his eyes than this trip to Pep Boys on Pico in West Los Angeles with Sug. He was beaming, but there was also a determined look on his face.

"I'm going to turn this around, Jean."

As the three of us sat there laughing and hugging, I remembered an incident with Kevin.

🐌 Kevin was very sick, but at home. He was recovering from the first surgery at UCLA. The one that lasted twelve hours. The one where they failed to clear the left carotid. The one where they didn't bother to cosmetically close the incision. He'd been home from the hospital only one day, was still on pain medication and antibiotics, was still weak, was sleeping a lot, and was confined to bed. But he'd had to spend most of the day alone. I was working and the children—three of them at that time—were in a day-care center.

It was around five in the afternoon. I'd picked up the children and hurried home to see how Kevin was doing. Only to discover he wasn't there.

I couldn't believe it. He'd obviously been there all day. The bed was cluttered with National Geographics and New Yorkers, a banana peel, note pads, and his tape recorder. But he wasn't in the house or in the backyard. When I'd left that morning, he was still wobbly, hanging onto things when he walked to the bathroom.

Now he was gone.

I didn't know what to do or what to think and ran around the house calling for him like my mother would say, "a chicken with her head off."

I was about to conclude he'd had a relapse, called himself an ambulance, and gone back to the hospital, when one of the children saw him, out the front window, walking down Olympic Boulevard. He was sauntering casually, the way he always did, loose-limbed and gangly, like a teenager coming out of a mini-market with a quart of Coke and without a care in the world.

"Here comes Daddy, Mama."

I ran out the front door and pulled up to a stop in front of him about a block from the house, huffing and puffing. "What have you been doing? Where have you been? I was scared to death."

He was the soul of innocence. "I haven't been anywhere. I just walked over to Gomi's to get some coffee."

"My God, Kevin, what's the matter with you? You can't just get up out of bed, after twelve hours of surgery, and go out for coffee."

"Yeah, well,…I was a little worried about the stitches, but I covered them up. I don't think anyone noticed." And he proceeded to unwind a large wool muffler that covered him loosely from shoulders to ears.

The incision in his neck was a ghastly-looking V, about four inches long on each side. I had opened like a flap during the surgery and they'd whipped it shut with huge black stitches like children make when they're learning to sew. The incision was so big, and the stitches so visible, it looked like someone had just sewn his head onto his neck, like the Frankenstein monster. It was a shocker until you got used to it.

"The incision's bad enough, but that's not the point. Kevin, you're sick."

"I got the fidgets. Why are you so upset?" He was shrugging his shoulders and raising his eyebrows as if he honestly didn't know why I was so excited. "All I did was go out for coffee. And," he winked at Chris, "I had a waffle."

Ed went to Pep Boys. Kevin went out for coffee.

Indeed, their spirits were so much in unison that in these months after Ed came home from Cedars, something began to happen that had never happened before. From time to time, they'd mix up in my mind. I'd mean Ed and say Kevin, and vice-versa.

Once or twice, I even got them mixed up in my dreams. I'd know I was dreaming about my husband who was sick, but I couldn't tell which one. ❧

November 7

ALICIA CAME ON SUNDAY, to give me some time out of the house. I was very grateful to her and left to run some errands. There were pictures of the Pebble Beach Concours Ed had left to be developed in August, which had never been picked up. I was going to do that and then just poke around the shops on Montana Avenue in Santa Monica, a street that I loved.

But as I left the house it started to rain, a wind-whippy, November, street-flooding kind of rain. I had a hard time seeing as I drove PCH toward Santa Monica. Then, when I got to the camera store, it was gone. In the months since we'd dropped off the pictures, the store had moved away, and I realized how long it had been since life had been normal and we'd done things like drop off pictures.

It was raining too hard to poke around Montana Avenue and I didn't know what to do. So I sat in my car and a thought began to envelop me like mud envelops a car when it slides off the cliffs and onto PCH in a slowly oozing mass of wet clay. It dawned on me that I was alone. I was alone in my car in the rain. And this was the way it was soon going to be. I wouldn't be able to turn to someone sitting beside me and say, "Let's go have lunch and listen to the rain."

It is terrible to be conscious of being alone. A bubble forms around you to mark you. You walk into a movie theater alone with your bubble around you and you hear people mocking, "she's alone, she's alone, she's alone." It's hard to see a weekend coming and know you're going to spend it alone. To eat by yourself on Sunday morning. To want to do something—take a trip, go out to dinner, go to a play, and know that first you have to find someone to do it with. It's hard to walk into a party alone. To come home after work to an empty house. To hear no one say, "How was your day?"

I think men hate to be alone even more than women, but they're better at combatting it. Men can sit at a bar, like they do in "Cheers," and find easy friendship. Or go pick up a game of basketball or baseball. Or just fall in with each other, or with a woman. Men go out and find people. Women don't as much. There's the social tradition as well as the very real problem of ending up in trouble like the bar-hopping school-teacher in *Looking for Mr. Goodbar.*

After Kevin died, I'd had my time of being alone. I'd paid my dues already. I didn't want to do it anymore. I shouted a profanity at the wind whistling past my car, then beat my head on the steering wheel and tried to cry.

But I couldn't.

November 8

EDDIE PHONED ON SUNDAY.
I told him I was so confused. Ed was up, then down. Things looked positive, then negative. I was strong, then defeated.

"I don't know what to say to people."

"You don't have to say anything."

"But people want to hear how Ed is doing. Even my family. My kids. They want to know what to feel, what to expect, and I don't know what to say. I don't know how he is myself. I don't know what I feel myself."

"Tell them," he said softly, "that there are good days and bad days. Tell yourself that. And take it one day at a time."

"There are good days and bad days," I said to Alan and Stacie when they came out that evening, bearing gifts and dinner. "We're taking it one day at a time."

November 11

WE WENT TO THE DOCTOR AGAIN.
Kresser/Craig was closed for Veteran's Day and I couldn't get help from the office; besides, I was beginning to feel it was enough. I couldn't ask

every week and needed to find some alternates. Chris was off from work, so he came out to Malibu to help, and Sug came with us as well.

Louise got a vein quickly this time and started the new drug, to Ed's enthusiastic approval.

I talked separately with Dr. Moore about Ed's lack of appetite. It had gotten so bad, there were days I didn't think he'd taken in more than 100 calories. Sug or I would sit by his bed for half an hour trying to get a spoonful or two of ice cream down him. Dr. Moore acknowledged the problem but didn't have much advice. Not eating is a big problem with cancer patients. You do what you can with high-protein, high-caloric foods. But a lot of it is banging your head against a wall.

When we got home, Chris, Sug, and I talked about it in the kitchen. The trip to the doctor had been hard. We were all tired. Sug was irritable.

"Mama, I'm tired of hearing about Ed not eating. If he won't eat, he won't eat. You should get it off your mind."

Then Chris, who'd been so quiet and steady through all of this, took a mental jog toward rage.

"I don't know why you don't force him to eat. Hold his mouth open or something and force it down. Or force feed him with tubes. If he doesn't eat he's going to die. Why don't you just make him eat? Or why don't they?"

Sug and I were both taken aback by his anger. I wasn't sure whether he was angry at Ed for jeopardizing himself or angry at Ed for causing strain on me and Sug. Chris had a black-and-white way of looking at things. Maybe he was thinking it would have been better for all of us if Ed had died at Cedars on the fifteenth of October. I could understand him feeling that way. There now seemed to be little use in a life that simply drained the life from others. But I didn't feel it myself. Not for a minute. And it caused me to remember my mother.

❧ *Mama was seventy-seven years old when she had her stroke. She was cooking dinner for herself and Grandpa Pat in their tidy little house on 34th Street in Oklahoma City, when she just crumpled to the floor. Pat ran and got a neighbor, who got an ambulance. Several hours later, I got a call from Howard.*

"It's bad news, Jeanie. Mama's in the hospital. She's had a stroke, there's going to be surgery, it doesn't look good."

But Mama was a fighter and she made it. Although she never walked again, never again had control of the left side of her body, never used the bathroom again, and never again washed her own hair, wrote a letter, or read a book.

After about a month in the hospital, we brought her home and between the five of us managed to keep her there. Mama lived bedridden at home with care around the clock for five years.

Her life span was notable in that it was twentieth-century America in miniature. She was a teenager in the teens; in her twenties as they roared; she was thirty-something during the '30s. Sometimes I think it's because of women like her, with values so deeply rooted in home, family, love of God, and fellow man, that we got through the Depression, won the War, and found prosperity in the '50s. Mama's father was a homesteader. He came to Oklahoma from Iowa in 1889 and made "The Run" when the Indian Territory was opened. Loretta was the eleventh of twelve children, born in 1904 in Lawton, Oklahoma near the Fort Sill army base, where the great Indian chief Geronimo was alive and well and living out his life. (He died there in 1929, in what I've always considered a great clash of nineteenth- and twentieth-century America.)

Loretta was a coquettish flapper in 1925, when she met Carl on a train she was taking from Shawnee to Oklahoma City. They were married in 1926. Bob came in 1927, Howard in 1928. Carl in 1932. Jean in 1937 and Marta in 1942. We grew up together in a house with five bedrooms but only one bath; we never had more than one car and had no car during the War; and we sweated through ninety-degree August nights, because Papa wouldn't let us run the attic fan since it ran up the electric bill. But we all went to college; indeed, it never entered our minds that we wouldn't. And Mama was the backbone of it all. Like so many women of her generation, she raised a family during the Depression and the War, then saw those children realize "the American Dream" in greater measure, perhaps, than any generation before or since.

It was difficult for us to see her in bed after her stroke. Crippled, slurring her words, spilling her food. And yet,…and yet….

She was a fighter during those years. She didn't want to die. And I believe that she enormously enriched all our lives, as she lay abed with her broken body. Indeed, she brought out things in all of us we might otherwise never have found. Etched into my mind forever are a hundred images. The tenderness of my cowboy-oilman brother Carl, as he changed his mother's diaper. The sweetness of my shy brother Bob, as he bent his six-foot-four-inch frame to pick his mother up and carry her to the car. The gentleness of my patriarchal brother Howard, as he'd listened quietly to his mother's advice, which he'd never stopped seeking. The Madonna-like serenity of my sister, Marta, that came from finally tending, I think, rather than being tended.

*There were Saturday evenings when I came to visit with my chil-
dren and Carl with his, when we'd sit around Mama's bed, play the guitar, and sing the cowboy songs she loved so much. "Red River Valley."
"The Streets of Laredo." I treasure those evenings as among the finest of
my life. And then, there were the moments with Uncle Ferdy.*

*He was her younger brother. Ferdinand Meis. A parish priest in the
diocese of Oklahoma City and Tulsa for forty-five years. Her sidekick
and buddy for seventy-five years. All of their lives, Loretta and Ferdy
were never far apart. And when she was bedridden, he'd come over
from the retirement home where he was living to say Mass on Saturday
afternoons. He'd set up his altar on her bed table—the chalice, the candles, the big Roman missal from which he'd read the prayers of the
Mass. His eyesight was failing and even with glasses, he still couldn't see
the words in the missal, so he'd bring a huge magnifying glass and, holding his glass and peering through his Coke-bottle lenses, he'd read the
prayers, and those of us crowded into her room and around her bed
would say the responses. Then Uncle Ferdy would give us all Com-
munion. Those moments, I believe, set in place a continuum that will
someday see me and my brother Carl together in some way after
seventy-five years and hopefully, Sug and her brother, Chris. My God,
what we all learned from Mama and Ferdy. And from each other and
about each other while Mama was in bed.*

*So while it may have seemed sometimes that it would have been
better if Mama had died swiftly and easily when she had the stroke
rather than spending her last five years imprisoned in a body that no
longer worked, bringing a rather inglorious end to a beautiful life, it
turned out instead to be a time of enrichment.* ❧

And I also felt that way about Ed.

As long as people are in a cognitive state and have the will to live,
there is life to be lived, there are lessons to be learned and there is love
to be had. I'm glad my mother lived those five years and that I got to
share them with her. I'm glad Ed came home from the hospital. Not for
one second would I have preferred he die at Cedars and get it over with.
Not for one second.

Besides, you don't get to choose.

"Try not to be mad at Ed," I said to Chris. "He is trying."

"He's trying so hard," said Sug, "it breaks your heart."

"I can't help it, Mom," said Chris. "All of this is so hard. I can't stand
to see him starve himself."

There are good days and bad days. Wednesday was a bad day.

November 15

SUNDAY WAS A GOOD DAY—SOFT AND WARM, with beautiful pink afternoon light, the way it gets in Malibu in the fall. Jimmy Buffett on the stereo. Tanning bodies on the deck. I set Ed up outside on a long lounge chair shaded by an umbrella, so he could watch while I fussed with my flowers. But, of course, he didn't really watch.

"You should put the Bird of Paradise in a larger pot, Jean."

"Jean, you should fertilize the Plumeria. No, not with Miracle Grow. You have to use the blood meal, Jean."

"Isn't the trumpet vine beautiful, Jean? I'm so glad you planted it up there where I suggested."

And all day long, the phone rang. Which it did a lot on weekends that fall. Carl would phone. And Maureen and Erin. Madeline. Eddie. Robin.

Sunday also became Visitors' Day at Cedars Malibu. I was touched by the parade of friends who took the time to come out to see Ed. I was also surprised from time to time by the friends who didn't. A lot of people are afraid to visit the terminally ill.

What do you talk about? they think. Well, . . . you talk about Monday-night football, what's going on in the advertising business, the Reagan administration. You talk about whatever people talk about.

But what if I stick my foot in my mouth? What if I mention next year when we all know the person won't be here next year? Don't worry about it. Talk about the future isn't upsetting. The mind likes to put the "ifs" of tomorrow away, and when a cancer patient is asked something like "Who do you think's going to win the World Series next year?" he is relieved you put the "ifs" in a drawer as well and are willing to treat him like a normal patient.

But I'm afraid to look at the person. I'm afraid I'll be shocked. I don't like to be around sickness.

Of course. Nobody likes to be around sickness. There are a lot of negatives involved; and fearing them is natural. But just by being you and showing up, you have an opportunity to make a very positive contribution. In the end, it's not negative at all, but fulfilling.

Kim and Mark started coming once a week. Ed's younger daughter seemed to glow in the flush of reconciliation with her father. The first time she came, she brought a childhood picture album Ed hadn't seen since the divorce and the two of them reminisced in soft, sweet tones about their family years in Armonk, New York, then later in Miami.

As I watched Kim and Mark and got to know them, I realized that by accident or design they were much a reflection of Ed. Mark, who was a former Dade County, Florida, police officer and was now working at Hughes Aircraft, started dating Kim when she was sixteen and he was already a rookie cop in one of the toughest law-enforcement counties in America. He had a protective, older-man demeanor toward Kim, who seemed to appreciate the attitude from him, even though she was an independent, strong-willed young woman, at home in the aggressiveness of advertising-agency media planning.

Like Ed, Mark wore loafers without socks and owned every camera lens known to man. Like Ed, he enjoyed cars. Like Ed, he was a student of architectural design and looked to the day he could start redoing a home.

Like Ed, Kim was a car freak and wanted to skew her advertising career toward working on a car account. Like Ed, she loved traveling, and she was accomplished in the same sports—fishing, diving, water sports. She'd picked up Ed's love of antiques and had started collecting things, like he'd collected authentic signatures of American presidents.

I saw Ed not just in the one of them, but in the two of them, and was charmed by the sweetness of their visits.

November 20

I PHONED LIFELINE HOMECARE LOOKING for Carol, in something of a panic. Ed hadn't eaten in twenty-four hours and he seemed to be gagging, even on water. He was lethargic and he hadn't had a bowel movement in three days. Carol had been to visit the day before and had been concerned, but not alarmed. By the morning, however, he seemed to have taken a turn for the worse. Lifeline found Carol through her beeper and she phoned me back.

"He still hasn't had a bowel movement, Carol."

"Did you give him the Dulcolax, Mrs. McNeilly?"

"I gave him everything you told me to give him, but nothing's happened and he hasn't urinated either. It's been about twelve hours. And he's so subdued and lethargic. It's like his body has shut down."

"I think you'd better phone Dr. Moore, Mrs. McNeilly, instead of waiting for me to make a visit. Why don't you phone right now."

Carol's tone was urgent, so I phoned Louise immediately and described the situation.

"Bring him in," she said briskly, "but you have to have him here by eleven-thirty."

I looked at my watch. It was ten A.M. I wasn't even dressed. Ed wasn't dressed. It was a forty-five-minute drive to the doctor's office. It took ten or fifteen minutes just to get his oxygen tanks ready.

"By 11:30? I don't know if I can make it by then."

"He has to be here by eleven-thirty or the doctor can't see him." Her tone was unequivocal.

I skipped my shower, I didn't even brush my teeth and got dressed in about two minutes, while Alicia, who was giving Georgetta the day off, dressed Ed. Then we filled his oxygen tanks, transferred him to the portable unit, gave him his medication, and packed his bag with the diapers, cough medicine, and tranquilizers he was afraid to be without. We jammed the wheelchair and the oxygen into the back seat of my car, because they wouldn't fit in the trunk. Then Alicia fitted herself in on top of the wheelchair, and with Ed and me in the front seat, we took off for West LA.

It was ten-thirty. If traffic was normal, we'd be at the medical building by eleven-fifteen. But when we turned off Rambla Pacifico onto PCH, my heart skipped. The traffic was backed up bumper-to-bumper. There's no way out of Malibu but PCH, and when it's bumper-to-bumper, you just get in it and creep.

"There must be an accident up ahead, Alicia."

"What're we going to do, Jean? Ed looks awful."

I picked up my car phone, asked information for the Malibu Sheriff's number, and punched it in.

"Could I have an escort, please, around the traffic on PCH? I have a seriously ill person in the car."

"You'll have to call the Highway Patrol for that."

So I got the number and called the Highway Patrol.

"I'm stuck in traffic on PCH."

"We know. The accident's at Topanga Canyon Boulevard."

"I don't want to know where the accident is, I want to get an escort around the traffic. I have a medical emergency."

"Oh, ... well, ... I don't know. I can't authorize that."

"May I speak to the officer of the day?"

"I'll have to put you on hold."

When she didn't come back after two minutes, I hung up and swung into the middle lane of PCH, the one that's reserved for left turns.

"To hell with it. We'll go around without an escort."

People honked and stared, but we got around the accident. Nevertheless, it was eleven-twenty-five when we pulled into the emergency-vehicle parking area at the medical building.

Alicia and I struggled to get Ed out of the car and into the wheelchair. She was pushing him toward the elevator in a near frenzy and I was running along behind, carrying the oxygen, when the parking-lot man called after me.

"Hey, you can't leave your car here."

"I'll be back down in a minute, but I have to get my husband upstairs."

"Okay, but you can't leave it here more than ten minutes or we'll tow it."

It was exactly eleven-thirty when we pushed Ed through the doors of Dr. Moore's office. Alicia looked like she had just crossed the finish line of a marathon and was going to collapse. Ed was catatonic. Louise was standing in the middle of the reception area, her hands on her hips, waiting for us.

"Hurry," she commanded. "I was just about to call your home. Hurry. Go immediately into the examining room."

"Alicia, you go with Ed," I said, "while I go down and move the car."

"You can't do that, Mrs. McNeilly," Louise said as if I didn't understand she'd just given me an order, "the doctor will want to speak with you."

"Look," I shouted, "it isn't my building, it's your building, and they told me I had to move the car."

"Then, hurry." She was undaunted.

I ran to the elevator and tried to make it come faster by jamming my finger clear through the lighted button. I ached while it stopped at each floor, rushed to the car, moved it to the parking garage, then rushed back up. Ed was in the examining room with Alicia.

The next thing that happened was that the three of us sat there for forty minutes. It was twelve-twenty when Dr. Moore finally walked into the room.

I couldn't even begin to tell him about not having a shower and not brushing my teeth, about the traffic jam on PCH and the police escort and Louise yelling at me. I mean, where do you start? With your husband sitting beside you gasping, what difference does it make anyway? We got him there. The doctor was going to see him.

I didn't have the energy then to try and change the medical profession. But I do now.

I believe Dr. Moore had no idea he caused a panic that morning. Louise caused the panic. But she did it because it was part of her job. Part of what Dr. Moore wanted from her.

It was up to her to keep Dr. Moore on a schedule, and her allegiance to that schedule was forged with the zeal of a patriot. She needed to have the last patient of the morning into the examining room by 11:30. And that's what she did no matter what. If there were inconveniences that had to be overcome by the patient, well that's the way it had to work. The doctor couldn't adapt his day to the needs of any one person, or the whole would suffer. It wasn't like he was going to play golf at the country club after the 11:30 patient, for Chrissakes, he was going to his rounds at Cedars.

That may be true.

It's no excuse.

The problem with medicine as it's practiced today is that it revolves around itself rather than the people it serves. There *are* some wonderful doctors, but the profession as a whole has become, in my opinion, self-absorbed, self-protective, and self-serving. Incidents that might go unremarked upon or unnoticed when a person sees a doctor twice a year or twice a decade, form a mosaic when a person sees a doctor for ten months or ten years. The mosaic I've pieced together is one of arrogance and elitism. A profession that's come to expect an entitlement it has no right to. A profession that fails to recognize the inestimable value of the human spirit.

More than anything else, the problem with doctors is that they treat disease, not people. Have you ever heard doctors chatting, like on an elevator? They talk about "the bypass down the hall," the "collapsed lung" on the third floor, the "edema" in post-op. It may be casual chitchat, but it's reflective of an attitude. They don't even say "the bypass patient" down the hall. It's all blood vessels, organs, tissue.

Forgive the pun, but it needs to become flesh and blood. The responsibility, in my opinion, isn't the narrow one of treating disease, but the larger one of caring for the sick.

Dr. Moore examined Ed but couldn't find anything the matter—any new problem, that is, causing the malaise. I wanted him to take X-rays, because I feared a blockage in the bowel or urinary tract, but he did not think this was the problem. Ed was looking less pale, as if the excitement had roused him. After a few minutes we left, relieved that Ed was okay but feeling somewhat bewildered by the whole experience.

"You shouldn't let that nurse talk to you that way, Jean," Alicia, who *is* aggressive by nature, told me on the way home. "If she talks to you like that in front of me, I'm going to tell her off, Jean."

That afternoon, Carol came and talked with Ed for a good hour. His speech was slow and labored and it took a great deal of patience to hear him out. He told her in painful detail every physical symptom he had.

After a while, Carol came and found me in the kitchen.

"Mrs. McNeilly, I think the problem is just that his bowels aren't working. We've tried everything else and now I have to give him an enema."

"He won't let you, Carol."

Ed had a fear of enemas that exceeded my own fear as a child of death at the hands of invaders from Mars. He'd gotten through fifteen months of cancer of the colon without one. Indeed, he'd gotten through his entire life without one. I didn't think he'd submit.

"But we have to give him one. Will you help me? I think it might be easier for him if you help me."

"Of course I'll help you."

I wonder if anyone has ever described the process surrounding an enema as touching. I doubt it. But that's the way it was that afternoon, in the living room with ocean view that had become Cedars Malibu. Ed ended up being submissive as a puppy. It was as if he knew we both loved him, understood him, and it wouldn't have come to this were there any other way. Carol and I spread lots of plastic garbage bags in case we didn't make it to the commode. Ed laid on his side in the bed and hung onto my hand, while I stroked his hair and Carol, in her skirt, stockings, and shoes with heels did the administering. She hung the enema bag from a floor lamp. Ed was naked, except for a T-shirt. But instead of being a ridiculous scene there was a dignity in it, because there was great compassion in Carol. Because there was still a great sense of self in Ed.

If there is a good from something as bad as cancer, it is, to me, the enriched understanding of the human spirit that comes from such remarkable and touching moments.

The "procedure" worked, and Dr. Carol was successful that day.

November 21

IT WAS GEORGETTA'S LAST DAY.
She gave me the purple-and-yellow doily.

November 22

ED WOKE UP COUGHING.
I didn't worry at first. Certainly there'd been a lot of coughing. We cracked jokes as I changed his bed and got him ready for his bath.

"You're going to cough up your socks, Ed."

"No. I'm trying to cough up the pumpkin pie Georgetta left."

I gave him all his medication early. I thought the morphine might calm the cough, along with the Ativan, which is a tranquilizer, and the Theodur, which helps dilate the passages in the lungs. We also had on hand a large bottle of prescription cough medicine and I gave him two tablespoons of that. But the coughing continued.

I fixed things for breakfast that I thought might soothe his throat. A dish of yogurt. Hot tea with lemon and honey. But he was coughing so frequently, he couldn't eat.

I'd never seen or heard anything like it. He coughed every twenty or thirty seconds. Sometimes as much as a minute would go by without a cough, but a minute was as long as it got. The coughs were big enough to shake his whole body. His shoulders would hunch, then bob up and down. The hernia in his abdomen was pouching out with each spasm. A month ago, the hernia had been the size of a grapefruit. Now it was the size of a cantaloupe.

At ten A.M., I decided we had a problem that wasn't going to go away, so I phoned Dr. Moore, but it was Sunday and I got the answering service.

"Is it an emergency?" the service asked.

"I don't know if it's an emergency or not. Tell Dr. Moore my husband has been coughing since seven A.M." But I caught myself. He has cancer in his lungs. Of course, he's going to cough. You'd have to be in the room to recognize that something different was going on. "No, don't tell him that. Just tell him that I need to talk with him, and to call me please." And the coughing continued. The stress of it was beginning to make Ed weak.

Medication wasn't due for another hour, but I decided to give it early. It didn't help. Sug, who'd been getting dressed to spend her Sunday with Julie, changed her plans.

"I'll stay here for a while, Mama, until we find out what's the matter. Just in case you need me."

And the coughing continued. We held his hand and stroked his forehead while he looked at us through bewildered eyes. He coughed so much he couldn't get words out. At eleven A.M., I phoned Dr. Moore again. But got the service again.

"He has the message. He'll call you as soon as he can."

Sug and I sat and stared at each other. It was a gray, winterlike day, with the wind whipping whitecaps on the slate-colored surface of the sea. We'd begun to be very frightened. Part of the fear was for Ed. Part of the fear was not knowing what to do. We tried to talk, but there was mostly a hollow silence, pierced by the howl of the wind and the hack of the cough.

At noon, I phoned Lifeline Homecare. I knew Carol wasn't on call on Sundays, but somebody would be. The nurse I spoke to listened very carefully and then advised me to take Ed to Emergency at Cedars.

I'd already thought of that. Indeed, I'd already agonized over it. But my instincts told me it was the wrong thing to do.

It was an hour's drive to Cedars. Ed would have to go onto portable oxygen and sit up in the car. There was the trauma of moving him, struggling to get him into the wheelchair, and taking him outside. Then there was the chaos that characterizes Emergency, and the fear and stress that go with it. When we got there, nobody would be familiar with Ed's case. They don't handle chronic cancer patients in Emergency; they handle knife wounds and automobile accidents. It was my fear that they wouldn't treat him, but instead admit him back into he hospital until his own doctor could take over. I had the certain feeling that if I took him to Cedars, he'd never come home again. If arrangements were under way to meet Dr. Moore there, it would be different.

"Can't someone come out?"

"Yes, but I don't know what we could do. If he needs medication, we can't prescribe. And if he needs a procedure, we can't do it. You better take him to Cedars, Mrs. McNeilly."

I hung up and talked to Sug.

"Do you think he's dying, Mama?" Ed had begun to hallucinate, but I thought it was stress and medication more than delirium. Sug's voice broke as she asked the question.

"I don't know, Sug. I don't think so. I wish we could find Dr. Moore. I think an antibiotic would help. I think it's another infection."

All morning long the situation had been reminding me of the other time he'd coughed so much. The time he'd had pneumonia. The cough sounded the same. Ed looked the same. It was just an instinct and it's hard to know where instincts come from, you just get them.

"I think we should take him to Emergency, Mama."

"I can't take him back to Cedars, Sug. I just can't." I was certain the trauma of the hospital would kill him. If he did die, I wanted him to die at home.

At noon, I phoned Dr. Moore again. And got the service again. I told them this time that it was an emergency.

And the coughing continued.

Sug canceled her plans for the day. Ed was now running a slight fever. We tried changing his position, putting his feet up, putting them down, lying him flat, sitting him bolt upright. We tried to amuse him. Tried to distract him.

And the coughing continued.

I called Dr. Moore at two P.M. And got the service. "Why hasn't he called me back?"

"I don't know, Mrs. McNeilly. He's gotten the messages. He must be handling an emergency."

"Do you know where?"

"No, I don't. We aren't putting calls through to him, he's phoning in."

At three P.M., I phoned Robin in Florida. She was a very good nurse and had often been able to help me assess a situation by phone and help me figure out how to handle things. But this time, she was quietly pessimistic.

"This may be the last crisis, Jean."

Sug and I held hands and listened to him cough and listened to him cough and listened to him cough while I doubted my decision and doubted my decision and doubted my decision.

Then, at five P.M., almost to the minute, the coughing stopped. It simply stopped. Ed had coughed for ten hours, from seven in the morning until five in the afternoon, but with the abruptness of switching off a blaring radio, it stopped. Sug and I were startled by the silence and unsure for the first few moments it would endure. I gave Ed some water. When he swallowed it without coughing, Sug started to cry.

With his brow still furrowed and his hands still clenched as if determination could ward off the return of the cough, Ed fell into a fitful sleep.

Dr. Moore finally phoned around six.

I tried to describe the day, but I knew I wasn't communicating what it had been like. The bottom line was that a lung-cancer patient had been coughing. There wasn't any way to get across how frantic it had been. And besides, it had stopped.

Dr. Moore listened and told me I should just continue to monitor him.

"Do you think I should take him to Cedars and meet you there?"

"No. There really isn't anything we can do at the hospital that you can't do at home."

"Should we start him on an antibiotic?"

"Since the coughing has stopped, let's see how he does tonight and you call me in the morning."

I hung up the phone, trying to figure out why every conversation with Dr. Moore left me so dismayed. I might just as well not have phoned him.

I thought he must have concluded the coughing was caused by the spread of the tumor; it was inevitable, unstoppable, and there wasn't anything he or anybody else could do about it. There was no point in bringing Ed to the hospital under the circumstances, or even in to see him. There simply wasn't anything anyone could do. That was all well and good. Except I didn't think he was entirely right.

I thought Ed had an infection.

November 23

IT WAS THE FIRST DAY OF MY LEAVE of absence from the advertising agency. I wasn't going back until January 4—the longest I'd been away from work since Maureen was born, in 1965. I was looking forward to it—to being with Ed, to being a housewife. I spent the day sitting beside his bed, polishing brass with the zeal of a downstairs maid in an English country melodrama.

Ed was still coughing, but it was normal, like people get when they have a cold.

Around midday, Carol phoned. It seemed whenever the doctor disappointed me, Carol rushed into the breach like the old White Knight from television soap commercials.

"I got a report that you called us yesterday, Mrs. McNeilly. Are you all right? Did you take Mr. McNeilly to Cedars?"

I babbled to her like a child who'd run to his mother with a scraped knee. She put a Band-aid on my bleeding emotions and soothed my fears. She told me she continued to think Ed had an infection and she'd phone the doctor.

Then she did me a kindness I knew was breaking the rules, but I loved her for it. She gave me her home phone number.

November 25

ALICIA AND I TOOK ED TO THE DOCTOR for his regular visit. Dr. Moore did a brief examination, listened with his stethoscope, asked him to "open wide and say ahhh," that sort of thing. When he finished he said, "I think Ed has an infection; let's start him on an antibiotic."

The incident was nothing new. It was a repetition of the pneumonia scenario in September. Doctors miss it once in a while. But most people don't see a doctor enough to realize it. Patterns emerge when the care is extended. You begin to get a feel for how a doctor works. You can tell when his staff is covering for him. You can tell when he hasn't read your lab reports until he walked into the room. You can sense "whoops" in his face.

Everybody in business wings it from time to time. I do. I've walked into more than one meeting with a client, unprepared. It's human. In a sense, it's easy to overlook. On the other hand, I wonder if winging it should be acceptable for doctors. Some professions have obligations others don't. Policemen can't strike. Airline pilots can't drink. Teachers and the clergy have unwritten obligations of service that will affect them all of their lives, as well as a clear understanding that they'll never make very much money.

Doctors aren't the only ones with out-sized obligations, and I don't think they should wing it.

November 26

THE FAMILY GATHERED ROUND FOR Thanksgiving. Maureen flew home from New York and Erin from Boston (without Rich, who had finals). Sug was there, of course. And

Chris. Plus Aunt Maureen. I always liked to serve Thanksgiving dinner at the table. But this year, we balanced our plates on our knees and clustered around Ed's bed. He was eating a little better. He commented, of course, that my stuffing wasn't up to his.

For years, we'd designated Aunt Maureen as the "Official Toast-maker" at family functions. Making a really sappy toast was one of her finer talents, and she wrung the last drop of emotion from the moment and brought us all to tears.

"To the love that binds a family," she said as she lifted her glass, "and brings peace to our hearts as no other love can."

"Hear, hear," Ed said softly from his bed.

November 27

SUG WAS EXPECTING HER LETTER from the California Bar Review Board and she was not expecting to pass. She paced up and down all morning watching for the mailman and when she saw him coming, she ran away to hide. Then she came back and sat on the front steps clutching the letter, afraid to open it. I was working in the yard nearby and when she finally tore it open, she looked at it, looked at me, and started to cry.

Since it was Sug, I knew that meant she had passed.

Later that afternoon, I stood on the deck overlooking the view that overlooks the Pacific and saw my three daughters down on the beach, walking along together arm in arm. Deirdre. Erin. Maureen. Kevin and I had discovered sometime after we did it that we'd given them rhyming middle names: Elise, Patrice, and Denise. "They can go on the road as an act," he'd laughed. "The Craig Sisters." Indeed, they looked like triplets, and they almost were, with only three years and three days separating the trio.

They weren't always the best of friends. All through junior high, Maureen couldn't stand Sug. I believe the feeling was mutual. And once, when I was moving furniture around in the walk-through bedrooms they shared on Benecia, I found a poem hidden behind a chest of drawers. Sug had written it when she was about twelve. Entitled "I Hate Erin," it was a great piece of work. Fine rhyming structure. Excellent imagery. As I recall, she made frequent and creative use of the word *snot*.

But somehow Deirdre Elise, Erin Patrice, and Maureen Denise had made it into adulthood on speaking terms.

What were they talking about down there on the beach? Men? Broken hearts? Erin's wedding? The Fireman? Me and Ed? Christmas? Me? Ed? Or the latest cover story in *People* magazine? Well, it was Sug's favored reading, despite passing the Bar.

There was one thing I felt for sure they weren't talking about this day after Thanksgiving in the year 1987, as I watched them from afar and Ed snoozed behind me in the middle of Cedars Malibu.

They weren't talking about death. None of us were.

November 28

ED WAS RESPONDING TO THE ANTIBIOTIC. He walked to his recliner. He asked about visiting the car wash.

Jim came down from San Francisco to make the circle of people complete. And the family just hung out together in the days following Thanksgiving. Watching football, playing Trivial Pursuit, making big breakfasts.

Nobody said we loved it. But we loved it.

November 30

I HEARD ED ON THE TELEPHONE. He'd never stopped using the telephone. "Penny Cumber? How's your wonderful island? This is Ed McNeilly."

After we came home from Grand Cayman in March, we'd put down a deposit on a rental house there for two weeks at Christmas. We thought we'd take the whole family—his kids, mine, everybody. It had been obvious long since that we wouldn't be able to go, but in the press of things we'd never canceled the booking. Now Ed was on the phone doing just that.

"We were looking forward to seeing you too, but unfortunately we have to cancel."

I was gathering laundry nearby and my heart skipped a beat as I heard him go on.

"We have a terminal illness in the family."

He'd never used the word *terminal* before, and I suddenly realized that the conversation about "90 days" that I'd been trying to decide to have or not to have wasn't necessary. He knew. Of course, he knew.

Yet he was looking ahead, making plans, thinking about Christmas. People need to realize that the terminally ill aren't dead.

Ed was calling to me. "Jean, I'm going to phone Gary Hill about painting the house this winter. Would you get me the number?"

December 1

SOMETHING GOOD WAS GOING ON. Something very good. Ed had energy. He was walking. During the past week, we'd loaded his wheelchair into the car and taken the trip to the car wash. We'd driven to Leo Carillo Beach and shared a picnic lunch in the sweet winter sunshine. He was eating like a horse. Asking for food. Demanding his TV clicker. Wanting coffee. He was even sitting at his drafting table and trying to work.

"Jean," he said to me as I was setting up the bedside table in the sunlight so he could brush his teeth and shave, "I want to talk to Simon about the car wash. Could you ask him to come out to the house? I want to see him."

Simon was going to Mexico to see his family and was going to be gone for three weeks in December. Joe, the assistant manager, would take over while he was gone. When I called Simon and asked him to come, he was a bit evasive.

"I'm leaving, you know, Señora. I don't have a lot of time."

I told Ed and he insisted. "I want to talk with him, Jean."

"About what?"

"Nothing, I just want to see him."

So I phoned again. "Take the time off from work, Simon. Ed really wants to see you, okay?"

"Okay," he said. "No problema."

I don't think he really wanted to come. He was uncomfortable with Malibu, uncomfortable coming to my home. But true to his word, he showed up.

I made coffee and we talked about the car wash, but mostly we talked about Simon and his family. I got out my old *National Geographic* atlas of the world and asked him to show me where he came from. He found it for me on the map, a small town outside of beautiful Guadalajara. Then I sat quietly and let the two men talk a little. Ed asked about cars piling up on the apron. He asked about crew costs and improving the signage. But underneath the chitchat, I felt something else was going on.

Ed wanted Simon to see. To see him with his hospital bed, his oxygen tanks, his portable commode. And he wanted Simon to see me.

"I can't take care of her anymore," he was trying to say. "She's going to need you. Don't let her down."

Of course, neither man said those words. But both men knew. And so did I.

December 4

"MRS. MCNEILLY?" CAROL HAD JUST finished up with Ed after her regular Friday visit. "I'm beginning to wonder if Mr. McNeilly needs oxygen anymore."

"You're kidding."

"No. I'm going to send the respiratory technician out to run the test, if it's okay with you."

So the technician came. When he was finished, he took the oxygen tubes out of Ed's nose, turned all the gauges and dials to "OFF," and switched off the motor in the huge tank that had hummed day and night beside Ed's bed.

"With that damned thing gone," said Ed, "I'll be able to smell the Christmas tree."

December 8

MADELINE PHONED. "I'm going to be in LA,...uh...I thought I might come out to see Ed. I mean, if it's okay...."

"That'd be great, Madeline."

"I'm not sure, I mean...well, when would be a good time?"

We made plans for her to come out to Malibu on Tuesday after a breakfast meeting she had in Century City. She arrived early—people always think it takes longer to get to Malibu than it actually does—and I was still in my PJs when she rang the bell just before ten A.M.

"Come on in. I'm a mess, but Ed isn't. He's shaved and everything."

Madeline tiptoed into Cedars Malibu, not knowing quite what to expect. But Ed was up and dressed, sitting in his chair. He greeted her warmly and they started babbling on about the advertising business,

ABC, changes in the media, new programming coming. I was trying to pick up the heaps of laundry scattered around and hoped to sneak out, comb my hair, and get dressed. But Madeline interrupted.

"Why don't you stop that housecleaning and come join us."

"But I'm in my pajamas."

"So what?"

So I joined them. And the three of us—me in my jammies, Madeline in her Anne Klein suit, and Ed in his best blue joggers—sat around and shot the breeze for an hour or so.

When I saw Madeline to the door, she confessed, "Jeanie, I was so afraid to come out here."

"You were?" Madeline, of all people, surprised me. She was so gutsy and sure of herself.

"It took everything I had to call you, but I'm really glad I did. I mean I'm really glad. For one thing, I saw a whole new side of Ed."

"You did?"

"There's a sweetness and a gentleness I never knew was there. It was very special to see. And it's not bad here, you know. I thought it would be awful. I'm really glad I came."

Madeline's visit made me understand how difficult it is for people to face illness. How morbid it must seem. How easy it is to rationalize avoidance. She and I had been friends for twenty-five years, yet it was hard for her to pick up the phone.

I'm really glad she came. I'm really, really glad. It gave me the chance to tell the story and show how it's not so bad after all. Sometimes—a lot of the time—it can even be good.

December 9

WHEN WE WENT TO THE DOCTOR THIS TIME, Ed walked in on his own two feet, without oxygen, without a wheelchair, without a couple of helpers.

Dr. Moore was shocked. With an embarrassed smile on his face, one of the few times he acknowledged Ed as a fighter, he shook his hand.

"It must be the chemo," he said.

No, I thought. It's Ed.

Dr. Moore hadn't expected Mycostatin to do anything, but obviously it was working. Ed was up, walking around, off oxygen, using the bathroom, bitching at me, giving orders—being Ed. When we got home, Carol was waiting for us and she was shocked as well.

"Mr. McNeilly, you look wonderful."

"I feel wonderful, but look here. My legs are swelling and I want you to do something about it because I have Christmas shopping to do."

"It's edema," she smiled. "I'll phone the doctor and get a prescription."

Still later, I overheard Ed phoning Sug at her office, asking her to pick up something at Tiffany's. I knew it was a Christmas present for me. My eyes drifted toward the merry-go-round horse that sat in our living room and I recalled a Christmas past.

❧ *I can't remember when I started to love merry-go-rounds, but it was firmly entrenched by the time I was six or seven. There was one at the Springlake Amusement Park in Oklahoma City and once when I was about seven my cousin from Chickasha, who was an only child and got to do such things, came to Oklahoma City on a Sunday afternoon to go to Springlake, and her parents stopped by our house to take me with them. But I was off somewhere playing "kick the can" or building forts in the Johnson grass on the empty lots behind our block, and no one could find me, so I didn't get to go.*

I stayed at home on Sunday afternoons for the next two years, hoping they'd come again so I could ride the merry-go-round. But they never did.

Maybe that's why merry-go-rounds became such a thing with me.

When Kevin and I got married and came to California in 1961, one of the first things I discovered was the merry-go-round on the Santa Monica pier. I loved that shoddy, seedy pier with the smell of fishermen cutting bait at one end and the mingled aromas of cotton candy, popcorn, and corn dogs on a stick at the other. And then there were the sounds. Baseballs knocking over bowling pins. Rifles shooting at targets. Bumper cars bumping. And always the calliope, rinky-tink sound of the merry-go-round as it started up and then, two minutes later, died down.

I rode the merry-go-round every single time I went to the pier. I have no idea why it made me so happy or why it still does. The innocence of childhood, I suppose. Blowing soap bubbles through a pipe. Chasing fireflies in the front yard. Climbing up an elm tree to sit on the roof of the garage and watch the boys play baseball.

After the children were born, going to ride the merry-go-round became a ritual. We went to the pier on a lot of Sunday afternoons. We went every Thanksgiving to pass the hours while the turkey cooked. In time, the children preferred the bumper cars and the giant slide, but we still always rode the merry-go-round.

"We have to humor your mother," Kevin would wink.

Somewhere along the line—during the 1960s—I became aware that merry-go-rounds were disappearing. I read an article in the Times one Sunday morning and almost shouted at Kevin.

"Listen to this. Did you know there are only four merry-go-rounds left in southern California? The one at Griffith Park, the one at NuPike in Long Beach, the one at Pacific Ocean Park, and ours at the Santa Monica pier?"

"No!" he shouted back, as if I'd just told him that dogs and small children were also disappearing.

After a while, the ones at NuPike and POP went away, along with the amusement parks themselves.

"They're taking down the merry-go-rounds," Kevin told me on another Sunday, looking up from another edition of the Times, "but they're saving the horses. They've become antiques. I wish we were back home. I could find you one."

Kevin knew a lot of antique dealers around Tulsa, dating back to the days when his family had money. But antiques weren't exactly what we were about in Los Angeles. Our furniture was early Sears, although we did have a rosewood dining-room buffet that was a period piece from the 1920s. Kevin had bought it for five dollars at the Salvation Army resale store in Santa Monica to gussy up the apartment he lived in before we were married.

Then one day—it was maybe 1970—he phoned me at work, all excited. "Hey," he said, "I was driving down Sunset in about the 5000-block and I saw this junky old used-furniture store, and they had a merry-go-round horse in there."

"You're kidding."

"No. I'm not. I might have even seen two. Why don't you meet me there at lunch?"

So I bolted from my typewriter at Foote, Cone & Belding and drove my VW van with the bashed-in top to meet him. They did have two of them, and they were beauties. A white horse with head held high, an arched tail, and a sweeping mane, carved so beautifully it made you ache. And the paint was barely chipped. The other horse was brown, with its front legs out in front and its rear legs stretched behind, as if in full gallop. Both horses were mounted on poles and were the ones that went up and down, rather than the ones on the outer rim of merry-go-rounds whose feet are on the ground and who remain stationary. The "jumpers," as I called them, were much more valuable.

But I was absolutely shocked when we priced them. One was 500 dollars and the other, 750. At the time, we still hadn't bought a color TV, a dishwasher, or an electric clothes dryer.

There was no way we could afford something so impractical. So we walked away, but Kevin told me he'd get back to Tulsa before long and find me one there. For a year or so, I drove down Sunset once in a while and saw the white horse on display on the sidewalk. Then one day I drove by and it was gone.

But I still rode the merry-go-round on the Santa Monica pier. As time went on and money became less of a problem, I regretted not spending the 500 dollars, in favor of a Kenmore two-cycle dryer. The horses were getting more and more rare. And more and more dear.

Years later, when I met Ed, one of the first things I did was drag him to the Carousel Pavilion on the pier. The merry-go-round had been renovated and the circular building brightly painted since it had been featured in the Paul Newman/Robert Redford movie The Sting.

"I can't ride a merry-go-round, Jean."

"Why not?"

"I'm too big. The horse will break."

"It will not. You're just embarrassed."

The ticket taker did look a little worried when Ed put his 240 pounds onto a black stallion with red jewels on the bridle. But the horse was strong and didn't falter. Ed did, however, and stood beside the lusty stallion while I rode round a second time.

And then, the first Christmas after Ed and I were married, it happened. That beautiful Christmas when he hung branches covered with twinkling lights from the ceiling. On that Christmas morning, he and my four all-grown-up children lugged a huge packing crate up from the garage. Inside was the most beautiful jumper ever carved, a silver stallion with a black mane and tail, a prancing head, a red-and-gold saddle. He'd come to me from a merry-go-round in Atlantic City, New Jersey, via a dealer Ed had found in Portland, Oregon.

Ed had taken the care he always took with Christmas gifts and researched antique horses all over the United States. He'd sent for catalogs and Polaroids. He'd learned the names of all the great carvers, the significance of original paint, and how the mane and tail couldn't be add-ons. The best horses were carved from a single block of wood and had become very prized. Great horses like the white one on Sunset now cost thousands and thousands of dollars.

Ed found the most perfect horse available at the dealer in Portland and paid to have it crated and shipped. It arrived the twenty-third of December, and he and the children formed a successful conspiracy to keep me out of the garage.

"I'll put your car away, Mom. You relax."

Or, "Gee whiz, Mom, you know I always take down the garbage."

When I saw the horse on Christmas morning, my hands shook and my knees wobbled.

I named him Mr. Ed, of course. He sits in a place of honor in our living room beloved by me, waiting with me for the grandchildren to be born. ❧

It's an altogether silly story for a person my age. But as I looked at Mr. Ed that afternoon, it didn't seem silly at all.

December 13

SUG HATCHED A PLOT TO GET ED a dog for Christmas. "He loves them so much, Mama. He watches the dogs play down on the beach and has names for all of them...."

"I know Sug, but...."

"I'll take care of it, I promise."

"I know Sug, but...."

"I'll take it to the vet and buy everything it needs. You won't have to do a thing, Mama."

"It isn't that. I think a puppy might be hard on Ed until it's trained."

"But see, I already thought of that. Lisa told me about the Miniature Schnauzer Breeder's Association. You can get dogs from them, Mama, that are eight or ten months old and already trained."

"You mean house trained and everything?"

"Yep. The owners keep them to see if they're going to be show dogs. If they aren't, they sell them after six months."

"Well...."

"I already talked to an owner in Anaheim. She has a dog ten months old. He's had all his shots. He's even been neutered. She said he's real sweet-tempered. I thought I'd go take a look at him. Is it okay?"

Miniature schnauzers were one of Ed's favorite breeds. I knew how much he loved dogs, although he and I had never had one, because the responsibility sometimes puts a damper on the spontaneity of life, which Ed also loved. But spontaneity wasn't much of an issue at the moment and I could see a doggie hopping onto Ed's bed to be petted. A dog could be company for him as well, after I went back to work.

"It's a wonderful idea, Sug."

So she drove to Anaheim after work and "interviewed" the dog. Actually, before she finished, she had driven all over Los Angeles county, looking at schnauzers.

"It's got to be the perfect dog. Not too feisty. It has to be a doggie who wants to be petted."

She finally settled on one owned by a breeder in Irvine and picked Sunday afternoon to go with Chris to get the pooch and bring him home. I told Kim and Mark, so they'd be present for the big arrival. Ed was settled in his recliner, chatting with his daughter and son-in-law when the doggie came through the front door on a red, Christmasy leash, with a big red bow on his neck. He was jet black with white paws and a white chest.

I looked at the dog and looked at him again. He certainly was a cutie. I can't say it was love at first sight, but I thought there was promise. The reaction from Ed, however, was strange.

"He's for you, Ed," Sug trilled. "He's your Christmas present from all of us." Ed smiled at her, looked at me, and petted the dog. "Here, boy."

I could tell there was something wrong, but nobody noticed in all the excitement. The dog was a sniffer and was busy checking out his new home, with Kim, Mark, Chris, and Sug following him around like a parade of wind-up tin men.

"You have to name him, Ed." Sug was so proud.

"Dad was always so good at naming dogs," chimed in Kim.

"I can't think very well today." Ed was stressed and nervous. So I helped come up with some names and we settled on "Tux," because the doggie looked like he was wearing a tuxedo.

After a while, I got ready to go out for some groceries at the Hughes Market and Ed asked if he could come with me. We loaded his wheelchair into the car and the minute we turned onto Pacific Coast Highway, he started to cry.

"What is it, Ed?"

"I love Sug so much, Jean. It was so thoughtful of her to want me to have a dog. But I can't, Jean . . . ."

"What do you mean?"

"I wouldn't want to hurt her for the world."

"What is it, Ed?"

"She has to take the dog back."

"Oh no, Sweetheart. No she doesn't. We'll take care of it . . . ."

"Jean, I can't love a dog right now. I have to focus on getting better. Dogs need love, Jean, and I can't make that commitment right now."

"Oh, Ed." I suddenly understood what was bothering him.

During all this time, Ed had never given up. He'd never complained of "why me," stopped talking about getting better, or expressed fear of the future. He was fighting. Still. With all his might and main. He couldn't be diverted or direct his attention to anything else. Everything he had to give was concentrated into a small, hard mass of will and determination. He was going to keep on. And on. And on. And on.

"It'll be okay, Ed."

"But I can't love the dog, Jean. And it isn't fair to him. Dogs need that."

"He'll be my dog. We won't tell Sug. But I'll love him for both of us, and you won't have to be responsible."

"Are you sure?"

"Yes."

"I'm sorry, Jean."

"Don't be sorry. The important thing is that you want to keep fighting."

"I can't stop fighting, Jean."

And so, I got a dog.

December 14

CEDARS MALIBU WAS ALIVE DURING DECEMBER. Eric and Mary came to visit a lot. With Kim and Mark, they helped us decorate the tree. Erin and Rich were home from school midmonth. Maureen scrounged a day or two extra away from her job. Ed and I were in and out doing a lot of Christmas shopping. He wanted to be involved in the selection of every gift. So we pushed his wheelchair up and down the Santa Monica Mall, as well as to more inaccessible places like Banana Republic and Abercrombie & Fitch.

He special-ordered a kiddy-car Porsche for Matthew and had it shipped from the manufacturer in New Hampshire to his grandson's home in Florida. We planned a party on Christmas Eve and Chris brought home the tree on top of the Mini-moke, Ed's silly little beachy jeep.

Among all the good moments, however, there were bad ones. Times when I felt not at the end of my rope, but at the end of a leash. And like a dog on a leash, I sometimes bared my teeth.

Ed and I were coming out of Feldmar Watch Co. on Pico, where we'd gone to pick out a lawyer's watch for Sug. We hadn't had a bad experience, it was just that the store was crowded, the wheelchair was bulky, and getting in and out was a pain. Then getting in and out of the car was a pain. Ed was giving me orders, as he sometimes did.

"You're hurting my leg, Jean. Stop it, right now."

I left him in his chair at the curb and ran halfway down the block. Running was an instinct, a way to vent the anger.

I felt like I was tied to that wheelchair, as if it had become an extension of my own body. I felt I could never be more than ten feet from it or five minutes from Ed. I had no identity of my own. I was leashed to cancer every bit as much as Ed was. So I ran for half a block and then, of course, I ran back.

"I'm sorry, Jean. I'd rather do anything than upset you. I love you so much."

I knew he did. It just took so much patience. So much patience. So much patience.

That day, Bob phoned. "Can somebody stay with Ed on the eighteenth?"

"Yeah, Erin's here. And Rich. Why?"

"The ARCO Christmas lunch is at noon and the company Christmas party is in the evening. I want you to come to both. I'm going to send a limousine for you, okay? You need to have some fun and everybody wants to see you. Besides, I miss you."

There is no way to put a value on the gestures people make toward one another. One human kindness can get you through a day, a week, a month. It was glorious to be away from cancer for a while and to forget about it. I loved being out and with people. Cameron Day, one of the young copywriters who'd worked for me but gone on, crashed the party, and he and I danced, laughed, and talked about the business.

People like Cameron who can talk past your crisis are wonderful. He knew what was going on in my life. In fact, in a wonderful mix of generations, he and Ed had been buddies when Ed worked at the agency on Daihatsu. But Cameron took my arm, whirled me onto the dance floor, and said, "Why don't you take your shoes off and let's go for it." We did.

I finally emerged from my limousine at the front door in Malibu, after midnight, a little drunk.

It was wonderful.

December 17

ED TOOK A BIT OF A DIVE.
Carol and I decided it was another infection. So she phoned the doctor;
I phoned Louise.

"Ed is running a fever," I told her.

"Yes, well, you should give him aspirin to bring that down."

"I've given him aspirin; there's still fever. There are also chills and
sweats."

"Do you want to bring him in?"

"No. I think he needs an antibiotic."

"Did the doctor order one?"

"No, the doctor hasn't returned my call. Or Carol's."

"Well, I can't conclude that the problem . . . ."

"Louise. He needs an antibiotic."

"Is that what you want from me, Mrs. McNeilly? An antibiotic?"

"Yes."

"If that's what you want, then we'll order one."

I hated Louise.

December 23

ONE OF THE MOST FASCINATING THINGS
about Christmas, to me, is the worldwide conspiracy between adults
and children.

It's an amazing suspension of disbelief. The children, who learn
that reindeer fly and that an old man named Santa Claus lives in a toy
factory at the North Pole, are told the story by adults, who either are in
league all over this earth to spread the myth among their young or believe it themselves in some way.

Every Christmas I can remember, since I was about seven, I've
watched *Miracle on 34th Street,* the movie about the department-store
Santa Claus at Macy's who claimed he really was Kris Kringle. I think
that he was. And, as an adult in this world, whether you live in Akron or
Zurich, you take on the responsibility of helping your children figure
out the truth of the matter, as well.

One year, for example, when Chris was about seven, he'd asked
Kevin how come Santa Claus knew he wanted the Hot Wheels
Model 734 Slot Car, when he'd told Santa Claus at the May Company he
wanted the Model 777 and then changed his mind.

"Well," Kevin said without missing a beat, "that's because *I* knew you wanted that slot car and I left a note in the fireplace for Santa's elves."

"You left a note in the fireplace?"

"Sure. Santa's elves go around picking up everybody's lists out of fireplaces. That's one of your jobs if you're an elf."

"Yeah?" said Chris.

"Yeah," said Kevin.

And so a little ritual began and continues to the present that has us all writing lists to put in the fireplace along about Thanksgiving, and sure enough, Santa's elves dutifully pick them up. Sometimes, little elf footprints have been left behind in the ashes of the fireplace. It's amazing.

But what few adults understand is that children are also working at it. I overheard an interesting conversation once shortly after Christmas between a six-year-old Sug and a four-year-old Erin, as they sat in the sandbox.

"If Santa got you 'Lina Ballerina,' how come I saw it in Mom's closet?" asked the younger child.

"Well, that's because Santa stores things in people's closets until he gets there," Sug said wisely, spinning a piece of logic that would fend off anything her sister might bring up. "See, he doesn't have room. And Lina Ballerina might break. And besides, he needs Mom to wrap it."

And so the minds of children compensate for adult blunders all the while the adults think they're the ones in charge. Fat chance.

Christmas has also caused us to share some fascinating gifts over the years. When she was eleven or twelve, Sug knew I had an interest in pretty lingerie. So she hand-embroidered me two pairs of panties. She went to Sears and got their best fifty-nine-cent nylon-tricot bikini briefs and embroidered her own designs. One pair had, as I recall, her interpretation of the sun on each cheek, with spires radiating from smiling sun faces. The other was filled with flowers. Zinnias. Fat, orange zinnias.

The embroidery was awkward and she'd used heavy cotton strands, but I loved the gift and wore one pair to work the day after Christmas, under gabardine slacks. I was stopped in my tracks on the way to lunch by a client named Joanne, who was walking behind me.

"Jean, do you have welts or something? Or...uh...are you wearing something odd? I mean, there's this design showing on your tush."

Sug's thick loops showed under my tight pants. I never wore them again, but I thought about framing them, except I couldn't figure out where to hang framed panties or how to explain why.

Baking is yet another ritual of Christmas that's worldwide. In December, the smell of cookies baking must radiate from the planet like fluorocarbons going into the ozone layer.

"Yep," they say on Mars, "it's Christmas again on Earth. I can smell it."

People make spritzer cookies in Copenhagen, Lebkuchen cookies in Hamburg, marzipan in Venice, and tollhouse in Kansas City. The Polish bake babka, the Hungarians have their nut rolls, the Italians their panettone, and the Germans their stollen. The sales of brown sugar worldwide must be staggering.

The first Christmas Ed and I were married, he baked fruitcakes as gifts to sent hither and yon and to have ready when the children came home. What but Christmas could send a fifty-five-year-old advertising executive, who drives a Porsche and drinks Jim Beam, into the kitchen to bake fruitcakes?

Don't tell me there's no Santa Claus.

Perhaps it was the memory of Ed up to his knees in batter and candied cherries that stirred up my own natural instincts.

"I gotta do a lot of baking this Christmas," I told Ed.

"Why?" he asked.

"I don't know. I just do. It means home, I think. It means everything is okay."

"I may not be able to eat it, Jean."

"I know. Maybe I'll make something I don't want anyone to eat, like a gingerbread house. I've always wanted to make a gingerbread house."

I was talking on the phone about it to Stacie one evening when she called in to check on Ed.

"I'm thinking of making one of those Christmas things you always think you're going to make, but never do, like a gingerbread house."

"Oh, yeah?" she said.

"Yeah," I said. "Or maybe marzipan cookies."

"Oh, yeah?" she said.

"Yeah," I said.

A couple of days later, Stacie phoned back.

"What we have to do," she said, "is make croquembouches."

"Croquembouches?"

"Yeah. They're the most wonderful, most beautiful Christmas thing ever."

And she described them to me. Bavarian in origin, they're made of dozens of tiny cream puffs, stacked on top of one another in the shape of a Christmas tree, then all held together with spun sugar.

"I saw one once at a Christmas party at the Waldorf in New York," she explained, "and I have the recipe in my gourmet cookbook."

So Stacie took an afternoon off the day before Christmas Eve to come out to the house, and together we made croquembouches.

We put Christmas music on the stereo and ran in and out of the kitchen to show batter and cream to Ed. We spun sugar all over the pans, the kitchen, and our hair. We were amazed when the puff pastries actually puffed. And cocky over the consistency of our cream filling. Stacie managed to build a better-shaped tree than me, but both croquembouches were stunning creations. We put them each on a silver tray lined with a doily. And Erin took our picture.

Alan came at the moment of triumph, and with Ed, Erin, and Rich, Maureen, Chris, and Sug in attendance, he toasted our efforts. Then, in the gallant gesture of a true Renaissance man, he made dinner. It was, I think, the best moment of Christmas.

Even though Stacie phoned me the next day. "Did yours fall down?" she asked.

"Yep," I said. "It collapsed during the night."

The cookbook failed to mention that spun sugar has its limitations and one can't expect croquembouches to be made days ahead.

"I don't really care," said Stacie.

"Neither do I," said I.

We both knew the point hadn't to do with eating croquembouches, but with making them.

But what I knew that Stacie didn't was one of the best presents I got that Christmas was a half day of her time spent with me as if Ed weren't sick, as if she and I hadn't a care in the world and had nothing better to do than spend hours in the kitchen.

And because of Stacie, whenever I think of Christmas 1987, I'll think of croquembouches. Not cancer.

December 31

ERIN AND RICH LEFT A DAY OR TWO after Christmas to go to Florida and visit Rich's parents; Sug flew up to San Francisco to spend New Year's with Jim; Maureen went back to New York and her job, as she'd used up all her vacation coming home when Ed was at Cedars; and Chris was away again on a field trip to

Arizona. So Ed and I were alone as New Year's approached. His energy was sapped, but I thought it was normal letdown after the excitement of Christmas. But when we went for our regular visit to Dr. Moore, the doctor immediately slapped Ed into the hospital for a blood transfusion. Chemo can wreak havoc on the red cells.

I thought there was some sense of "whoops" in Dr. Moore's face when he sent us to the hospital. Weekly blood tests had been routine at the City of Hope. I felt perhaps the less frequent monitoring in a private-practice scenario was insufficient.

Then, when Louise put me on the phone to the hospital, it was made grumpily clear that we should be at Admitting at six the following morning. I was told about five times "don't be late." We "made room" for your husband, the implication being if we weren't there on time, the room would go to someone else.

So we weren't late. Even though it meant getting Ed up and dressed at four-thirty A.M. It was black outside and chilly. I tried to warm him with tea before we left but didn't give him breakfast, because that would have meant getting him up even earlier. But when we got to the hospital at ten minutes till six, there wasn't anybody in Admitting. The waiting area was pitch dark. Nobody showed up to open the Admitting desk until six-forty-five. Ed sat in his wheelchair and waited. He couldn't read. Indeed, he hadn't been able to read at any time since he'd left Cedars, because he couldn't seem to focus his eyes well enough, probably because of the morphine. He couldn't walk around. I sat with him and held his hand and we tried to talk. It was only an hour, but it was very, very difficult.

Then, when we got Ed to his room, the nurse said, "What are you doing here? Why are you here so early?"

The blood hadn't even been ordered yet. What's more, they were in the middle of changing shifts and hadn't time for Ed, so nothing happened, including breakfast, except that we waited some more, until after nine.

And it all happened because somebody in Admitting had a schedule. She thought if she told us six, she'd be sure to have us there when she opened at seven. She was correct. We were there. And the travail she caused us was not as important to her as meeting the needs of herself and her hospital.

I quarreled with the lady in Admitting. And I snapped back at the nurse on the floor when she snapped because we'd arrived during shift change.

But after a while, you just give up.

January 1, 1988

THE TRANSFUSION HELPED ED.
His color, which had gone to yellow, was back to pink. His energy level came back up. He was still able to walk around the house on his own, or to the car. He was still off oxygen. He was lucid and strong-willed. He was not in pain beyond what small steady doses of morphine could handle.

But his weight had continued to fall and, despite occasional flurries of real appetite, he was down to 180 pounds. I'd hug him from time to time and feel bones where before I'd been enveloped in the warmth and comfort of his big bear embrace. The hernia on his stomach continued to grow. His attention span was short and he was often jittery. Although he couldn't read, he could play cards. So we played gin rummy in the afternoons, and he begged me to take him to movies.

We'd load up his wheelchair and take off for the theaters in the Marina. We'd fold up the chair and park it in the lobby, and he'd let me help him to a seat. People stared a little because he looked so frail, but if he noticed, he didn't care. On New Year's Day we saw *Good Morning Vietnam,* which Ed just loved.

I watched him laughing at Robin Williams playing the movie's hero, an indomitable American soldier who fought the war in Vietnam in his own way, by being an irreverent, irrepressible deejay on Armed Forces Radio. No wonder Ed loves the movie, I thought to myself. He's the same kind of man.

It made me realize that the reservoir of strength Ed drew on day after day is within all of us if we dig deep enough for it. It's part of the American character. We're optimists. We like to crack jokes in the face of danger. We're taught from birth to admire "rugged individualism." We're taught from birth to believe any one of us can accomplish whatever we put our minds to. "Yes. You can grow up to be President," our children are told. And they can.

When Ed was born in 1927, people were still alive who'd crossed the country in covered wagons. His own family was part of the second great western migration to escape the dust bowl in the '30s. There's a belief passed down from generation to generation that we can overcome the odds, that we can achieve, that there is nothing on earth like American guts and ingenuity. Indeed, the American dream is nothing more or less than the idea that ordinary people can succeed in extraordinary ways.

It's a simplistic, perhaps, but powerful legacy. Middle America. Home. Family. Belief in God. Do the right thing. Laugh. Be irreverent. Don't be afraid to break the rules. And never give up. It settled a nation. Won us a couple of world wars. And was getting Edward R. McNeilly through cancer. The "right stuff," Tom Wolfe called it.

Ed had it in greater measure than some, but it's in the character of all of us.

January 15

I WENT BACK TO WORK, which wasn't a decision, really. I had to go back to work. Sitting out in Malibu, I'd already begun to feel a subtle shift at the office. I took strong stands on things at Kresser/Craig, and it provided a focus. Bob went off on entrepreneurial tangents from time to time, some brilliant, some just awful. I had a more clearly defined set of business principles that were boring at times and intractable at others, but a clear reference point nonetheless. It was a great combination. Those kinds of intangibles are what make a company tick. And I was beginning to sense a drift because I wasn't around. One of the young account execs told me, in a backhanded kind of compliment, "When you aren't there to argue in meetings, no one's sure."

So I went back. But I was unprepared for how hard work/home were going to be this time and in addition, I got hit in the face with a crisis over nursing care as complicated as an episode of "LA Law."

With the help of Aunt Maureen, I'd found a new nursing service and set about bringing in a practical nurse, five days a week.

It wasn't until then that Aetna realized there were two nursing services involved: Lifeline, where we got Carol, and Norrell, whom I'd contacted for the five-day-a-week nurse.

Aetna wasn't inclined to pay for two—it was against their policy—even though Carol came for only an hour or so twice a week, and even though they'd double-paid before, for Carol and Jessie, then Carol and Georgetta. Lifeline had been slow in billing, actually, and by the time their billing was processed, I'd taken over from Georgetta and the double team wasn't apparent.

Anyway, it was apparent now and I didn't know what the hell to do.

"I have to have Carol, Jean," Ed told me, as I knew he would. "I have to have Carol." Doing without her was simply not an option.

"I'll pay the nurses myself," I told Aetna, "until we get it straightened out."

I was absolutely floored by Aetna's response: "No, Mrs. McNeilly, we'll pay until everything's straightened out. We don't know what we're going to do exactly, but we can make exceptions and we'll work with you and sort it out."

I'd been conditioned all my life to hate and mistrust insurance companies, but here was the insurance company stepping in like a friend. You never know.

But the situation was terribly complex. It came to light that the maximum coverage for home nursing during any one calendar year was 126 units, with every four hours counting as a unit. At that rate, we'd use up the nursing coverage in about sixty eight-hour working days. If we subtracted for Carol, the coverage would be gone in about forty-five days. If I kept to a normal working schedule, which meant I left the house around eight and got home around six, it was a ten-hour day, not an eight-hour day, and the coverage would be gone in about thirty days.

If the insurance ran out, the combination of Carol and a second nurse from eight to six, five days a week, would cost 5,000 dollars per month. And of course, that was with me and Sug doing nights, evenings, and weekends, which I also didn't know if we'd be able to handle long-term. She was a beginning attorney, for heaven's sake, and I had a company with its problems.

I made a lot of money, but I didn't make enough to handle 5,000 dollars a month, without borrowing or something. All of Ed's resources —everything he had—had gone into the car wash, which at that moment was sudsing away in the background. In the red.

Carol brought up hospice care, and I thought about it but I didn't like it. The only reason I could see to take Ed away from home was pain. If he began to have the kind of pain I'd heard about, and I couldn't handle intravenous morphine or whatever it took at home, then a hospital or hospice might be better. But hospice wasn't a good option for me until that happened, if it ever did.

I didn't know what to do and Ed wasn't helping. Indeed, he took an already difficult situation and compounded it.

Strong-willed personalities like Ed will try to retain control. But when their resources have dwindled and they don't have much to fight with, they use whatever they have. They refuse to eat. They refuse to swallow medication. They use their bodies. That's all they've got.

I came home one night to learn the nurse we'd had for a few days had given her notice. She'd stay until we got someone, but she found Ed too hard to deal with.

"She told me," Sug said later on in the kitchen, "that he urinated on her."

"On purpose?"

"Yep."

I didn't doubt it. I also didn't confront Ed with it. He was struggling, and he shouldn't be belittled. On the other hand, I didn't blame the nurse for quitting.

I was sitting on his bed later in the evening, exhausted by the whole thing, indeed feeling defeated. I really didn't know what to do.

Ed had taken on a demeanor, a shift in personality that was becoming more and more childlike. He'd respond to his food by smacking his lips and clapping his hands. "That tastes so good, Jean. Can I have some more?" He'd tug on my sleeve for attention. "Could you read to me before bed?" There was an innocence in his eyes and his voice. I'd noticed the same thing in my mother during the bedridden years after her stroke.

Ed picked my hand up off the bed and spoke to me in his childlike tone. "Jean," he said, "can I have Alicia?"

"What do you mean, Ed?"

"Can I have Alicia to be my nurse?" His tone was that of a ten-year-old asking for the red bicycle in the Sears catalog.

I hesitated for Alicia's sake. "She'd have to quit her other jobs, Ed."

"Please, Jean, I want Alicia."

"I don't know if I can ask her . . . ."

"Please, Jean. She said she would."

Then I hesitated for my own sake. "You know she's not a real nurse." I was afraid if things got really bad, they might be beyond her. I also knew she couldn't work a full day and I didn't know if I could handle things without full-time help.

"Please, Jean. I want Alicia. I love her and she loves me."

When he said that, it became a simple decision. Skill from a nurse who was a stranger wasn't as important as love from someone who cared. Insofar as Alicia working part-time, we'd manage.

And so I spoke to Alicia, knowing that the twenty-nine-year-old mother of three, who already had a six-night-a-week job and two other housekeeping obligations during the day, was carrying a load that would stagger most people.

But when I asked her, her tone seemed to say, "It's about time."

"I can take better care of him, Jean. I know I can."

"Alicia, . . . about quitting your other jobs, . . . I'll make it up to you later on."

"It's no problem, Jean. It's not for the rest of my life. I'll be fine."

But she couldn't quit her night job at the nursing home, so we worked it out so she'd come every morning at eight—after the nursing home—and stay with Ed until three in the afternoon. I'd work a shortened day and relieve her at three. Jocelyn would continue at Kresser/Craig indefinitely.

We even worked it out with Aetna. They agreed to classify Alicia as a nurse's aide because of her nursing-home experience, and they further agreed to cover both her and Carol for an indefinite period of time—no units counting up—as long as Alicia's hours didn't exceed thirty or thirty-five a week.

And so Alicia Lopez became Ed's nurse, taking her place at Cedars Malibu with me, my daughter, and my son.

My only regret is that I didn't have her do it sooner. She was incredible with Ed. She swooped in and just took him over. She cut his hair and trimmed his moustache. She rubbed him down every morning with creams to salve his flaking skin. She put flowers by his bed and played music in the room. She cooked lunches so packed with nutrition they practically walked off the stove on their own. She brought half a dozen different teas into the house. Teas to calm. Teas to medicate. Teas to help him sleep. She had no compunction whatever about loading him into the car and taking him out. Alicia stood about five feet tall. I don't know where she got the strength to shove his wheelchair into her Ford Pinto, but she did.

I had some problems getting away every day at two to be home by three. People would forget and schedule late-afternoon meetings. But mostly, the working day just didn't want to be snipped at early afternoon. There was stress on the Century City end. But on the Malibu end, I loved it. I loved coming home and spending a quiet couple of hours with Ed in the softness of late afternoon. He'd gotten comfortable enough to let me go out for ten or fifteen minutes and I'd walk the dog, look at the ocean, and collect myself.

Sometimes it hurt. This was the life Ed and I had been thinking about when he bought the car wash. We'd both work less and spend more time at home in our beloved Malibu. We'd talked so often of days filled with simple things. "I'll terrace the back of the lot, Jean, so you can put in a vegetable garden." We'd talked of buying a small boat so we could go fishing on June mornings, right off the beach near our home. I'd talked of writing. He'd talked of sketching. We'd talked of working together on projects that I would write and he would photograph or illustrate. "Let's learn Spanish together," he'd say one day. "Let's learn astronomy," I'd say another. "Jean, I think I can put a third story on the house." For the grandchildren. That's the kind of life we'd seen. And I longed for it.

But along with the hurt was a good feeling. There was a sense of peacefulness that's hard to explain. I knew we were doing a good job for Ed, and it calmed the fears in my heart and drove away the speculations about an empty tomorrow.

January 18

ED WAS HOLDING HIS OWN. He was still off oxygen and walking around the house under his own power. He was eating okay. And not coughing too much.

We went to see Dr. Moore, who took me aside and changed the ninety-day prognosis he'd given me at Cedars to six months. But before we left, Ed got very angry at the young oncologist. I didn't confront, but he did.

"You took X-rays when I was here two weeks ago," Ed said accusingly. "What did they show?"

"Let me get the file, Ed."

Dr. Moore pulled the file and began to read aloud from the X-ray technician's report. It seemed to me he'd never seen the report before.

"Did you compare these X-rays to the last ones?" Ed wanted to know.

"Uh, . . . no."

"Then how do you know what's happening?"

"I can tell from the technician's report, Ed."

"But it's not the same as comparing. Could you get the previous X-rays and compare them?"

"We'll have to pull the file, Ed. We'll have them ready next time."

He then asked the doctor to check PDQ, the Physician's Data Query from the National Cancer Institute, to find out if there was any new experimentation going on with colon cancer. It was through PDQ that Ed had first found the City of Hope. But Dr. Moore didn't subscribe to PDQ. I told him "never mind" about PDQ or checking with NCI; I'd do it myself.

When we were driving home, Ed was deeply frustrated. "They were prepared for me to die," he said, "but not for me to live."

January 19

PUSHING ED IN HIS WHEELCHAIR through the Santa Monica Mall, into the Hughes Market, across the street to Malibu Cinema—all of it was a revelation to me of what it's like to be handicapped.

I don't know what people did before they cut ramps into curbs. It's simply not possible to get a grown person in a wheelchair over a curb without a ramp. And thank goodness for handicapped parking spaces. Trying to get a wheelchair out of a car, and a person into the wheelchair in a busy parking lot, is taking your life in your hands, unless you're in a handicapped space.

To get a wheelchair into a supermarket, you have to push it through one of the aisles where the cashier stands. If all the cashiers are busy, you have to ask one of them to let you through and the chair barely fits. There's about an inch on each side. The chair has plenty of room in the main aisles of department stores, but it's a tight squeeze in the side aisles.

Restaurants are a real problem. There's just no room for a wheelchair. If the person can walk a few steps, you can leave the chair at the door, but if he can't, it's too bad. It's the same with movies. There's no place to tuck in a wheelchair. If people are comfortable sitting in the aisle, it works. If they don't like to attract that kind of attention, it doesn't.

We managed to do a lot with Ed in his chair, but everything we did took four times longer. In the huge Santa Monica Mall, there's only one elevator. To go up or down a level, we'd have to go the length of the mall to get to it. It's a struggle to open doors to get in or out of a store. The pusher has to turn around and shove himself backward through the door, with the wheelchair following and the door banging on the patient.

Thanks to changes made in the last decade or so, people in wheelchairs can use public bathrooms. But they can't use public phones, since they can't reach them, nor public transportation, unless the street car or bus has a lift, and most of them don't.

And the wheelchair itself…well,…I'll bet it hasn't changed or been improved in a hundred years. It weighs a ton. I'm tall, healthy, and strong. But it was all I could do to lift Ed's chair in and out of the car. Once in a while, a man would see me struggling and come help. But more often than not, people were embarrassed and walked past me, pretending not to see.

I'd pretended myself in the past, but I don't do it anymore. People can't always stop to help and that's okay. They have a right to be in a hurry, have their own problems, or just not be up to getting involved at that moment. But looking at someone because you're curious, then pretending not to see is really rude. It makes the one being stared past feel like a nonperson.

One afternoon at the Santa Monica Mall, Ed needed to use the men's room. So we parked the chair outside the door, he went in under his own steam, and I plopped down in the chair to wait, because I was pooped. And the strangest thing happened.

Suddenly, I was handicapped.

I felt people staring at me, past me, through me. Trying to surreptitiously figure out my problem. I sat there and watched myself being looked at for about ten minutes until Ed reappeared and I'll never forget what it felt like. I saw split-second looks of distaste as people searched for the withered leg, the twisted torso, the missing limb—and when they didn't find it, split-second looks of curiosity sometimes followed by downright staring. "What's the matter with her?"

I wanted to shout, as I'll bet handicapped people do all the time, "There's nothing the matter with me. It isn't my body that makes me a person, it's what's inside." It was my Great Wheelchair Lesson.

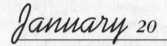

January 20

I GOT A BOOK FOR CHRISTMAS entitled *Love, Medicine & Miracles,* written by a New York cancer specialist named Bernie Siegel. I'd never heard of it but looked it up in the *New York Times Book Review* and discovered it had been on the bestseller list for thirty-seven weeks. I devoured the book in one evening, on a long Saturday night.

Dr. Siegel wrote about what he called "exceptional patients"— people who had taken control of their illness in order to heal themselves. Patients who had the courage to work with their doctors to participate in and influence the course of their disease.

Most of Dr. Siegel's patients had cancer. Some of them had miraculous recoveries. All of them reminded me of Ed.

They were people who wouldn't give up. Who had spirit, heart, and courage, like Ed. And the doctor, himself, expressed a philosophy rooted in a set of beliefs not unlike those of Norman Cousins, whose book had encouraged us at the onset of Ed's illness.

"Medicine is not only a science," wrote Dr. Siegel, "but also the art of letting our own individuality interact with the individuality of the patient."

As I read the book, I cried. I ached for a doctor like Bernie Siegel. I sat on the couch beside Ed's bed and grieved for one.

Where was a doctor who could see the courage in Ed's eyes, the hope that blossomed in his heart? Where was a doctor who would give him his dignity as he struggled? Who would make Ed feel there was a partnership between physician and patient and that the partnership was a bond that was never broken, no matter how terminal the patient became? Where was a doctor who was still a doctor? Where were you, Bernie Siegel?

The book gave me renewed hope that there *were* other doctors like him. I decided, right then and there, to put aside my earlier defeatism and find an oncologist somewhere in Los Angeles who was not Everydoctor but who was like Bernie Siegel.

I decided not to worry anymore whether it was medically problematic. If it was, I didn't care. I suddenly knew that what I was looking for was a way to help Ed die well. It's not that I'd given up. I hadn't. But like soldiers in battle, like the men of the first wave who went ashore at Normandy, or Tennyson's Light Brigade, you know your odds are terrible. But all the while you fight like hell. And you want to march in holding your head up.

I thought Ed had a right to that. To keep fighting if he chose, no matter now bad the odds. And thus, by his standards, to die well. Surely a doctor somewhere would understand. And I now had hope I could find him.

January 21

I PHONED AUNT MAUREEN AT ST. JOHN'S. "Listen, would you ask around for me. The nurses. The other nuns. And see if you can find the name of a cancer specialist who's known for being involved with his patients?"

"What's the matter?"

"Nothing's the matter. I just want to change doctors."

"Jean, I'm so glad. I've wished all along Ed was with a doctor at St. John's. Me and the nuns could be involved. Like family. Let me see what I can find out."

"I don't want just anybody. Do you know what I'm trying to do, Maureen? I know he's going to die. But until he does, I want a doctor who's working with him. Do you understand what I mean?"

"I understand. I'm glad you called me. I'll get back to you in a day or so."

Bernie Siegel, LA version, here we come.

January 23

ROBIN AND MATTHEW CAME FROM FLORIDA to visit. Robin was pregnant, expecting a baby in June. She'd come when Ed was at Cedars and had stayed in close touch all fall and winter. I knew it was hard to cross the country with three-year-old Matthew, even to see a dying father, but it didn't go well.

Ed had just had chemo and unlike the two previous injections of Mycostatin, it knocked him out. He spent most of each day in a deep, drugged sleep, hardly aware that Robin and Matthew were there.

Robin wanted the visit for Matthew so he'd have a good memory of his grandfather and she was upset.

"Why couldn't chemo have waited until after our visit?"

I wished we'd put chemo off for a few days too, but the treatments had never knocked Ed out before and I couldn't have presupposed they would. I didn't know if Ed would have allowed it anyway. He was just too focused on not backing off.

Ed roused himself toward the end and on Saturday we crammed the wheelchair into the trunk of my car, which I had to tie shut with a rope, and drove to the Santa Monica pier to give Matthew a ride on the merry-go-round. But after we got Ed and the chair and Matthew and his stroller and Robin and me out of the car, out of the parking lot, and onto the pier, we found the carousel was closed for repairs.

Shit.

Robin and Matthew went home, with the visit lingering not as a warm and emotional memory, but as a strained four days.

Life is real. There are good days. And bad days.

IN BERNIE SIEGEL'S BOOK,
I had read about Dr. O. Carl Simonton and the Simonton Cancer Center
in Pacific Palisades. Dr. Siegel was mightily influenced by Dr. Simonton
and explained that his practice of medicine changed in 1978 as a result
of meeting Dr. Simonton, who with psychologist Stephanie Matthews
(then his wife) were the first Western practitioners to use imaging
techniques against cancer.

The Simontons used meditation and imaging—calling up pictures
in the mind—to enlist the patient's inner self in the fight against disease.
Their techniques are controversial in the medical establishment.
Bernie Siegel described his first session with the Simontons like this:

> When I looked around during the first workshop session, I was
> amazed and angered to find that I was the only "body doctor"
> there. There were a psychiatrist and a holistic practitioner, but
> not one other primary-care physician out of seventy-five par-
> ticipants. Those attending were mostly social workers, pa-
> tients, and psychologists. I became even angrier when many of
> the participants told me they already knew about these tech-
> niques, because the things I was learning hadn't even been
> hinted at in my medical education. Here I was, an M.D., a
> Medical Deity, and I didn't know what went on in the head at
> all! The literature on mind-body interaction was separate, and
> therefore unknown to specialists in other areas. I realized for
> the first time how far ahead theology, psychology, and holistic
> medicine are in this respect.

People come to the Simonton Cancer Center from all over the
world to learn the meditative techniques, and the center tells of success with patients, ranging from apparent miracle cures, to regression,
to lengthening the predicted survival time.

I didn't know if I believed in imaging techniques, but I did believe
that the mind interacted with the body. I'd seen it too many times with
Kevin and Ed. I'd listened to Alan Fogelman tell me Kevin lived the last
five years "because he decided to." So I began reading the Simontons'
book *Getting Well Again*.

It was their theory that disease enters the body when the body's
immune system breaks down, due to stress, fatigue, or other emotional

factors. And that the mind and emotions can be used to put the immune system to work to drive disease back out.

The results at the Simonton Center were mostly what the medical establishment calls "anecdotal," not scientific. Yes, there were some success stories, but they were mostly stories about flukes. This is what Bernie Siegel had to say about that:

If a "miracle" such as permanent remission of cancer happens once, it is valid and must not be dismissed as a fluke. If one patient can do it, there's no reason others can't. I realized that medicine has been studying its failures when it should have been learning from its successes. We should be paying more attention to the exceptional patients, those who get well unexpectedly, instead of staring bleakly at those who die in the usual pattern.

I called the Simonton Center and talked to them about Ed. Their course was a week long, and patients were required to live there along with their primary caretaker, which by that time was out of the question. But I ordered their audio tapes, and Ed and I sat together in the afternoons and listened to them. Ed couldn't focus enough to do imaging and I still didn't know if I believed in it. But there was such comfort and peace in the Simonton approach. The tapes began by asking that you concentrate on the positive emotions of faith, hope, love, and trust. To search inside yourself for quietude and strength. To forget your fears and focus on the life that still existed in your inner self.

I realized that most people would interpret both the Simonton Center and what I was doing as clutching at straws. I remembered Dr. Richmond from so many months before: "Don't do a Steve McQueen, Ed."

But that wasn't it at all. I wasn't looking for a miracle so much as I was looking for a unification of mind and body. I was looking for practitioners who understood the effect of mind and emotions on physical well-being. I was looking for people who would understand Ed and appreciate the fight he'd been making.

A lot of the world has enormous success on a daily basis with medical techniques that are not practiced in the Western world. Carl Simonton is not a quack. You have only to read his book or listen to his tapes to know that.

I thought, what would the harm be in giving him an hour sometime at an AMA convention? Then, at least, people handling cancer, like myself and Ed, could find out about his approach and make a choice. It is not the purview of medicine to make that choice. It is the purview of the individual. And it is the responsibility, in my opinion, of the medical community to be aware and make their patients aware of treatments that are available, whether or not they agree with all of them.

It is unfair to lump Carl Simonton with the people grinding up apricot pits in Mexico, and it is unfair of the medical community to be underinformed when a responsible resource like the Simonton Center exists.

I wish I'd found it sooner. That I didn't is one of my few regrets.

January 26

AUNT MAUREEN PHONED AND GAVE ME the name of a doctor. Martin Blum.

"Everybody I asked gave me two or three names," she said, "and everybody... everybody... included him."

I began referring to him in my mind as "the great-white-hope doctor." I began to see images of him on a giant white stallion charging in with his lance to save Ed from indignity.

But somehow, I didn't have the courage to phone him. I didn't know if it was the right thing to do. I didn't know if I could drag Ed into a new environment. I wasn't sure. I just wasn't sure.

I was reading Gore Vidal's great novel *Lincoln* and every night when I turned to it, I was comforted by Vidal's stories about the President. So many of his decisions made just before and during the Civil War—decisions that now seem obvious and sure—were uncertain at the time. Whether or not to keep the capital in Washington, which was really a southern city. Whether or not to defend the border states. In fact, whether or not to sign the Emancipation Proclamation. Even great people making great decisions can guess, be unsure, go on instinct.

Or, like me at that moment, they could even do nothing.

January 29

IT WAS SATURDAY MORNING. I was humming and sort of singing to myself as I made up my bed on the couch, happy not to be at the office, looking forward to the weekend. People like Bob kept saying to me, "It's good you're working. It lets you get away, it keeps some balance." But I knew that the best place in the world for me to be was here.

Suddenly, I heard Ed, sitting in his recliner across the room, lose his breakfast. I turned and recognized what was happening as projectile vomiting—a term I first read in Dr. Spock, when the children were babies. It comes up like a rocket being fired from the stomach.

I though Ed was nauseous from "Lord-knows-what" and gave him some Compazene to settle his stomach.

About noon, I gave him some lunch and he threw up again. An hour or so later, I tried to give him some water and he threw that up. He was also starting to hallucinate and talk in jumbled sentences.

I called Dr. Moore and got the answering service. He was out of the city, but his associate Dr. Aaron was on call. I left a message for Dr. Aaron to phone, and she did, around three in the afternoon.

"What's up?" she said briskly, precluding niceties and chitchat. I could tell she was on her car phone, probably just leaving Cedars, in a hurry to get somewhere. I explained about the vomiting and told her I had the feeling something strange was going on.

"Try the Compazene again and call me back in two or three hours if it doesn't work."

So I gave Ed Compazene and he threw it up. Then the chills and fever started. He would shake and rattle his teeth under a four-foot pile of blankets. A few minutes later, he'd be sweating. And there was a strange aura about the whole thing. It wasn't that Ed was delirious or unconscious; he wasn't making sense. He was seeing things that weren't there. He was asking strange questions. "Did Robin take Matthew for a drive in the Porsche today?" And there were mood swings. He'd be nervous and jittery. Then he'd lapse into a dazed sort of numbness.

I made a call to Dr. Aaron at six. Then again at seven-thirty. Then again sometime later. I made the last call at eleven. She never called back.

Ed fell into a fitful sleep and as I made up my bed on the couch beside him, I racked my brain trying to figure out what was going on. The pieces of the puzzle just didn't fit together and I couldn't make sense out of the combination of symptoms. I went to sleep thinking about it and sometime around four in the morning, I woke up with a start.

"It's the morphine," I said aloud to no one. "It's the morphine. I'll bet anything it's the morphine."

A couple of days before, Carol thought Ed was doing so well we could cut back on the morphine. So we gave him half dosage for a day and then nothing at all. All day Saturday, he hadn't had any morphine.

I waited for morning, and at seven-thirty I phoned the service and told them to get Dr. Aaron out of bed. She phoned me back in five minutes and I heard a guilty tone in her voice, from not calling me back the night before.

I told her I thought Ed might be having morphine withdrawal and she screamed into the phone.

"Why did you take him off morphine?"

"I didn't take him off," I shouted back. "The nurse did."

She lowered her voice and changed her tone. "Well, put him back on immediately."

I did. And the vomiting stopped. He held down a little breakfast. But the chills and fever continued. I stayed with him constantly until about noon, when I made my own diagnosis. In addition to morphine withdrawal, if that's what it had been, he had the flu. I could hear it in his cough and see it in his face. I'd held back some Ampicillin, an antibiotic, from an earlier incident and started him on it, but I'd need some more. I didn't want to go through it the next day with Louise. I didn't want to go through it with Dr. Aaron either. But I decided she was the best of two evils and called the service. When she called me back, I didn't ask her for anything—I just told her I needed some Ampicillin. She didn't even ask my why; she just took the pharmacy's number, called them, and that was that.

Carol felt terrible about the incident and so did I. But not because of Carol. I felt terrible because I couldn't get the doctor's attention. She, too, was Everydoctor and I just couldn't stand it anymore. I was going to phone the great-white-hope doctor. I didn't care anymore that Ed was eighteen months into a terminal illness. I was going to get him a Bernie Siegel.

January 31

STRAIN WAS SHOWING FROM TIME to time around the edges of Sug's eyes and in the measured tone of her voice. She'd been in the middle of all of it. The diarrhea and vomiting. The urine-stained sheets. The coaxing to eat. Oxygen, morphine, injections, coughing, emptying the portable commode. Trips to the doctor. Stays in the hospital. Chills and fever. Disorientation. Irritability. The yelling at her. The yelling at me. Worry. Fear. Fear for Ed. Fear for me.

"I worry about you, Mama, more even than Ed. There's not much more we can do for Ed than we're doing. But nobody's doing anything for you."

God, I love her.

February 1 was her birthday. Hers and Chris's. Twenty-six years old. I wanted to do something special. Because they just took their place in all of this without being asked. And because it had been so hard. But there wasn't a lot I could do at that moment. There wasn't time for shopping or even time for thinking about shopping. So I resorted to what mothers often do in a pinch. I went to the kitchen.

I dug through my shelves of cookbooks, looking for my vintage Betty Crocker, circa 1960. My mother had given me that cookbook when I was married. It was a dog-eared, grease-stained loose-leaf classic. Whenever I wanted to do good old-fashioned American cooking, out came Betty, wearing her silly apron on the flyleaf and holding her wooden spoon, ready to direct me to meat loaf, macaroni and cheese, pot roast, and fried chicken. Betty had seen better days, but no cookbook before or since has ever equaled her chocolate cake.

I made a three-layer triumph and frosted it with the only real choice—Betty's all-time great, seven-minute frosting, which you make in a double boiler.

Aunt Maureen came for the occasion, along with Sug's best friend, Pam.

"Let's have some fun, Jean," Ed said from his bed. "Light the candles and have a parade."

So I lit the twenty-six candles and came in from the kitchen to the darkened living room, while the others sang. Then Sug blew and I marched in again for Chris, we sang again, and he blew, because we'd made it a point over the years to let them each have the moment. And it was fun and it made me remember the best birthday present I ever got.

  "We've got to get you a better watch, Jean."

My watch irritated the hell out of Ed.

"There's nothing the matter with this watch. I like it."

"It's a piece of junk, Jean. It doesn't suit you."

It was a Timex.

"I like it because I can garden with it on and not worry about it. Or wash the car and not worry about it. I don't like fancy watches I have to worry about."

"Good and fancy are not the same. You should only be wearing good things."

My concept of good and Ed's concept of good were quite different at that time. We weren't married yet and were still discovering each other.

"You need a new front door," he'd said to me a few weeks earlier. "My grandmother could kick in your front door. A strong wind could break the lock. It's a disgrace, Jean. You're going to get killed or robbed."

So he took me to a door store, picked out what he thought was a great door for my house, and told me to buy it.

"My God, Ed, that door costs nine hundred dollars."

"It's a good door."

"It's nine hundred dollars."

"Damn it, Jean. You live in a three-hundred-thousand-dollar house."

"I can't afford a nine-hundred-dollar door."

"Buy the door, Jean."

I bought it. He installed it. It's one of the few things we brought with us when we moved to Malibu. It's now the front door in Malibu, and my concept of good has become remarkably similar to Ed's.

Anyway, my watch really irritated him but I didn't want to be pushed around, so I kept wearing the Timex. Then one day, shortly before my birthday in June, he called me for lunch.

"Sure. Where should we meet?"

"Mr. Chow."

It was a Mandarin restaurant in Beverly Hills and I thought the choice a little odd, because Ed had never taken me there before or even mentioned it. But I didn't think about it too much and we went. When lunch was over, he said, "I ate too much. Let's take a walk."

"Okay," I said.

And so we walked around the corner onto Wilshire Boulevard and suddenly he was steering me into the front door of Tiffany's. "I want to look at watches with you. Just in case you ever decide to get rid of that piece of junk."

"Well, . . . okay."

So we went to a counter filled exclusively with Rolex watches that say "Tiffany" on the face.

"You can't hurt a Rolex, Jean. You can garden in it, wash the car in it, snorkel in it, shower in it. Even you can't hurt a Rolex, Jean."

"But they cost so much."

"They're good."

"I know they're good, but . . . ."

"If you were ever to have a Rolex, which one do you think you'd like?"

"Well, gee, I don't know," I said. And I stared at them through the glass counter. The sales clerk wandered over and I asked him to take one out for me. But I didn't really like it the best and he put it back. I looked at another one. I thought I saw the sales clerk smiling at Ed.

I finally decided that the classic Rolex had to be my favorite. Their original design that combined steel with gold in the linked band. It was waterproof, with a sweep second hand and the white face with the gold Roman numerals. Ed himself had one like it that he'd worn for twenty years.

"That's my favorite," I said, pointing to the classic.

"Are you sure?" Ed asked.

"I'm sure," I said.

Ed smiled at the clerk, who took the watch out of the case and handed it to me. I studied it carefully. It was beautiful.

"Turn it over," said Ed. "Look at the back."

I did. And I couldn't believe what I saw. The watch I'd picked out of the counter was already engraved on the back. It said:

> Jean.
> 6-1-83
> Love,
> Ed

"How did you know that'd be the one I wanted?" I asked as we left the store.

"I just knew," he grinned.

There's something wonderful about having your best birthday present when you're all the way to forty-six years old. ❧

February 2

''DOCTOR'S OFFICE,'' THE VOICE ON the other end of the phone gave the anonymous identifier they all seem to use these days.

"I'd like to make an appointment with Dr. Blum."

"Are you a new patient?"

"Well, I'm not actually the patient. I'm phoning for my husband, and before I make the appointment, I'd like to talk to Dr. Blum."

"Oh?"

I thought I'd better play an ace. "I was referred by the nuns at St. John's."

The tone changed a little. "How can we help you?"

"My husband has been a cancer patient for eighteen months. He's been treated at the City of Hope and he's now under the care of a private doctor, but we're unhappy with the doctor." I felt my voice getting thick with emotion and my mouth getting dry with nervousness. "I made a lot of inquiries and Dr. Blum was very highly recommended. But I want to tell him about my husband and sort of explain things, before I just bring him in. I mean, he's very sick."

"Do you feel he hasn't been getting good care?"

"No. It isn't that exactly. I feel he hasn't been getting understanding care. I feel he's become a low-priority patient. Everyone I talked with told me that Dr. Blum was just wonderful with people."

The voice at the other end of the phone raised a decibel or two in the flush of pride. "Oh, yes. Everybody loves Dr. Blum. All of his patients do. He's just a wonderful man."

I felt myself relaxing a little. "Yes, everyone has told me that. But I thought I should talk to him first. He may not want to take a patient as far along as my husband, and it may not be medically wise to change doctors at this point. Anyway, that's why I wanted to speak with him first. I thought I'd just make an appointment for myself and come see him and talk."

"What is your name, please?"

"Jean McNeilly."

"Mrs. McNeilly, why don't I have Dr. Blum call you. You can talk to him on the phone and see if you can work things out and that would save you the trouble of coming to the office."

"That would be terrific."

She took my number at home and told me that Dr. Blum would call that evening. I wanted to hug her through the phone.

"Thank you for listening and for being so helpful."

"You're quite welcome, Mrs. McNeilly. I'm sure you're going to be delighted with Dr. Blum. All his patients are."

I hung up feeling a surge of relief. Maybe the great-white-hope doctor could put our hearts at ease.

February 3

ED WAS VERY, VERY SPACEY.
He couldn't remember what to call things. He picked up his knife and tried to use it like a fork. And he was sleeping a lot. When I got home to relieve Alicia at three in the afternoon, we compared notes before she left.

"I'm worried about him, Jean. He didn't eat. He's got no energy."

"Were there any phone calls, Alicia?"

"Ed phoned Carol and she called him back."

"Did a Dr. Blum phone?"

"No. Nobody but Carol, Jean."

February 5

LINDA CHANDLER, A FREELANCE WRITER,
was working at the advertising agency. She'd been creative director at Della Femina when Ed was there, and they were fond of each other. She came into my office to ask about him, which people at my office seemed uncomfortable about doing. I suppose no one knew what to say. Or they were afraid.

But Linda walked into my office to talk and after I told her a little about things at home, we traded stories about Ed. When she turned to leave, she said, "Perfection is fleeting, Jean."

I loved her for it.

But the comment stayed with me. It was, indeed, fleeting. Ed was getting ready to leave. I could see it. I found myself talking to him, trying to pull from him the memories that I wanted to keep.

"Tell me about your mother, Ed."

"Tell me about the time your grandfather fell from the horse."

"Tell me what it was like in the early days at DDB."

I also tried to pull his ideas from him, so I wouldn't forget. "How were you going to move the big sign at the car wash, Ed? How do you want me to landscape? Do you remember your ideas about adding another story to the house? Could you tell me about it again?"

It was like a giant book I couldn't stop from closing. Or a candle I couldn't stop from going out. It was driving me crazy. I'd hold his hand after he fell asleep and stare at him and say, "Don't go, Ed." But I knew he was going and there was nothing on earth I could do about it except feel helpless, worthless, and afraid.

February 6

I PHONED DR. BLUM'S OFFICE AGAIN. "I'm Jean McNeilly. I called a couple of days ago about my husband."

"Oh yes, Mrs. McNeilly."

"Dr. Blum hasn't phoned yet and I wonder if he got the message."

"He hasn't?" She was genuinely surprised. "I'm really sorry. I talked to him about you and gave him your number. I'll tell him again. He'll phone."

"Thank you. Tell him I need him."

"Don't worry, Mrs. McNeilly. I'll make sure he phones."

February 8

ALICIA AND I TOOK ED TO THE DOCTOR for a regular visit, and Dr. Moore put him immediately into the hospital.

"It's a metabolic problem," he told me.

"What are you going to do while he's hospitalized?" I asked.

"We're going to give him some medicine," he answered absently without looking up from the chart he was writing.

"Some medicine? What kind of an answer is that?"

He looked at me, surprised.

"Don't just tell me it's medicine. Tell me what it is. Tell me what you're going to do." I couldn't believe that after all this time, he was still talking to me in euphemisms. "I'm going to give you some medicine" is what you tell a second-grader you want to swallow Pepto-Bismol.

"It's medicine for his liver. His liver isn't working well."

Dr. Moore simply had no comprehension that his patronizing manner offended people. I'm sure somebody told him in medical school to put things in simple terms and that's what he did, no matter what. He was simply not a people person and didn't pick up on vibes.

"Are you going to run a CAT-scan?"

"On his liver?"

"Yes."

"We'll see."

I turned in frustration and went back to my office, leaving Alicia with Ed. He was still in his wheelchair, waiting for them to make up a room.

"I'll be back in about an hour," I told Alicia. I needed to pick up my briefcase and cancel a couple of meetings I had scheduled for later in the day. Half an hour later, she called me from a pay phone in the hall.

"You better get over here, Jean."

"What's the matter?"

"These people don't give a damn. I don't like what's going on here, Jean."

"What is it, Alicia?"

"You better come, Jean. Right now."

When I got there, Ed was in a room and Alicia was strutting up and down the corridor like an angry bantam rooster. Her chin was thrust forward and there was venom in her eyes. "Look at where they put him, Jean. There's a man dying in there. They have no business putting Ed there. They told him he could have his own room."

I tiptoed in. It was a huge room. One of the very expensive suitelike rooms they have in the hospital. In one corner, a very old man was crying out and moaning in delirium. He was quite alone. Ed's bed was off to itself in the other corner.

"And look what they tried to give him for lunch, Jean. I told them to take it out of here. He can't eat that."

It was fried chicken and she was quite right. Ed hadn't had much but soft food in months.

The floor nurse explained to me they had an emergency and Ed's room was going to someone coming up from surgery. As soon as another room opened up, they'd move him. In the meantime, this was the best she could do.

"Why does the other patient get priority?" I asked.

"You'll have to talk to the doctor," she said briskly as she walked away.

So we spent the afternoon, Ed, me and Alicia, in the midst of a swirl of technicians and nurses setting Ed up with IVs, getting him ready for a transfusion, taking his vitals, while the old man in the corner—completely alone and largely unattended by the staff—moaned, and then retched, and then shouted, and then moaned. Alicia ran to get help a couple of times when he gagged. It was a grisly few hours.

Around three o'clock, I walked down the hall to the room Ed was supposed to have, the one going to the man coming up from surgery. It was empty. I checked it again, around six. It was still empty. Around eight, they moved Ed to a private room, but not that one.

When I left, at ten-thirty, the room was still empty. When I returned at eight in the morning, it was still empty.

"We can't leave Ed alone here, Jean," Alicia said when she got back in the morning.

"I know." And I remembered my fear of leaving him alone at Cedars and the week I'd spent sleeping on a cot in his room.

I asked one of the nurses what had happened to the man who was supposed to be coming up from surgery.

"What man? I don't know anything about it. This isn't a surgery floor."

She was able to tell me, however, that the old man had died during the night.

February 12

ED WAS IN THE HOSPITAL FOR THREE DAYS. He got two liters of blood and some "green medicine" for his liver. They never ran a CAT-scan or took X-rays of any kind.

"I don't understand," I said to Sug. "What can an X-ray hurt? Don't they want to know what's going on inside? Are there tumors in his liver or is it failing or what?"

Actually, I did understand. There was no medical reason to X-ray or run a CAT-scan because there wasn't anything they could do with the information. It didn't make any difference what was causing the problem in his liver, because whether it was tumors or something else, he was too sick for them to treat it.

But nobody told me that. Nobody shared that opinion with me. I figured it out for myself. I also found it arrogant. The "it-doesn't-make-any-difference" syndrome is fine for the doctors. It isn't so fine for the patients and their families. The doctor may not give a damn whether it's tumors or liver failure that's causing the metabolic problem, but I did. And Ed did. Not knowing left a feeling of being less than human, like a piece of meat. Of being cast aside, of not being important anymore. An X-ray wouldn't have hurt Ed. No matter how dire the situation it exposed, it couldn't have been more dire than what we already knew.

And it would have given him his dignity.

It would have given him his dignity.

When we got Ed home, I decided to call the great-white-hope doctor once more. This time, his nurse covered her embarrassment with briskness.

"He never called you? Well, he's been awfully busy. Yes, I'll give him your message again."

February 18

IT CROSSED MY MIND TO CALL Harper & Row in New York, Bernie Siegel's publisher, get his number, and phone him to find out if he knew of any doctor in southern California who was like him.

But I didn't have the nerve to do it.

February 20

EVERY TUESDAY AND EVERY FRIDAY, Carol came. And every time I'd get dragged down, dismayed, or disheartened by the doctors, this remarkable nurse would give me hope.

Carol's job for Lifeline Homecare took her all over Los Angeles County. She'd visit about five patients a day, jockeying her beat-up brown Chevy through the LA Freeway system in between stops. Like a lot of modern medicos, she wore a beeper on her belt so she could be paged at any point in time. Every time she was paged, she'd have to pull off the freeway, get to a pay phone, phone Lifeline, find out where the problem was, and then phone the patient.

One day, Ed had her beeped five times. All over his malfunctioning bowels. Each of the five times, she got to a pay phone and called him. She talked to him, soothed him, calmed him, never got mad at him. Never asked him not to phone. When I found out, I apologized for him.

"It's okay, Mrs. McNeilly." Then she grinned. "We all talk about Ed at the Monday morning staff meetings. We're supposed to bond with our patients. But everybody laughs. Carol, you've gone too far."

"I know. Bonding is one thing. Crazy glue is another."

"No. It's okay, really. I've never had a patient like him. He's so in control. I want him to be, you know what I mean?"

I knew what she meant.

With time, patience, and understanding, Carol found a regimen for Ed that kept him more or less regular. He had a severe fixation with his bowels. I'm told that a lot of sick people do, I suppose because their thoughts and feelings are all focused inward and bodily functions take control of consciousness.

Diarrhea and constipation are not my favorite subjects, and Ed drove me nuts with them. There were times when I thought he'd lost his ability to ever speak again about anything else.

But Carol never lost her patience. And because she understood the importance of the problem to Ed, she didn't quit trying things until she found something that worked. Believe it or not, what did it in the end was milk of magnesia. Carol dumped all the prescription drugs, capsules, suppositories, herbal mixtures, witches remedies, and strange brews offered up by Alicia and put him on a twice-daily dosage of MOM. The confidence toward Carol that welled up in Ed when that regimen began working was a touching thing to see.

"I need Carol, Jean," Ed would tell me. "Whatever we do about nurses, I need Carol."

"Don't worry, Darling. We'll always have Carol."

"I think I love Carol, Jean. You don't mind, do you?"

He'd gotten so childlike, he'd bring tears to my eyes. There was such a trusting tone in his voice. Yet it wasn't as if I'd become his mother. It was more as if he'd put himself completely in my hands, given himself over to me, allowed himself to be dependent. Ed and I didn't talk about the sacrifices the family and I were making on his behalf because it was a matter of trust, not gratitude. I'm not sure gratitude belongs in a marriage. The giving that flows back and forth should be given freely. "I don't want anything back for this" is love at its finest hour.

Ed would say to me, from time to time, listening to my daughters on the phone, "Young people position themselves in a relationship. Isn't it wonderful we don't have to do that anymore?"

And we didn't. We never mentally counted who ran more errands, worked harder that week at the office, cooked more meals. And unlike today's liberated couples, it didn't bother me to iron an occasional shirt for Ed or to let him get my car washed.

"I just love doing for you," he'd say.

And that's what our marriage was about. Each of us would do for the other with no strings attached. To speak of gratitude during this time of crisis would have been demeaning.

It was, instead, a time of trust. We always knew we'd do for the other, no matter what. And that's what we did.

Carol also saw that we managed the pain, although Ed never suffered to the extent that many cancer patients do. It never got so bad he had to go onto morphine injections or intravenous morphine.

I'm convinced that had to do with the fact that we removed the colon tumor those many months before. If the tumor had remained—to grow, spread, block, entwine, strangle, or rupture—Lord knows what Ed might have endured. But because of Dr. Ewen at the City of Hope, who didn't acknowledge the conventional wisdom to leave it alone, that tumor was gone.

Carol also did something that no doctor save Alan Fogelman had ever done. While the patient was my husband, a hand was also extended to me.

"Is there anything you need, Mrs. McNeilly?" she'd ask. "If you're having trouble sleeping, if you need sedatives or anything like that, let me know."

She also took the time to talk. "Are you and your family okay? I know this is hard. I've been trained in hospice care," she told me. "If anybody needs to just talk...or let it out, you know,...anything,...maybe I can help."

I talked to her about my feelings toward Dr. Moore and confided in her that I was considering a different doctor. When I used the words *low-priority patient,* a look darkened her already serious eyes. I knew I'd uncovered a phrase the medical profession used only among themselves within the tight inner sanctum of their own community, and I knew she agreed with my use of the word, although she was careful not to criticize the doctor.

I told her about Dr. Moore's staff protecting him from his patients. About Louise and her linebacker tactics when it came to running things. About the fact that their office was constantly too busy and how they constantly let you know it. And how I wished someone would explain to me why doctors take on too many patients. I told her how they distanced themselves and were careful not to get involved at a people level. About how Dr. Moore was not always up to speed on what was going on with Ed and how Louise tried to cover for him. And how obvious that was to me. How they tried to avoid questions, and how patronizing their answers were. Insultingly, offensively patronizing.

We'd been going to see Dr. Moore for nine months. During that time, Ed had gone from a robust, twinkling giant who'd had the guts to buy a business and run it with a Heparin lock in his arm and a bag of chemical dripping into his veins, to a tall, frail old man, but the guts were still there and so, by God, was the twinkle when he could manage it.

And during those nine months, Ed had come there once every ten days or so, sometimes in a wheelchair and sometimes hobbling in on a walker, hanging onto me or Alicia, with oxygen tubes in his nose, edema in his legs, and a hernia in his stomach that was now the size of a basketball. And in all that time, they had never once made gestures to Ed of warmth, kindness, or special caring.

They never saw that he didn't have to wait, or helped him to a chair, or got a pillow for his back, or asked if he was hot or cold or if he would like a blanket. No one ever put an arm around his waist to steady him while he walked. Or took his hands to help ease him into a chair. No one ever even walked to the door with me to help me get the wheelchair through. Week after week, I struggled through that door by myself, banging Ed's knees as I backed us out. No one, not once, not ever, sat down beside him for a moment to talk, to ask him how he was doing on an emotional level. To make human contact. No one ever said anything. They never said, "Ed, we're proud of you. We're glad to be working with you." They never said, "How can we make this easier for you, Ed? How can we make it better for you, Ed?" Nobody ever said, "Is there anything we can do for you, Mrs. McNeilly?" Nobody ever asked me what it was like at home. Were there children around, was there family around, were we doing okay? Nobody in Dr. Moore's office ever said one personal word to either one of us.

One day, Carmen, the technician who took blood, noticed that Ed was having a lot of trouble because he'd had to wait a long time, and he was starting to sweat and look faint. So she went and got him a glass of water.

That is the one, sole, single, solitary human gesture that anyone in that office ever made to my husband and it stuck like glue in my brain because it was the only one.

I told Carol all of those feelings. I told her I was keeping a journal and I was going to write a book about it when it was all over.

"Write your book, Jean," she said. "It's important." There were tears in her eyes and in mine.

It was the only time she ever called me Jean.

February 25

ALICIA PHONED ME AT THE OFFICE. "Jean, I got to do something about Ed's hernia. It's awful, Jean. It's as big as a basketball. It makes him bend over when he walks."

"I know it's awful. Carol's worried too. I don't know what to do. I called the doctor but he didn't call me back."

"I'm going to take him out and get him a truss."

"A what?"

"A truss. You don't know what a truss is?"

"I guess I don't."

"A lot of old men at the nursing home wear 'em, Jean. It'll help."

"Okay."

"I found a place in Santa Monica and I called them and made an appointment. But I don't have any money. Can you meet me there, Jean?"

God, I love Alicia.

I found her and her beat-up Ford Pinto in front of California Prosthetic Devices about an hour later. Ed was sitting in her little car and his wheelchair was lying in the hatchback.

We took him inside and they fitted him with a band of elastic, about sixteen inches wide, that closed with Velcro. If he wore it around his waist, it kept the hernia from sagging, although it still poofed right through the thick elastic every time he coughed. It wasn't perfect, but it was a help.

"I guess you've got another old man on your hands, Alicia," Ed said with a wan smile.

February 26

KIMI PULLED ME OUT OF A MEETING in the agency's conference room. "There's a Dr. Blum on the phone. I thought it might be important."

"Dr. Blum?"

"Yeah."

"Oh, my goodness."

It was the great-white-hope doctor. But as I ran to my office, I couldn't figure out how he knew to find me at the advertising agency.

I'd never given his nurse the office number. Indeed, I'd never even given her my office name—Jean Craig—but had identified myself as Jean McNeilly.

By the time I got to my desk, I recognized the fine hand of Aunt Maureen. She'd asked me a couple of days before if I'd gotten in touch with Martin Blum and I'd told her about the unreturned phone calls. I guessed she'd asked one of the nursing nuns to phone him.

I didn't get his attention. But that did.

Never mind. I was just glad he phoned.

I talked to him for about ten minutes, and as soon as I got off the phone, I wrote down the conversation, because I didn't want to forget it. I gave him a brief review of Ed's case. Then it went like this:

"I'm a compassionate man, but I'm a pessimist. I don't offer hope when there isn't any."

"I'm not looking for hope. I'm looking for support."

"Well, what is your doctor doing that makes you feel you're not getting it?"

"He doesn't return my phone calls. He's quit taking X-rays and blood tests. He put Ed in the hospital for a liver problem, but never took an X-ray to find out what was really going on."

"I probably wouldn't have either."

"Wouldn't you even have been curious to know if it was a tumor or the liver failing for other reasons?"

"Look, your doctor's right. He couldn't treat it anyway. He's giving him all there is to give him."

"He's taking care of his body, but what about his spirit? Look, Ed knows he didn't get an X-ray, and he isn't stupid; he knows what that means. It means he isn't worth the effort. He's a low-priority patient. And I just don't think that's fair. People have a right to die in the hands of people they feel are pulling for them."

"Mrs. McNeilly, I can't tell you that you'll come to my office and feel better when you leave. I'm honest. I tell people the truth. I don't believe in giving a couple of months just to have a couple of months. Especially when there's pain."

"You don't understand, Doctor. I'm not trying to buy time and I believe in the truth. What I'm after is the right to die with people who are on your team."

There was a brief silence; then Dr. Blum continued.

"There's a doctor at Cedars. Michael Melvin. He's more of a fighter. Maybe you should talk to him."

He was telling me the conversation was over. I hung up the phone feeling as empty as I'd ever felt in my life. The great-white-hope doctor had no idea what I was talking about.

He, too, was Everydoctor.

I wasn't fighting for time. I wasn't trying to get a month or two. And I certainly wasn't running from the truth. For God's sake, I'd been trying to get truth, honesty, and open communication out of the doctors since this started.

What I was fighting for—asking for—was human dignity. What I wanted for Ed was so simple. A doctor who would help him die well. Who would offer him not hope, but trust and confidence. A doctor who would say, "I'm still with you, Ed." I think a person has a right to that.

What Ed said, himself, so many months before, kept ringing in my mind. "Nobody wants to take responsibility."

And also what Robin had said: "Doctors leave the dying to the nurses."

I didn't want sympathy. I wasn't asking for emotional involvement. I simply wanted a doctor for my husband who wouldn't abandon him.

March 1

ED'S CLOTHES WERE FALLING OFF OF HIM, so I went up to the attic where he had another whole wardrobe stored. From time to time over the years he'd lost weight, so he had a second wardrobe of clothes in smaller sizes. I was poking through boxes of bags looking for pajamas and underwear when a newspaper clipping fell out.

It was dated August 10, 1971, and it was from the Elmira, New York *Star-Gazette.* Here's what it said, in its entirety.

People come from far and wide to dine at Moretti's Restaurant in Elmira, but not many come from 250 miles for a take-out order.

A man named McNeilly did. He came from New York City for eight pizzas with everything.

Joe Moretti said the man stopped in for dinner while at the Can-Am races at Watkins Glen a couple weekends ago. He had a pizza. Evidently it left a lasting impression on him.

Last weekend McNeilly (Joe didn't get his first name) and some friends decided to have a party and show films of the Glen races. McNeilly figured a few pizzas would enliven the party.

He wanted Moretti pizzas. Nothing else would do. So he called the Hatch St. restaurant Saturday afternoon from New York and ordered the $40 worth of pizzas—to go. The pizzas were ready by 6:30 and McNeilly was there.

He caught a Mohawk flight to the Chemung County Airport, rented a car, drove to Moretti's, picked up the pizzas, returned to the airport, and caught another flight back to New York.

This was the hallmark of a man who walked through life with more gusto than the rest of us, and who made life for those around him, like me, so much more fun. I came downstairs with the clipping.

"Do you remember the pizzas, Ed, the ones you flew all the way to Elmira to get?"

"From Moretti's. After the races at Watkins Glen."

"You never told me that story."

"You would've loved those pizzas, Jean." Then, as wistfully as a child remembering a Christmas past, he said, "I wish I could live all of my life over with you in it."

March 6

IT WAS SUNDAY. THE DAY STARTED easily enough. Breakfast. Watching "Sunday Morning" on CBS. But around eleven o'clock, the chills and fever started. Ed's fever shot up to 102 and an hour later I couldn't get enough blankets on him to stop him shaking from cold.

I called the doctor but got the answering service. So I started Ed on Ampicillin myself. He seemed to respond to the antibiotic, but he couldn't eat and he seemed very weak. I sat with him all afternoon. The chills and fever started again. Monty and Ginny phoned to ask if they could come by, but I told them Ed was too sick.

He didn't talk much all day. He didn't seem to have the energy. I wrapped him in blankets because he was so cold and wondered if I should phone Kim and Mark and ask them to come. I called. They weren't home.

Around seven in the evening, I took Ed's temperature and it read

92. I was shocked. I'd never seen a body temperature that low and didn't know what it meant. I took it three times. Every time it read 92. I phoned the service again.

Around ten o'clock Dr. Moore phoned. He said to continue the antibiotic, that the low temperature didn't necessarily mean anything, and to call him in the morning.

Ed had been sitting up in his E-Z Boy and when it came time to get him into bed, I had to call Sug to help. He couldn't walk by himself, and when he got into bed, he didn't have the strength to scoot his head onto the pillow.

His breathing seemed labored and I was very worried, but he fell asleep. I sat beside him for a long time with the light on, reading a book, listening to his breathing, and looking at him. His body had become an absolute wreck. The face was drawn and gaunt and his big frame was so thin. Most of his hair was gone, his color was sallow, and the huge hernia hung from his stomach like a pitiful testament to his struggle. His body was gone, but his spirit was whole. He'd never lost his dignity. He'e never stopped being a man.

I finally put the light out about two in the morning and went to sleep myself on the couch beside his bed, where I'd been sleeping since he came home from Cedars.

When I woke up at six-thirty in the morning, I knew that Ed was gone before I opened my eyes.

I lay there on the couch, afraid to move, afraid to look, but I knew he was gone. It wasn't just that I couldn't hear him breathe. His presence was gone.

Sug came downstairs to put coffee on. I sat up. She saw Ed and came to me.

"I think Ed's gone, Mama," she said ever so softly.

I got up and took his hand. His head was turned toward the picture window, looking out over the ocean. I thought he looked as if he saw something coming from across the sea.

Sug put her arm around me.

"Aren't you just a little bit relieved, Mama?"

"No," I said. "No, I'm not, Sug."

I'd thought I would be. So much of it had been so hard. And the outcome was inevitable. But I wasn't. I think all those people who are still in love with someone when death comes will understand.

There is no relief.

There is just loss.

Ed died.

Epilogue, December 31, 1989

I'M SITTING ON THE PORCH OF THE HOUSE Ed and I rented on the Grand Cayman Islands in the Caribbean. The wind has been blowing all night, so the surf is pounding the reef and spewing up a high, white froth. I'm here with Carl, Jacque, and Maureen. We spent Christmas together. Carl and I got Scuba certified. It's a help, not a hurt, to be where Ed and I were happy together.

Sometime today, tomorrow, or the next day, the phone will ring and we'll get the news that Erin and Rich's baby has been born. Their wedding was beautiful and touching. Thirty-seven members of the family—Howard and Carl's children, and their children—trooped from Texas and Oklahoma in a sweet and loving display of support. Bob performed the marriage ceremony, even though he isn't a priest anymore and we weren't sure it was kosher.

Sug stayed with me for six months after Ed died, then moved back to San Francisco. She's practicing law there and still seeing The Fireman, though their relationship seems bumpy at times. My fondest hope right now is that life is good to her, as she has been so good to the people around her, especially me.

Chris comes out to Malibu most Sunday afternoons for dinner. We talk. We watch Laker games. He puts gas in my car before he leaves. These days, he also picks me up at the airport.

Three months after Ed died, Maureen moved home to Malibu from New York. She stuck her Phi Beta Kappa key into a drawer and went to work at Robertson Car Wash. In a year's time, she's become a skillful small-business manager. She knows the books, the suppliers, the equipment, the crew, and the profit and loss. She and Simon are great friends. He still calls me Señora, but he calls her "Mi Amore." She won't stay at the car wash forever, but I look upon her time there as a gift to me and Ed.

Alicia took over a lot of my life these past months, so I could write this book. Like Erin, she's expecting a baby. Robin had a little girl last June. We see a lot of Kim and Mark.

Kresser/Craig is growing and prospering. Bob and I had some bad moments after Ed died. I was out of focus, and I think he was afraid I'd move to Australia or something. But it's okay now. Indeed, the agency is on the precipice of enormous success. (The other day, however, Bob and I went to a formal function at The Music Center of Los Angeles, and he had on brown socks with his tux.)

I've become great friends with Tux, my dog. He and I go on long walks down the Malibu beach or up Carbon Canyon. There's a vacant lot sitting on a bluff at the opening of the canyon. Sometimes Tux and I climb up there. I can sit and look out across the Coast Highway, over the tops of the homes on the beach, and out to sea. He chases butterflies. I think a lot.

I think I'll miss Ed every day of my life. I was lucky to have had him and he enriched my life immeasurably. At this moment I'm content and at peace. We did our best for Ed. One day—perhaps soon—I'll be happy again. I know he would want that for me. I know he would expect that of me.

As for Kevin and Ed, I realize of course that neither of them won.

On the other hand, no one could ever convince me that they didn't triumph.